made INCREDIBLY EASY!

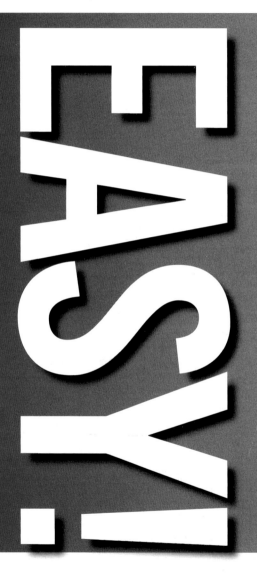

Clinical Skills

Adapted for the UK by
Mhairi Hastings, RGN
Local Health Partnership Manager
Dumfries and Galloway NHS Board;
formerly Clinical Skills Tutor, Whipps
Cross University Hospital NHS Trust
and London South Bank University

First UK Edition

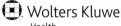 Wolters Kluwer | Lippincott Williams & Wilkins
Health
Philadelphia • Baltimore • New York • London
Buenos Aires • Hong Kong • Sydney • Tokyo

Staff

Director, Global Publishing
Cathy Peck

Production Director
Chris Curtis

Senior Production Manager
Richard Owen

Production Editor
Laura Maguire

Academic Marketing Executive
Alison Major

Copy Editor
Linda Antoniw

Proofreader
Stella Morris

Illustrator
Bot Roda

© 2009 by Lippincott Williams & Wilkins. All rights reserved. This book is protected by copyright. No part of it may be reproduced, stored in a retrieval system, or transmitted, in any form or by any means—electronic, mechanical, photocopy, recording or otherwise—without prior written permission of the publisher.

Printed in the UK by Stephens & George Ltd, Merthyr Tydfil, Wales. Typeset by Macmillan Publishing Solutions, New Delhi, India.

For information, write Lippincott Williams & Wilkins, 250 Waterloo Road, London SE1 8RD

British Library Cataloguing in Publication Data. A catalogue record for this book is available from the British Library.

ISBN13 978-1-901831-05-4
ISBN10 1-901831-05-1

Contents

Acknowledgements

Reviewers of the UK edition

Jeremy Finch, RGN, BA (Hons), MA
Senior Lecturer in Nursing, Manchester Metropolitan University

Karen Fritz, RN, BSc, MSc
Senior Lecturer, University of York

Carol Purcell, PhD, MSc, BSc (Hons), RGN
Director of Centre for Clinical Skills/Lecturer, University of Hull

Waterlow Pressure Ulcer Risk Assessment/Prevention Policy Tool (p.21) reproduced with permission from Judy Waterlow.

Patient Assessment Early Warning System Scoring Card (p.40) reproduced with permission from Whipps Cross University Hospital NHS Trust.

Contributions

Mhari Hastings would like to acknowledge the support received from the Non Medical Education and Practice Division, The Clinical Skills Service and the Nursing Staff of Whipps Cross University Hospital, Leytonstone, London.

Foreword

The ability to perform nursing procedures with skill and confidence is the essence of nursing care. Whether you're a nursing student or an experienced nurse, you need clear, reliable, up-to-date information to perform procedures safely and accurately. Although you can find some of this information in procedure manuals and manufacturers' instructions, you may not have access to these materials when you need them most. Or—even more likely—these manuals may lack many of the crucial guidelines you're seeking.

Staying current on all procedures requires continuous effort. With the rapid pace of technological advances and the increasing importance of maintaining professional standards, keeping pace with procedural changes is a real challenge. *Clinical Skills Made Incredibly Easy!* provides the most up-to-date information about the ever-changing topic. You'll find it comprehensive yet concise, enjoyable yet educational. Its light-hearted approach will help you attain procedural perfection.

The book is set out in chapters relating to specific episodes of care. Starting at the beginning with Fundamental procedures, such as taking care of patient's hygiene requirements, and then, chapter by chapter, building up to more difficult and complex care skills.

To help you use this book, each nursing procedure appears in the same easy-to-follow format, with short paragraphs and bulleted lists that let you skim an entire entry quickly to pinpoint instantly the specific information you need. Each procedure starts with a brief description. Next you'll find sections listing:
- the equipment you'll need to perform the procedure
- instructions for preparing the patient and the equipment, where necessary
- step-by-step instructions for carrying out the procedure
- practice pointers covering additional concerns, such as ways to avoid common complications, variations in performing procedure and warnings.
- Essential Skills Clusters Mapping. Each clinical skill (or set of skills where applicable) is mapped to the NMC Essential Skills Clusters, ensuring that you and your mentor are taking the correct course of action to meet NMC standards and maintain them.

Throughout the book, a playful cast of cartoon characters takes the tedium out of learning. Within each chapter, special features enhance your understanding. Chapters 1–9 start with a summary of key topics and Chapters 1–8 end with a quick quiz (which includes answers and rationales) to reinforce learning. Special logos highlight important points:

'Warning' alerts to possible dangers, risks, complications or contraindications associated with specific skills.

 'Home care connection' gives tips for adapting the procedure to the home care setting.

 'Ages and stages' highlighting important age-related variations in performing a particular skill.

 'Write it down' features essential points to document for each procedure.

Please take time to fully acquaint yourself with *Clinical Skills Made Incredibly Easy!*, UK edition. The more familiar you become with this refreshingly original book, the more confident and competent you will be in performing clinical skills, both independently and when working under supervision of your mentor. Your patients, too, sensing your confidence and expertise, will feel more confident and comfortable in your care.

Mhairi Hastings, RGN
Local Health Partnership Manager –
Hospitals for Wigtownshire LHP, Dumfries
and Galloway NHS Board; *formerly* Clinical
Skills Tutor, Clinical Skills Service, Whipps
Cross University Hospital NHS Trust and
London South Bank University.

Contributors and consultants to the US edition

Susan E Appling, RN, MS, CRNP
Assistant Professor
Johns Hopkins University School of
 Nursing
Baltimore

**Deborah Becker, RN, MSN, CCRN,
CRNP, CS**
Assistant Program Director
Adult Critical Care Nurse Practitioner
 Program
University of Pennsylvania School of
 Nursing
Philadelphia

Darlene Nebel Cantu, RN, C, MSN
Director
Baptist Health System School of
 Professional Nursing
San Antonio, Tex.
Adjunct Faculty
San Antonio College

Janice T Chussil, RN, C, MSN, ANP
Nurse Practitioner
Dermatology Associates
Portland, Ore.

Jean Sheerin Coffey, RN, MS, PNP
Unit Leader—Pediatrics
Children's Hospital at Dartmouth
Dartmouth Hitchcock Medical Center
Lebanon, N.H.

**Colleen M Fries, RN, MSN, CCRN,
CRNP**
Family Nurse Practitioner
Private Practice
Voorhees, N.J.

Rebecca Crews Gruener, RN, MS
Associate Professor of Nursing
Louisiana State University at
 Alexandria

Sandra Hamilton, RN, MEd, CRNI
Western Director of Pharmacy
 Nursing Services
Vencare Pharmacy
Boise, Idaho

Dr Joyce Lyne Heise, MSN, EdD
Associate Professor of Nursing
Kent State University
East Liverpool, Ohio

Lucy J Hood, RN, DNSc
Associate Professor
Saint Luke's College
Kansas City, Mo.

Mary Ellen Kelly, RN, BSN
Director of Staff Development
Infection Control Coordinator
John L. Montgomery Care Center
Freehold, N.J.

Susan M Leininger, RN, MSN
Advanced Practice Nurse
Allegheny General Hospital
Pittsburgh

Catherine Todd Magel, RN,C, EdD
Assistant Professor
Villanova (Pa.) University College of
 Nursing

**Donna Nielsen, RN, MSN, CCRN,
CEN, MICN**
Nursing Instructor
Pasadena (Calif.) City College

**Ruthie Robinson, RN, MSN,
CCRN, CEN**
Instructor
Lamar University
Beaumont, Tex.

Lisa Salamon, RN,C, MSN, CNS
Clinical Nurse Specialist
The Greens Adult Living Community
Lyndhurst, Ohio

Cynthia C Small, RN, MSN
Nursing Instructor
Lake Michigan College
Benton Harbor, Mich.

1 Fundamental procedures

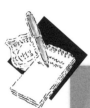

Just the facts

In this chapter, you'll learn:

♦ about achieving the standards set for pre-registration nurse education

♦ about standard infection control procedures (SICPs)

♦ about fundamental procedures and how to perform them without complications

♦ about essential documentation.

Setting standards

One of the many roles and responsibilities of The Nursing and Midwifery Council (NMC) is to identify the patients' and clients' expectations of nurses. Once these are identified, they also have a duty under the Nursing and Midwifery Order (2001) to set standards for education programmes and to review these. To enable them to address potential areas of deficit found from the *Review of fitness for practice at the point of registration* (2006) and to provide reassurance to the public that their expectations for care are being addressed, essential skills clusters (ESCs) must be incorporated into pre-registration nurse education from September 2008. Your university will have taken this on board and throughout your training will give you practice documents full of learning outcomes you need to achieve to meet these standards, for both entry to branch training and entry to the NMC register at the end of your training. You are responsible, with your mentor, for completing these documents; they will then provide the evidence you require to demonstrate that you have achieved these learning outcomes and are ready to progress to branch training and entry to the register. This book is cross-referenced to the ESCs to assist both you and your mentor in achieving the standards.

Focus

ESCs do not provide a definitive training programme; instead, your university will use the ESC document as an addendum to the Nursing Standards document from the NMC to establish this. The ESCs are therefore generic and applicable to all branches of nursing, not just adult nursing. ESCs are being introduced for the following areas and aspects of care: Communication, Organizational aspects of care, Infection prevention and control, Nutrition and fluid management, Medicines management, and Care and compassion. Each topic in this book has a 'practice pointers' section. In this section, or at the beginning of each chapter, you will find the relevant standard number in order that you can cross-reference to the *ESCs for pre-registration nursing programmes* document (2007) and read this book in conjunction with it. The ESC document is available on the NMC website.

Joining them up

The ESC document will provide you with further information and background about the reasons for their introduction and also about how they have been used by your university. To use them in conjunction with this book as an education tool, follow this procedure: note the relevant standard number(s) in the practice pointers section, open the ESC document and read the information given in the first column for each number (1–42), this is what the public and patients expect of a nurse; in order that you can demonstrate this you must achieve the outcomes in either of the next two columns, depending on whether you are meeting the outcome for entry to branch or the NMC register. At the bottom of the second and third columns of outcomes you will also find a list of numbers. These relate to two further NMC documents, which you must be aware of: *Standards of proficiency for pre-registration nursing education* (2004) and the all-important *Code of professional conduct* (2004). You can also cross-reference this book with these documents and guides, giving you a complete guide to both the practical skill and the core, professional values required to achieve competency in it.

Hand hygiene

Hand hygiene is the single most important SICP for preventing the transfer of microorganisms—and thus for preventing infection. To protect patients from healthcare-acquired infections (HCAI), hand hygiene must be performed routinely and thoroughly. In effect, clean and healthy hands with intact skin, short fingernails, no jewellery or clothing below the elbow will minimize the risk of contamination.

What you need

Soap or detergent ✳ warm, running water ✳ paper towels ✳ optional: alcohol hand gel, plastic sponge brush and plastic cuticle stick.

How you do it

- Wash your hands before and after giving patient care or having contact with contaminated objects, even when you have worn gloves.
- Remove rings and jewellery as local policy dictates, because they harbour dirt and skin microorganisms. Remove your watch—preferably wear a fob watch.
- Clothing should not be worn below the elbow when working in the clinical environment.
- Artificial fingernails and nail polish should not be worn as they have the potential to harbour microorganisms. Check local policy.
- Wet your hands and wrists with warm water, and then apply soap from a dispenser. Avoid using bar soap to prevent cross-contamination. Hold your hands below elbow level to prevent water from running up your arms and back down, thus contaminating clean areas. (See *Proper hand-washing technique.*)

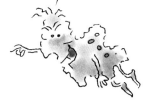

Ha, ha, ha! I love it when nurses forget to wash their hands!

Lather it up

- Work up a generous lather by rubbing your hands together vigorously for about 10 seconds. Soap and warm water reduce surface tension and this, aided by friction, loosens surface microorganisms, which wash away in the lather.
- Pay special attention to the area under your fingernails (use a disposable orange stick to remove dirt from this area rather than a nailbrush, which harbours bacteria) and around the cuticles, and to your thumbs, knuckles, palms and sides of your fingers and hands, because microorganisms thrive in these protected or overlooked areas. If you do not remove your wedding ring, move it up and down your finger to clean beneath it.
- Avoid splashing water on yourself or the floor, because microorganisms spread more easily on wet surfaces. Avoid touching the sink or taps, because they are considered contaminated.

Rinse and dry

- Rinse hands and wrists well, because running water flushes soil, soap or detergent, and microorganisms away.
- Pat hands and wrists dry with a paper towel. Avoid rubbing, which can cause abrasion and chaffing.

Proper hand-washing technique

To minimize the spread of infection, follow these basic hand-washing instructions. With your hands angled downward under the tap, adjust the water temperature until it's comfortably warm.

Lather up

Wet your hands under the running water. Apply soap and work up a generous lather by covering all areas of your hands, rub all surfaces of lathered hands for 10–15 seconds. Make sure you clean beneath your fingernails, around your knuckles, and along the sides of your fingers and thumbs, and don't forget the palms of your hands.

Six-step hand-washing technique

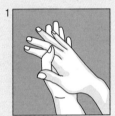

1

Palm to palm.

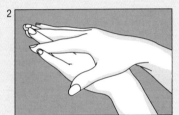

2

Right palm over left dorsum and left palm over right dorsum.

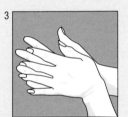

3

Palm to palm fingers interlaced.

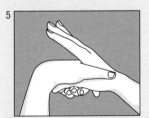

4

Fingers to palm

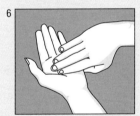

5

Rotational rubbing of right thumb clasped in left palm and vice versa.

6

Centre of palm with fingertips

Pat dry

Rinse your hands under running water to wash away residual soap and microorganisms. Dry thoroughly with a paper towel using the same six steps. To prevent recontaminating your hands on the taps, cover each one with a dry paper towel when turning off the water, if they do not have elbow levers.

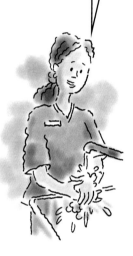

It's simple! Washing your hands is the single most important procedure for preventing the spread of infection.

- If the sink is not equipped with elbow controls, turn off the taps by gripping them with a dry paper towel to avoid recontaminating your hands.
- Dispose of paper towels in the waste bin (as per local policy), using a foot pedal to open the bin.

Practice pointers

- Follow local policy concerning how to decontaminate your hands (when to wash with soap or antiseptic hand wash and when to use an alcohol-based hand rub). Ideally, you'll wash with hand wash and water when beginning your shift; before and after direct or indirect patient contact; between each episode of patient care; before and after performing any body functions, such as blowing your nose or using the bathroom; before preparing or serving food; before preparing or administering medications; after removing gloves or other personal protective equipment; and after completing your shift.
- Use an alcohol-based hand rub when soap and water is unavailable to you. However, alcohol hand rubs are not appropriate if your hands are visibly soiled, and be aware that the manufacturers of some hand gels advise that they should be used a maximum of three times before you use hand wash and water (or if you experience a build-up of residue on your hands).
- Hand washing with soap and water must be used when caring for patients with *Clostridium difficile*, as alcohol-based hand rubs and gels are insufficient to kill this microorganism.
- If you are providing care in the patient's home, ideally bring your own supply of hand wash and disposable paper towels. If there is no running water, disinfect your hands with an alcohol-based hand rub.
- You must always remember to allow alcohol-based products time to dry; it is the drying of the alcohol that reduces the bacterial count.
- For further information regarding hand washing, visit the Royal College of Nursing website and their 'Wipe it out campaign'.
- ESCs specific to standard numbers 21–26 (Infection prevention and control) plus in accordance with 1–9 (Care, compassion and communication) and 10–11 (Organizational aspects of care).

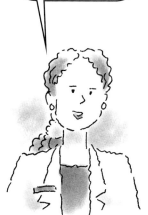

Soap will do for most situations. But before performing an invasive procedure, wound care or dressing change, use an antiseptic cleaner.

Personal protective equipment

Personal protective equipment (PPE) will be provided by your employer to assist in protecting both you and your patients from HCAIs. It is important to be aware of what is available to you and when to use it.

Cues to use

Generally, you will have access to the following PPE:

- *Uniforms*, short sleeved for wearing in the clinical area. These should be laundered after each shift. If your Trust does not provide laundering facilities, then you should wash your uniform separately from other clothes and on a high-temperature wash cycle, this will remove soiling and reduce the colonization of bacteria. This should be followed by steam ironing and/or tumble drying as the heat from these will eliminate pathogens.
- *Gloves* (non-sterile and sterile; latex and latex-free) prevent gross contamination of your hands and should never be used as a substitute for hand hygiene. Non-sterile gloves should be worn when dealing directly with body fluids, or when you are at risk of coming into contact with body fluids and, of course, when you have any open cuts or abrasions on your own hands. You should change your gloves at the same intervals/or frequency as for hand-washing guidelines, i.e. when possible (non-visible) contamination has occurred or visible contamination has occurred. Sterile gloves must be worn when performing an aseptic technique or practice. See *Latex allergy management* for use of latex and non-latex gloves.
- *Aprons*, usually plastic and in various colours for different roles (see local policies), assist in preventing the transfer of bacteria from your uniform or personal clothing to the patient, or vice versa. The apron must be changed between separate aspects of care (i.e. oral hygiene and perineal care!) and always between patients.
- *Goggles, glasses or face shields* are designed to protect your eyes against foreign bodies, splashes and aerosols. In other words, wear them when you are at risk of contamination from body fluids or blood through splashing. This would include when you are manually decontaminating reusable instruments, irrigating wounds, removing urinary catheters, giving oral care and during airway suctioning.

Practice pointers

- Follow local policy and procedure guidelines.
- ESCs specific to standard numbers 21–26 (Infection prevention and control) plus in accordance with 1–9 (Care, compassion and communication) and 10–17 (Organizational aspects of care).

Latex allergy management

Although latex is commonly used to make all sorts of products, it is used widely in the healthcare setting because it gives good protection against infections. However, many people have an allergy to it.

You must be on guard! Those at increased risk include people who have had, or will undergo, multiple surgical procedures, healthcare workers, employees who manufacture latex and latex-containing products, and people with a genetic predisposition to latex allergy.

Tell-tale foods

People who are allergic to certain foods—including apricots, cherries, grapes, kiwis, passion fruit, bananas, avocados, chestnuts, tomatoes and peaches—may also be allergic to latex. This is due to the proteins in latex being very similar to the proteins found in these foods, and they can cross-react. The allergic response to these foods will be similar to that produced when the person comes into contact with latex. Remember though, that any food that has been handled by someone wearing latex will cause a reaction!

Itching, sneezing, coughing

Latex allergy can cause various signs and symptoms, including generalized itching (on the hands and arms, for example); itchy, watery and burning eyes; sneezing and coughing (hay fever-type signs); rash; hives; bronchial asthma, scratchy throat and difficulty breathing; oedema of the face, hands and neck; and anaphylaxis.

Letting history speak for itself

To help identify people at risk for latex allergy, ask latex allergy-specific questions during the history-taking process. (See *Latex allergy screening*.)

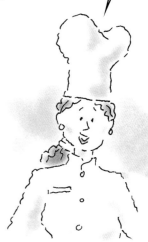

Allergies to certain foods—such as grapes, kiwis, bananas, or peaches—may indicate latex allergy.

Latex allergy screening

To determine if your patient has a latex sensitivity or allergy, ask the following screening questions:

- Do you have a history of allergies, dermatitis, or asthma? If so, what type of reaction do you have?
- Do you have any congenital abnormalities? If yes, explain.
- Do you have any food allergies? If so, what specific allergies do you have? Describe your reaction.
- Do you experience shortness of breath or wheezing when blowing up latex balloons? If so, describe your reaction.
- Have you had previous surgical procedures? Did you experience associated complications? If so, describe them.
- Have you had previous dental procedures? Did complications result? If so, describe them.
- Are you exposed to latex in your work? Have you experienced a reaction to latex products at work? If so, describe your reaction.

If the patient's history reveals a latex sensitivity, the doctor assigns him to one of three categories based on the extent of his sensitization. Group 1 patients have a history of anaphylaxis or a systemic reaction when exposed to a natural latex product. Group 2 patients have a clear history of a non-systemic allergic reaction. Group 3 patients do not have a previous history of latex hypersensitivity, but are designated as high risk because of an associated medical condition, occupation or 'cross-reactive' allergy.

Going latex-free

If your patient is sensitive to latex, make sure that he doesn't come in contact with latex because such contact could result in a life-threatening hypersensitivity reaction. Creating a latex-free environment is the only way to safeguard your patient. Healthcare providers must now provide latex-free equipment, both for use if you have a latex allergy and for your patients who have a latex allergy. (See *Choosing the right glove*.)

Choosing the right glove

Healthcare workers may develop allergic reactions as a result of their exposure to latex gloves and other products containing natural rubber latex. Patients may also have latex sensitivity.

General precautions

Take the following steps to protect yourself and your patient from allergic reactions to latex:

- Use non-latex (for example, vinyl or synthetic) gloves for activities that aren't likely to involve contact with infectious materials (food preparation, routine cleaning, and so forth).
- Use appropriate barrier protection when handling infectious materials. If you choose latex gloves, use powder-free gloves with reduced protein content.
- After wearing and removing gloves, wash your hands with soap and dry them thoroughly.
- When wearing latex gloves, don't use oil-based hand creams or lotions (which can cause gloves to deteriorate) unless they've been shown to maintain glove barrier protection.
- Refer to the material safety data sheet for the appropriate glove to wear when handling chemicals.

- Learn procedures for preventing latex allergy, and learn how to recognize the signs and symptoms of latex allergy: skin rashes; hives; flushing; itching; nasal, eye, or sinus symptoms; asthma; and shock.
- If you have (or suspect you have) a latex sensitivity, use non-latex gloves, avoid contact with latex gloves and other latex-containing products, and consult your Occupational Health Department.

If you know you're allergic

If you have latex allergy, consider these precautions:

- Avoid contact with latex gloves and other products that contain latex.
- Avoid areas where you might inhale the powder from latex gloves worn by other workers.
- Inform your employers and your healthcare providers (doctors, nurses, dentists and others).
- Wear a medical identification bracelet.
- Follow your doctor's instructions for dealing with allergic reactions to latex.

What you need

Latex allergy identified on notes and patient ID wristband ✳ latex-free equipment, including room contents ✳ anaphylaxis kit.

Getting ready

After you've determined that the patient has a latex allergy or is sensitive to latex, arrange for him to be placed in a private room. If that isn't possible, make the room latex-free to prevent the spread of airborne particles from latex products used on the other patients.

How you do it

- Check for latex allergy in all patients being admitted to the clinical area.
- If a patient has a latex allergy, ensure you have latex-free equipment by his bedside.
- Document the allergy on the patient's nursing and medical notes, according to local policy. If policy requires the patient to wear an allergy identification wristband, place it on him immediately.

Write big

- If the patient will be receiving anaesthesia, make sure that 'latex allergy' is clearly visible on the front of his notes. (See *Anaesthesia induction and latex allergy.*) This, as well as ensuring that you verbally hand over the information during any patient transfer between clinical areas, will assist in ensuring that all multidisciplinary team members are aware that the patient has a latex allergy.
- If the patient is to have an I.V. line, make sure that it's inserted using latex-free products. Apply a latex allergy sign on the I.V. tubing to prevent access of the line with latex products.

First flush

- Flush I.V. tubing with 50 ml of I.V. solution, because of latex ports in the I.V. tubing.
- Place a warning label on I.V. bags that says 'Don't use latex injection ports'.
- Use a non-latex tourniquet. If none are available, use a latex tourniquet over clothing.
- Remove the vial stopper to mix and draw medications.
- Use latex-free oxygen administration equipment. Remove the elastic, and tie equipment on with gauze.
- Wrap your stethoscope with a non-latex product to protect the patient from latex contact.

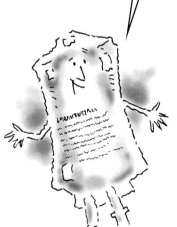

I need a warning label that says 'Don't use latex injection ports'.

Anaesthesia induction and latex allergy

Intraoperative latex reaction may be caused by latex contact with the mucous membrane, inhalation of particles during anaesthesia, or injection through latex ports. Here are signs and symptoms in conscious and anaesthetized patients.

Conscious patient

- Abdominal cramping
- Anxiety
- Bronchoconstriction
- Diarrhoea
- Feeling of faintness
- Pruritus
- Itchy eyes
- Nausea
- Shortness of breath
- Swelling of soft tissue
- Vomiting

Anaesthetized patient

- Bronchospasm
- Cardiopulmonary arrest
- Facial oedema
- Flushing
- Hypotension
- Laryngeal oedema
- Tachycardia
- Urticaria
- Wheezing

- Wrap Tegaderm over the patient's finger before using pulse oximetry.
- Use latex-free syringes when administering medication through a syringe.
- Keep an anaphylaxis kit nearby. If the patient has an allergic reaction to latex, treat him immediately.

Practice pointers

- Remember that signs and symptoms of latex allergy usually occur within 30 minutes of anaesthesia induction. However, the time of onset can range from 10 minutes to 5 hours.
- Don't forget that, as a healthcare worker, you can develop a latex hypersensitivity. If you suspect that you're sensitive to latex, contact the occupational health department concerning local policy for latex-sensitive employees. Use latex-free products whenever possible to help reduce your exposure to latex.
- ESCs specific to numbers 21–26 (Infection prevention and control) and numbers 36, 41 and 42 (Medicines management); plus in accordance with numbers 1–9 (Care, compassion and communication).

Looks can deceive

- Don't assume that if something doesn't look like rubber it isn't latex. Latex can be found, for example, in electrocardiograph leads, oral and nasal airway tubing, tourniquets, nerve stimulation pads, temperature strips, and blood pressure cuffs.

Isolation nursing

What you need

Aprons ✳ gloves ✳ goggles ✳ masks ✳ specially marked laundry bags (and water-soluble laundry bags, if used) ✳ plastic waste bags.

A trolley may be used outside the patient's room. It should include a work area (such as a pull-out shelf), drawers or a cupboard area for holding isolation equipment. A door card announcing that isolation precautions are in effect should also be posted, according to local policy.

Getting ready

Remove the cover from the isolation equipment trolley if necessary, and set up the work area. Check the trolley to ensure that there is sufficient equipment and supplies for the designated isolation category. The following isolation categories will each have a local policy to follow: Contact isolation, Respiratory isolation, Enteric isolation and Protective isolation.

How you do it

• Remove jewellery and watches, according to local policy. These actions help to prevent the spread of microorganisms.
• Wash your hands with an antiseptic cleaner to prevent the growth of microorganisms under gloves.

Putting on personal protective equipment
• Put the apron on and wrap it around the back of your uniform. Tie the strings to secure the apron at the waist. The apron should cover the majority of the front of your uniform.
• If necessary place a mask snugly over your nose and mouth. Secure ear loops around your ears or tie the strings behind your head high enough so the mask will not slip off. If the mask has a metal strip, squeeze it to fit your nose firmly but comfortably. (See *Putting on a face mask*.) If you wear glasses, tuck the mask under their lower edge.
• Put on goggles, if necessary. If you wear glasses, you may choose not to wear goggles. However, this will usually depend on how much protection your glasses will give to your eyes, i.e. how large they are. If you wear small glasses that offer little to no protection, you may choose to wear goggles over your glasses.
• Put on the gloves.

Putting on a face mask

To avoid spreading airborne particles, wear a sterile or non-sterile face mask as indicated. Position the mask to cover your nose and mouth, and secure it high enough to ensure stability.

Get all tied up

Tie the top strings at the back of your head above the ears. Then tie the bottom strings at the base of your neck. Adjust the metal nose strip if the mask has one.

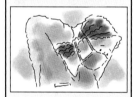

Removing personal protective equipment

- Remember that the outside surfaces of your PPEs are contaminated.
- With your gloved left hand, remove the right glove by pulling on the cuff, turning the glove inside out as you pull. Don't touch any skin with the outside of either glove. (See *Removing contaminated gloves*.) Then remove the left glove by wedging one or two fingers of your right hand inside the glove and pulling it off, turning it inside out as you remove it. Discard the gloves in the clinical waste bin.

Mask can be last

- Untie your mask, holding it only by the strings. Discard the mask in the clinical waste bin. If the patient has an infection that's spread by airborne pathogens, you may prefer to remove the mask last.
- To remove your apron, grasp the neck straps of the apron and tear apart, untie or break the plastic ties at the waist and then fold the apron down in front of you to avoid carrying it over your head and spreading any pathogens collected on it.
- Discard it in the clinical waste bin.

Washing up

- If the sink is inside the patient's room, wash your hands and forearms with soap or antiseptic cleaner before leaving the room. Turn off the tap using a paper towel and discard the towel in the room. Grasp the door handle with a clean paper towel to open it,

---

Removing contaminated gloves

Proper removal techniques are essential for preventing the spread of pathogens from gloves to your skin surface. Follow these steps carefully:

Using your non-dominant hand, pinch the opposite glove near the top. Avoid allowing the glove's outer surface to fold inward against your wrist/arm.

Pull downward, allowing the glove to turn inside out as it comes off. Keep the dominant-hand glove in your non-dominant hand after removing it.

Now insert the first two fingers of your ungloved non-dominant hand under the edge of the dominant-hand glove. Avoid touching the glove's outer surface or folding it against your wrist.

Pull downward so that the glove turns inside out as it comes off. Continue pulling until the glove completely encloses the other one and its uncontaminated inner surface is facing out.

and discard the towel in the clinical waste container inside the room. Close the door from the outside with your bare hand.
- If the sink is outside the isolation room, wash your hands and forearms with soap or antiseptic cleaner after leaving the room.

Practice pointers

- Use gowns, gloves, goggles and masks only once, and discard them in the appropriate container before leaving a contaminated area. If your mask is reusable, clean it and retain it for further use unless it's damaged. Refer to manufacturer's instructions or local policy for cleaning instructions.
- Always maintain a high standard of cleanliness in the patient's room.
- Ensure that the patient and his visitors are aware of the need for isolation and the precautions they must take to prevent the spread of infection.
- ESCs specific to standard numbers 21–26 (Infection prevention and control) plus in accordance with 1–9 (Care, compassion and communication).

Decontaminate the area

- After patient transfer, discharge or death, return the isolation equipment trolley to the appropriate area for cleaning and restocking of supplies. A dedicated isolation room or other room prepared for isolation purposes must be thoroughly cleaned and disinfected before use by another patient. This is usually done by a domestic team, specifically trained in this procedure.
- At the end of your shift, restock used items for the next person. (See *Documenting isolation equipment use*.)

> **Write it down**
>
> ## Document-ing isolation equipment use
>
> Record any special needs for isolation precautions on the nursing care plan and as otherwise indicated by local policy.

Patient hygiene

Maintaining personal hygiene is a basic human right (Young, 1991), you know you would want to be clean if in hospital! Thus assisting patients to meet these needs is a fundamental part of nursing care. *The National Service framework for older people* (Department of Health, 2000) states that service users and carers should be able to expect that personal hygiene needs are met sensitively and in privacy; who would want to be stripped naked and embarrassed in front of all the other patients—not me! This is emphasized in the

Essence of Care (Department of Health, 2001) with the following benchmark for practice:

> Patients/clients have access to an environment that is safe and acceptable to the individual.

> Areas of hygiene that need to be considered are:

- eye care
- mouth care
- total care
- perineal care
- foot care.

Eye care

When paralysis or coma impairs or eliminates the corneal reflex, frequent eye care aims to keep the exposed cornea moist, preventing ulceration and inflammation. Application of saline-saturated gauze pads over the eyelids moistens the eyes. Commercially available eye ointments and artificial tears also lubricate the corneas, but a doctor's prescription is required for their use.

Eye care is a clean procedure, your aim is to clean the eye and prevent cross-infection. Therefore, you wear non-sterile gloves and use a non-touch technique to reduce the risk.

What you need

Sterile galley pot ✳ gloves and apron ✳ sterile towel ✳ sterile normal saline solution ✳ sterile low-linting gauze swabs ✳ artificial tears or eye ointment (if prescribed).

Getting ready

Assemble the equipment at the patient's bedside. Open the sterile towel and open all sterile equipment on to this. Pour a small amount of saline solution into the galley pot. Open the sterile gauze using an aseptic technique and place on the sterile towel.

How you do it

- Wash your hands thoroughly, put on gloves and apron, and inform the patient of what you would like to do, in order to gain consent. Inform the patient even if he's comatose or appears unresponsive.

Clean . . .

- To remove secretions or crusts adhering to the eyelids and eyelashes, first soak gauze in sterile normal saline solution. Then gently wipe the patient's eye with the moistened gauze, working

from the inner canthus to the outer canthus to prevent debris and fluid from entering the nasolacrimal (tear) duct.
• To prevent cross-contamination, use a fresh piece of gauze for each wipe until the eye is clean. To prevent irritation, avoid using soap to clean the eyes. Repeat the procedure for the other eye.

. . . and lubricate

• After cleaning the eyes, instil artificial tears or apply eye ointment, as prescribed, to keep them moist.

Finishing up

• After giving eye care, dispose of the galley pot, apron and gloves. Use new equipment for each care episode. (See *Documenting eye care*.)

Practice pointers

• ESCs specific to standard numbers 21–26 (Infection prevention and control) plus in accordance with 1–9 (Care, compassion and communication), 10–20 (Organizational aspects of care) and 33–42 (Medicines management).

> **Write it down**
> ## Documenting eye care
> Record the time and type of eye care in your notes. If applicable, record administration of eyedrops or ointment in the patient's medication chart. Document unusual crusting or excessive or coloured drainage and report findings as appropriate.

Mouth care

Given as many times as is necessary (but specifically in the morning, at bedtime or after meals), mouth care entails inspecting the mouth and giving care as necessary, i.e. brushing the teeth and oral cavity. It removes soft plaque deposits and calculus from the teeth, cleans and massages the gums, reduces mouth odour, and helps prevent infection. By freshening the patient's mouth, mouth care also enhances appreciation of food, thereby aiding appetite and nutrition.

Although an ambulatory patient can usually perform mouth care alone, a bedridden patient may require partial or full assistance. A comatose patient requires use of suction equipment to prevent aspiration during oral care.

What you need

Towel and/or disposable soft cloths ✳ disposable bowl ✳ waste bag ✳ mouthwash ✳ toothbrush and toothpaste ✳ jug and glass ✳ drinking straw ✳ gloves, goggles and apron ✳ small, free-standing mirror ✳ tongue depressor ✳ pen torch.

Getting ready

Fill a jug with water, and bring it and other equipment to the patient's bedside. If you'll be using oral suction

> Mouth care is not just for morning, bedtime and after meals, but as required!

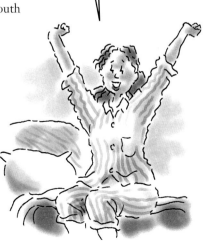

equipment, connect the tubing to the suction bottle and suction catheter, insert the plug into an outlet, and check for correct operation.

How you do it

• Wash your hands thoroughly, put on gloves and apron (you may wish to wear goggles to prevent splashing into your eyes), explain the procedure to the patient, and provide privacy.

Supervising mouth care

• If the patient is bedridden but capable of self-care, encourage him to perform his own mouth care.
• If allowed, assist the patient into an upright position. Place the over-bed table in front of him with the mirror angled to allow the patient to view his face; arrange the rest of equipment on the table, ensuring that everything is within reach of the patient.
• Drape a towel over the patient's chest to protect his clothing.
• Mix mouthwash and water in a glass, place a straw in it if necessary, and position the disposable bowl nearby.
• Instruct him to brush his teeth and gums while looking into the mirror. Encourage him to rinse frequently during brushing, and provide facial tissues or soft cloths for him to wipe his mouth.
• Ensure all areas of the mouth are cleaned—teeth, palate, buccal surfaces, gums and tongue—and all with a soft toothbrush to clean the mucosa and stimulate circulation.
• Check for irritated areas or sores and report and administer prescribed treatment as instructed.

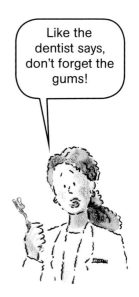

Like the dentist says, don't forget the gums!

Performing mouth care

• If the patient is comatose or conscious but incapable of self-care, perform mouth care on him. If he wears dentures, clean them thoroughly. (See *Dealing with dentures*.)
• Some patients may benefit from the use of an oral irrigating device and the use of these is becoming more commonplace. (See *Using an oral irrigating device*.)

Prepping the patient

• Raise the bed to a comfortable working height to prevent back strain. If a patient is unconscious, then lower the head of the bed and position the patient on his side, with his face extended over the edge of the pillow to facilitate drainage and prevent fluid aspiration. The conscious patient should be assisted into an upright position.
• Arrange the equipment on the over-bed table or bed locker, including the oral suction equipment, if necessary. Turn on the machine.

Dealing with dentures

Dentures require proper care to remove soft plaque deposits and calculus and to reduce mouth odour. Such care involves removing and rinsing dentures after meals, daily brushing and removal of tenacious deposits, and soaking in a denture-cleaning agent. Dentures must be removed from the comatose or pre-surgical patient to prevent possible airway obstruction.

Equipment and preparation

Start by assembling the following equipment at the patient's bedside: ✳ disposable bowl ✳ labelled denture pot ✳ toothbrush or denture brush ✳ gloves and apron ✳ toothpaste ✳ denture-cleaning agent if available ✳ paper towel ✳ mouthwash ✳ gauze.

Wash your hands, put on gloves and an apron.

Removing dentures

- Obtain the patient's cooperation and consent. The patient may request not to be seen by anyone while he does not have his dentures in; comply and care for the patient's psychological needs as well as his physical needs.
- To remove a full upper denture, grasp the front and palatal surfaces of the denture with your thumb and forefinger. Position the index finger of your opposite hand over the upper border of the denture, and press to break the seal between denture and palate. Grasp the denture with gauze because saliva can make it slippery.
- To remove a full lower denture, grasp the front and lingual surfaces of the denture with your thumb and index finger, and gently lift up.
- To remove partial dentures, first ask the patient or caregiver how the prosthesis is retained and how to remove it. If the partial denture is held in place with clips or snaps, then exert equal pressure on the border of each side of the denture. Avoid lifting the clasps, which can easily bend or break.

Oral and denture care

- After removing dentures, place them in a properly labelled denture pot. Add warm water and denture cleaning agent (if available) to remove stains and hardened deposits. Follow package directions. Avoid soaking dentures in mouthwash containing alcohol because it may damage a soft liner.
- Instruct the patient to rinse with mouthwash to remove food particles and reduce mouth odour. Then stroke the palate, buccal surfaces, gums, and tongue with a soft toothbrush to clean the mucosa and stimulate circulation. Check for irritated areas or sores because they may indicate a poorly fitting denture.
- Carry the denture pot, disposable bowl, toothbrush, and toothpaste to the sink. After lining the basin with a paper towel, fill it with water to cushion the dentures in case you drop them. Hold the dentures over the basin, wet them with warm water, and apply toothpaste to a denture brush or long-bristled toothbrush. Clean the dentures using only moderate pressure to prevent scratches and warm water to prevent distortion.
- Clean the denture pot, and place the dentures in it. Rinse the brush, and clean and dispose of the bowl in the clinical waste. Return all equipment to the patient's locker.

Wearing dentures

- If the patient desires, apply adhesive liner to the dentures. Moisten them with water, if necessary, to reduce friction and ease insertion.
- Encourage the patient to wear his dentures to enhance his appearance, facilitate eating and speaking, and prevent changes in the gum line that may affect denture fit.

Using an oral irrigating device

An oral irrigating device, such as the Water Pik, directs a pulsating jet of water around the teeth to massage gums and remove debris and food particles. It's especially useful for cleaning areas missed by brushing, such as around bridgework, crowns, and dental wires. Because this device enhances oral hygiene, it benefits patients undergoing head and neck irradiation, which can damage teeth. The device also maintains oral hygiene in a patient with a fractured jaw or with mouth injuries that limit standard mouth care.

Equipment and preparation

To use the device, first assemble the following equipment: oral irrigating device ✳ gloves ✳ towel ✳ disposable kidney bowl ✳ pharyngeal suction apparatus ✳ salt solution or mouthwash, if ordered ✳ soap.

Implementation

- Wash your hands, put on gloves and an apron.
- Turn the patient to his side to prevent aspiration of water. Then place a towel under his chin and a kidney bowl next to his cheek to absorb or catch drainage.
- Insert the plug of the oral irrigating device into a nearby electrical socket. Remove the device's cover, turn it upside down, and fill it with lukewarm water or with a mouthwash or salt solution, as instructed by manufacturer's or physician's instructions.
- Secure the cover to the base of the device. Remove the water hose handle from the base, and snap the jet tip into place. If necessary, wet the grooved end of the

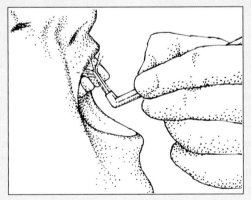

tip to ease insertion. Adjust the pressure dial to the setting most comfortable for the patient. If his gums are tender and prone to bleed, choose a low setting.
- Adjust the knurled knob on the handle to direct the water jet, place the jet tip in the patient's mouth, and turn on the device. Instruct the patient to keep his lips partially closed to avoid spraying water.
- Direct the water at a right angle to the gum line of each tooth and between teeth. Avoid directing water under the patient's tongue because this may injure sensitive tissue.
- After irrigating each tooth, pause briefly and instruct the patient to expectorate the water or solution into the kidney bowl. If he can't do so, suction it from the sides of the mouth with the pharyngeal suction apparatus. After irrigating all teeth, turn off the device, and remove the jet tip from his mouth.
- Empty the remaining water or solution from the cover, remove the jet tip from the handle, and return the handle to the base. Clean the jet tip with soap and water, rinse the cover, dry them, and return them to storage.

- Place a soft disposable cloth under the patient's chin and a disposable kidney bowl near his cheek to absorb or catch drainage.
- Lubricate the patient's lips with water or petroleum-free balm to prevent dryness and cracking. Reapply lubricant, as needed, during oral care.
- If necessary, use a tongue depressor to hold the patient's tongue flat during the procedure.

Brushing them clean

- Wet the toothbrush with water. If necessary, use hot water to soften the bristles. Apply toothpaste.
- Brush the patient's lower teeth from the gum line up; the upper teeth, from the gum line down.
- Place the brush at a 45-degree angle to the gum line, and press the bristles gently into the gingival sulcus. Using short, gentle strokes to prevent gum damage, brush the buccal surfaces (toward the cheek) and the lingual surfaces (toward the tongue) of the bottom teeth; use just the tip of the brush for the lingual surfaces of the front teeth. Using the same technique, brush the buccal and lingual surfaces of the top teeth. Brush the biting surfaces of the bottom and top teeth, using a back and forth motion.
- Hold the disposable kidney bowl steady under the patient's cheek, and wipe his mouth and cheeks with tissues/soft cloth as needed. Use suction as required and remember to only apply suction when withdrawing the suction catheter from the mouth.

Follow up with a swab

- After brushing the patient's teeth, dip a cotton-tipped mouth swab into the mouthwash solution or warm water. Press the swab against the side of the glass to remove excess moisture. Gently stroke the gums, buccal surfaces, palate, and tongue to clean the mucosa and stimulate circulation.

After mouth care

- Assess the patient's mouth for cleanliness and tooth and tissue condition.
- Rinse the toothbrush and glass, dispose of the kidney bowl.
- Empty and clean the suction bottle, if used, and place a clean Yanker suction catheter on the tubing.
- Remove your gloves and apron, return reusable equipment to the appropriate storage location, and discard disposable equipment in the clinical waste or household waste as per local policy. Wash your hands. (See *Documenting mouth care*.)

Practice pointers

- Factors compromising oral health: poor nutritional status, drug therapy, age, oxygen therapy and physical dexterity problems.
- For further information on oral care visit the British Dental Health Foundation website: www.dentalhealth.org.uk
- ESCs specific to standard numbers 27–32 (Nutrition and fluid management), 21–26 (Infection prevention and control) plus in accordance with 1–9 (Care, compassion and communication), 10–20 (Organizational aspects of care) and 33–42 (Medicines management).

Write it down

Documenting mouth care

In your nursing care plan document:

- date and time of mouth care and sign
- the condition, such as: dry, bleeding, oedema, mouth odour, excessive secretions or plaque on the tongue
- the care that you administered.

Total care

The skin has many functions, including:
* protection from friction, shear, dehydration, UV light and radiation
* perception of temperature, pain and touch
* excretion of salts and perspiration
* synthesis of vitamin D
* prevention of water and electrolyte balance deficits and
* maintenance of body temperature.

It is therefore extremely important that we keep the skin intact and in good health. When assisting or administering hygiene care to a patient you will have the opportunity to fully assess the skin condition. Use of the Waterlow Score (see *Waterlow scoring*) and National Institute for Clinical Excellence (NICE) guidelines on pressure ulcer risk assessment and prevention will assist with this assessment and care planning.

> Good thing I'm learning about skin and back care!

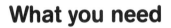

What you need

Basin ✳ soap ✳ blankets ✳ bath towel ✳ washcloths ✳ prescribed lotions ✳ gloves, if the patient has open lesions or has been incontinent ✳ fresh linen ✳ apron.

Getting ready

Explain the procedure to the patient and gain consent. Remember that this care should be given when the patient wishes it to happen and this is not necessarily before breakfast. Ensure privacy for the patient by drawing the bed curtains if in an open ward.

How you do it

* Assemble the equipment at the patient's bedside. Lastly, fill the basin two-thirds full with warm water to prevent it from getting cold.
* Explain the procedure to the patient, and provide privacy. Ask him to tell you if you're applying too much or too little pressure.
* Adjust the bed to a comfortable working height. Wash your hands and put on gloves, if applicable, and an apron.
* In the first instance place the patient on his back
* Untie the patient's gown and expose his chest and arms, now cover with a bath towel to prevent chills and minimize exposure. Place a bath towel behind him to protect bed linen from moisture.

Waterlow scoring

WATERLOW PRESSURE ULCER PREVENTION/TREATMENT POLICY

RING SCORES IN TABLE, ADD TOTAL. MORE THAN 1 SCORE/CATEGORY CAN BE USED

BUILD/WEIGHT FOR HEIGHT	◆	SKIN TYPE VISUAL RISK AREAS	◆	SEX AGE	◆	MALNUTRITION SCREENING TOOL (MST) (Nutrition Vol.15, No.6 1999–Australia		
AVERAGE		HEALTHY	0	MALE	1	A– HAS PATIENT LOST WEIGHT RECENTLY	B–WEIGHT LOSS SCORE	
BMI = 20–24.9	0	TISSUE PAPER	1	FEMALE	2		0.5–5kg = 1	
ABOVE AVERAGE		DRY	1	14–49	1	YES –GO TO B	5–10kg = 2	
BMI = 25–29.9	1	OEDEMATOUS	1	50–64	2	NO –GO TO C	10–15kg = 3	
OBESE		CLAMMY, PYREXIA	1	65–74	3	UNSURE –GO TO C	> 15kg = 4	
BMI > 30	2	DISCOLOURED		75–80	4	AND	unsure = 2	
BELOW AVERAGE		GRADE 1	2	81 +	5	SCORE 2		
BMI < 20	3	BROKEN/SPOTS				C–PATIENT EATING POORLY	NUTRITION SCORE	
BMI = Wt(Kg)/Ht (m)^2		GRADE 2–4	3			OR LACK OF APPETITE	If > 2 refer for nutrition	
						'NO' = 0; 'YES' SCORE = 1	assessment / intervention	

CONTINENCE	◆	MOBILITY	◆	SPECIAL RISKS				
COMPLETE/		FULLY	0	TISSUE MALNUTRITION	◆	NEUROLOGICAL DEFICIT		◆
CATHETERIZED	0	RESTLESS/FIDGETY	1	TERMINAL CACHEXIA	8	DIABETES, MS, CVA		4–6
URINE INCONT.	1	APATHETIC	2	MULTIPLE ORGAN FAILURE	8	MOTOR/SENSORY		4–6
FAECAL INCONT.	2	RESTRICTED	3	SINGLE ORGAN FAILURE		PARAPLEGIA (MAX OF 6)		4–6
URINARY + FAECAL		BEDBOUND		(RESP, RENAL, CARDIAC,)	5	MAJOR SURGERY or TRAUMA		
INCONTINENCE	3	e.g. TRACTION	4	PERIPHERAL VASCULAR		ORTHOPAEDIC/SPINAL		5
		CHAIRBOUND		DISEASE	5	ON TABLE > 2 HR#		5
		e.g. WHEELCHAIR	5	ANAEMIA (Hb < 8)	2	ON TABLE > 6 HR#		8
				SMOKING	1			

SCORE

10+ AT RISK

15+ HIGH RISK

20+ VERY HIGH RISK

MEDICATION—CYTOTOXICS, LONG TERM/HIGH DOSE STEROIDS, ANTI-INFLAMMATORY   MAX OF 4

Scores can be discounted after 48 hours provided patient is recovering normally

© J Waterlow 1985 Revised 2005*

Obtainable from the Nook, Stoke Road, Henlade TAUNTON TA3 5LX

* The 2005 revision incorporates the research undertaken by Queensland Health.

REMEMBER TISSUE DAMAGE MAY START PRIOR TO ADMISSION, IN CASUALTY. A SEATED PATIENT IS AT RISK
ASSESSMENT: IF THE PATIENT FALLS INTO ANY OF THE RISK CATEGORIES, THEN PREVENTATIVE NURSING IS REQUIRED. A COMBINATION OF GOOD NURSING TECHNIQUES AND PREVENTATIVE AIDS WILL BE NECESSARY

<u>ALL ACTIONS MUST BE DOCUMENTED</u>

PREVENTION
PRESSURE

REDUCING AIDS
Special

Mattress/beds:	10+ Overlays or specialist foam mattresses.
	15+ Alternating pressure overlays, mattresses and bed systems
	20+ Bed systems: Fluidized bead, low air loss and alternating pressure mattresses
	Note: Preventative aids cover a wide spectrum of specialist features. Efficacy should be judged, if possible, on the basis of independent evidence.
Cushions:	No person should sit in a wheelchair without some form of cushioning. If nothing else is available - use the person's own pillow. (Consider infection risk)
	10+ 100mm foam cushion
	15+ Specialist Gel and/or foam cushion
	20+ Specialized cushion, adjustable to individual person.
Bed clothing:	Avoid plastic draw sheets, inco pads and tightly tucked in sheet/sheet covers, especially when using specialist bed and mattress overlay systems
	Use duvet - plus vapour permeable membrane.

NURSING CARE

General	HAND WASHING, frequent changes of position, lying, sitting. Use of pillows
Pain	Appropriate pain control

Nutrition	High protein, vitamins and minerals
Patient Handling	Correct lifting technique - hoists - monkey poles Transfer devices
Patient Comfort Aids	Real Sheepskin - bed cradle
Operating Table	
Theatre/A&E Trolley	100mm(4ins) cover plus adequate protection
Skin Care	General hygene, NO rubbing, cover with an appropriate dressing

WOUND GUIDELINES

Assessment	odour, exudate, measure/photograph position

WOUND CLASSIFICATION - EPUAP

GRADE 1	Discolouration of intact skin not affected by light finger pressure (non-blanching erythema)
	This may be difficult to identify in darkly pigmented skin
GRADE 2	Partial thickness skin loss or damage involving epidermis and/or dermis
	The pressure ulcer is superficial and presents clinically as an abrasion, blister or shallow crater
GRADE 3	Full thickness skin loss involving damage of subcutaneous tissue but not extending to the underlying fascia
	The pressure ulcer presents clinically as a deep crater with or without undermining of adjacent tissue
GRADE 4	Full thickness skin loss with extensive destruction and necrosis extending to underlying tissue.
Dressing Guide	Use Local dressings formulary and/or www.worldwidewounds

IF TREATMENT IS REQUIRED, FIRST REMOVE PRESSURE

Make it into a mitt

- Fold the washcloth around your hand to form a mitt. This prevents the loose ends of the cloth from dripping water on to the patient and keeps the cloth warm longer.
- Work up lather with soap. Using long, firm strokes, bathe the patient's chest, beginning at the neck and shoulders and moving downward to the waist, then move to the arms. Expose small areas at a time to prevent chills and maintain dignity.

Rinse and dry

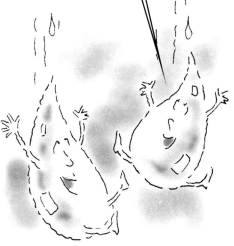

Dry well because trapped moisture can cause chaffing.

- Rinse and dry well because any moisture trapped can cause chaffing and predispose the patient to pressure ulcers.
- While giving total care, closely examine the patient's skin, especially the bony prominences of the shoulders, the scapulae, and the coccyx, for redness or abrasions.

Patient first, bed last

- Take any prescribed lotion and pour a small amount into your palm. Rub your hands together to distribute the lotion.
- Apply the lotion to the patient's chest, using long, firm strokes. The lotion reduces friction, making application easier. Add lotion as prescribed.
- Finish the application by using long, firm strokes, and blot any excess lotion from the patient's chest and arms with a towel.
- Repeat the process for the patient's legs, ensuring the chest, shoulders and genitals are covered with a blanket. See *Perineal care* of the male and female patient (below) for further details of administering perineal and genital hygiene.
- Cover the patient with a blanket again and assist him on to his side.
- Untie the patient's gown, and expose his back, shoulders and buttocks. Then drape the patient with a blanket to prevent chills and minimize exposure. Place a bath towel next to, or under, his side to protect bed linen from moisture
- Repeat the process for the neck and back, then buttocks, perineum and legs, ensuring the buttocks, legs and genitals are covered as necessary. See *Perineal care* of the male and female patient (below) for further details of administering perineal and genital hygiene.
- Once this has been completed, with the patient still on his side, begin to remove the bottom sheet from the bed, roll it inwards on the bed towards the patient's back.

- Take a clean sheet and open it out along the length of the bed behind the patient. Using hospital corners, tuck the sheet under the mattress to secure it in position and roll the excess sheet towards the old sheet and the patient's back.
- Roll the patient on to his back over the ends of both the old and new sheet and on to their opposite side.
- You will now be able to remove the old sheet and pull the clean sheet through and secure under the mattress on the other side of the bed, again using hospital corners.
- Assist the patient into a comfortable position and change the top linen, without exposing the patient to cold and maintaining his dignity at all times. Lastly, assist the patient into a fresh gown or pyjamas.

When you're done

- Return the bed to its original position, and make the patient comfortable. Empty and clean the basin.
- Dispose of gloves, if used, dispose of apron, and return equipment to the appropriate storage area.

Practice pointers

- Before giving total care, assess the patient's body structure and skin condition and read the nursing care plan.
- Give special attention to bony prominences because pressure ulcers are common in these areas.
- ESCs specific to standard numbers 1–9 (Care, compassion and communication), 21–26 (Infection prevention and control) plus in accordance with 10–20 (Organizational aspects of care) and 33–42 (Medicines management).

Perineal care

Perineal care, which includes care of the external genitalia and the anal area, should be performed during the daily bath and, if necessary, at bedtime and after urination and bowel movements. The procedure promotes cleanliness and prevents infection. It also removes irritating and odour-emitting secretions, such as smegma, a cheese-like substance that collects under the foreskin of the penis and on the inner surface of the labia.

For the patient with perineal skin breakdown, frequent bathing followed by application of an ointment or cream aids healing. Always follow standard precautions when providing perineal care.

What you need

Gloves and apron ✳ washcloths ✳ clean basin ✳ mild soap ✳ bath towel ✳ blanket ✳ toilet tissue ✳ clinical waste bag ✳ optional: bedpan, urine bottle, antiseptic soap, prescribed ointments/creams.

Following genital or rectal surgery, you may need to use sterile supplies, including sterile gloves, gauze pads, and/or low-linting gauze balls.

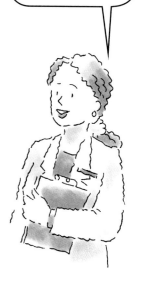

Always follow standard precautions when providing perineal care.

Getting ready

Obtain ointment or cream as prescribed. Fill the basin two-thirds full with warm water.

How you do it

- Explain to the patient the care you are offering and gain permission.
- Assemble equipment at the patient's bedside and provide privacy.
- Wash your hands thoroughly, put on gloves and apron.
- Adjust the bed to a comfortable working height to prevent back strain.
- Provide privacy and help the patient to a supine position. Place a towel under the patient's buttocks to protect the bed from stains and moisture.

Caring for the female patient

- To minimize the patient's exposure and embarrassment, place the blanket over her with corners head to foot and side to side. Wrap each leg with a side corner, tucking it under the hip. Then fold back the corner between the legs to expose the perineum.

Front to back

- Ask the patient to bend her knees slightly and to part her legs. Separate her labia with one hand and wash with the other, using gentle downward strokes from front to back of the perineum to prevent intestinal organisms from contaminating the urethra or vagina. Avoid the area around the anus, and use a clean disposable washcloth for each stroke to prevent the spread of contaminated secretions or discharge.
- Using a clean washcloth, rinse thoroughly from front to back, and then pat the area dry with a bath towel to prevent soap residue and moisture from irritating the skin. Apply prescribed ointments or creams.

- Turn the patient on to her side, if possible, to expose the anal area.
- Clean, rinse and dry the anal area, starting at the posterior vaginal opening and wiping from front to back.

Caring for the male patient
- Drape the patient's legs to minimize exposure and embarrassment and to expose the genital area.

Make it a circular motion

- Hold the shaft of the penis with one hand and wash with the other, beginning at the tip and working in a circular motion from the centre to the periphery to avoid introducing microorganisms into the urethra. Use a clean section of washcloth for each stroke to prevent the spread of contaminated secretions or discharge.
- For the uncircumcised patient, gently retract the foreskin and clean beneath it. Rinse well but don't dry because moisture provides lubrication and prevents friction when replacing the foreskin. Replace the foreskin to avoid constriction of the penis, which causes oedema and tissue damage.
- Rinse thoroughly, using the same circular motion.

Hitting all the necessary spots

- Wash the rest of the penis, using downward strokes toward the scrotum. Rinse well, and pat dry with a towel.
- Clean the top and sides of the scrotum. Rinse well, and pat dry. Handle the scrotum gently to avoid causing discomfort.
- Turn the patient on his side. Clean the bottom of the scrotum and the anal area. Rinse well, and pat dry.

After perineal care
- Reposition the patient and make him/her comfortable. Remove the blanket and towel, and then replace the bed linens.
- Clean and return the basin and dispose of soiled articles including gloves and apron in the clinical waste bag. (See *Documenting skin assessment and care*.)

Practice pointers

- Give perineal care to all patients in a matter-of-fact way to minimize embarrassment.
- ESCs specific to standard numbers 1–9 (Care, compassion and communication), 21–26 (Infection prevention and control) plus in accordance with 10–20 (Organizational aspects of care) and 33–42 (Medicines management).

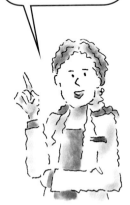

When performing perineal care, minimizing exposure and embarrassment is very important.

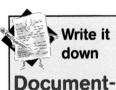

Write it down

Documenting skin assessment and care

Record perineal care and special treatment in your notes. Document the need for continued treatment and changes to your plan of care as necessary. Describe general skin condition, discharges and odour.

When incontinence is a factor

- If the patient is incontinent, first remove excess faeces with toilet tissue. Then position him/her on a bedpan, and add a small amount of antiseptic soap to a urine bottle or jug to eliminate odour and soften faeces. Irrigate the perineal area to remove any remaining faecal matter.
- For management of the patient with continence problems, seek advice from the Continence Advisory Service in your locality.

Foot care

Daily bathing of feet and regular trimming of toenails promotes cleanliness, prevents infection, stimulates peripheral circulation, and controls odour by removing debris and skin flora from skin, between toes and under toenails.

This type of care is particularly important for bedridden patients and those especially susceptible to foot infection, such as patients with peripheral vascular disease, diabetes mellitus, poor nutritional status, arthritis, or a condition that impairs peripheral circulation. In such patients, proper foot care should include meticulous cleanliness and regular observation for signs of skin breakdown. (See *Foot care for diabetic patients*.)

Foot care for diabetic patients

Because diabetes mellitus can reduce blood supply to the feet, normally minor foot injuries can lead to dangerous infection. When caring for a diabetic patient, keep these foot care guidelines in mind:

- Exercising the feet daily can help improve circulation. While the patient is sitting on the edge of the bed, ask him to point his toes upward, then downward, 10 times. Then have him make a circle with each foot 10 times.
- A diabetic patient's shoes must fit properly. Instruct the patient to break in new shoes gradually by increasing wearing time by 30 minutes each day. Also, tell him to check old shoes frequently in case they develop rough spots in the lining.
- Tell the patient to wear clean socks daily and to avoid socks with holes, darned spots, or rough, irritating seams.
- Advise and refer the patient to see a doctor, podiatrist or chiropodist if you are concerned about the condition of his feet.

- Tell the patient to wear warm socks or slippers and use extra blankets *to avoid cold feet.* The patient shouldn't use heating pads and hot water bottles because these can cause burns when sensory perception is impaired.
- Teach the patient to inspect the skin on the feet regularly for cuts, cracks, blisters and red, swollen areas. Even slight cuts on the feet should receive a doctor's attention. As a first-aid measure, tell him to wash the cut thoroughly and apply a mild antiseptic. Urge the patient to avoid harsh antiseptics, such as iodine, because they can damage tissue.
- Advise the diabetic patient to avoid tight-fitting garments or activities that can decrease circulation. He should especially avoid sitting with his knees crossed, touching or tampering with sores or rough spots on his feet, walking barefoot, or applying adhesive tape to the skin on his feet.

What you need

Blanket ✳ large basin ✳ soap ✳ towel ✳ pillow ✳ washcloth ✳ cotton ✳ lotion ✳ gloves, if the patient has open lesions ✳ an apron ✳ optional: cotton-tipped applicator, gauze pads or cotton balls.

Getting ready

Fill the basin half way with warm water. Test water temperature with a thermometer because patients with diminished peripheral sensation could burn their feet in excessively hot water (over 40.6°C) without feeling any warning pain. If a thermometer isn't available, test the water by inserting your elbow. The water temperature should feel comfortably warm.

How you do it

• Ask the patient if he would like his feet washed, and gain permission/consent.
• Assemble equipment at the patient's bedside. Wash your hands and put on gloves if necessary.
• Cover the patient with a blanket if in a chair. Fold the top linen back to mid calf if the patient is in bed.
• Remove anti-embolism stockings or footwear.
• Place a towel under the patient's feet, if in bed this should keep the bottom linen dry and if the patient is in a chair it will prevent slips, trips and falls. Then position the basin on the towel.
• Insert a pillow beneath the patient's knee to provide support if the patient is in bed, and cushion the rim of the basin with the edge of the towel to prevent pressure.

Soak, rinse, dry, detail and moisturize

• Immerse one foot in the basin and wash it with soap, and then allow the foot to soak for about 5 minutes. Soaking softens the skin, loosens debris under toenails, and comforts and refreshes the patient.
• After soaking the foot, rinse it with a washcloth, remove it from the basin, and place it on the towel.
• Dry the foot thoroughly, especially between the toes, to prevent skin breakdown. Blot gently to dry because harsh rubbing may damage the skin.
• Empty the basin, refill it with warm water, and clean and soak the other foot.

Soak one foot, clean the other

• While the second foot is soaking, assess the first one. Using the cotton-tipped applicator, carefully clean the toenails.

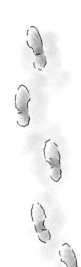

- Refer to a podiatrist or chiropodist if nails need trimming.
- Rinse the foot that has been soaking, dry it thoroughly, and repeat the process.
- Apply lotion to moisten dry skin.
- Re-apply anti-embolism stockings if prescribed to encourage vascular return, or patient's footwear to prevent chills.
- Remove and clean all equipment, and dispose of gloves as per local policy. (See *Documenting foot care*.)

Practice pointers

- While providing foot care, observe the colour, shape and texture of the toenails. If you see redness, drying, cracking, blisters, discoloration, or other signs of traumatic injury, especially in patients with impaired peripheral circulation, notify the doctor. Because such patients are vulnerable to infection, they need prompt treatment and referral to the chiropodist or podiatrist must be made.
- ESCs specific to standard numbers 1–9 (Care, compassion and communication), 21–26 (Infection prevention and control) plus in accordance with 10–20 (Organizational aspects of care) and 33–42 (Medicines management).

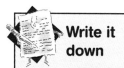

Write it down

Document-ing foot care

Record the date and time of foot care in your nursing care plan. Record and report abnormal findings and actions you take. Sign.

Care of the dying patient

A patient needs intensive physical and emotional support as he approaches death. Signs and symptoms of impending death include reduced respiratory rate and depth, decreased or absent blood pressure, weak or erratic pulse rate, lowered skin temperature, decreased level of consciousness (LOC), diminished sensory perception and neuromuscular control, diaphoresis, pallor, cyanosis and mottling.

Emotional support for the dying patient and his family usually involves reassuring them and being there to help ease fear and loneliness. More intense support is important at earlier stages, especially for a patient with a long-term progressive illness, who can work through the stages of dying. (See *Five stages of dying*.)

What you need

Clean bed linen ✳ clean patient clothing ✳ gloves ✳ apron ✳ basin ✳ soap ✳ washcloths ✳ towels ✳ medication ✳ water ✳ suction and resuscitation equipment, if necessary ✳ optional: indwelling urinary catheter, analgesia, intravenous fluids, incontinence aids.

Five stages of dying

According to Elisabeth Kübler-Ross, author of *On death and dying,* the dying patient may progress through five psychological stages in preparation for death. Although each patient experiences these stages differently, and not necessarily in this order, understanding the stages will help you meet your patient's needs.

Denial

When the patient first learns of his terminal illness, he'll refuse to accept the diagnosis. He may experience physical signs and symptoms similar to a stress reaction—shock, fainting, pallor, sweating, tachycardia, nausea and GI disorders.

During this stage, be honest with the patient but not blunt or callous. Maintain communication with him so he can discuss his feelings when he accepts the reality of his impending death. Don't force him to confront this reality.

Anger

When the patient stops denying his impending death, he may show deep resentment toward anyone who will live on after he dies. Although you may instinctively draw back from the patient or even resent this behaviour, remember that he's dying and that he has a right to be angry. After you accept his anger, you can help him find ways to express it and can help his family understand it.

Bargaining

Although the patient acknowledges his impending death, he attempts to bargain with God or fate for more time. He will probably strike this bargain secretly. If he does confide in you, don't urge him to keep his promises.

Depression

In this stage, the patient may first experience regrets about his past and then grieve about his condition. He may withdraw from his friends, family, doctor and you. He may suffer from anorexia, increased fatigue or self-neglect. You may find him sitting alone, in tears. Accept the patient's sorrow, and if he talks to you, listen. Provide comfort by touch, as appropriate. Resist the temptation to make optimistic remarks or cheerful small talk.

Acceptance

In this last stage, the patient accepts the inevitability and imminence of his death—without emotion. The patient may simply desire the quiet company of a family member or friend. If, for some reason, a family member or friend can't be present, stay with the patient to satisfy his final need. Remember, however, that many patients die before reaching this stage.

How you do it

- Assemble equipment at the patient's bedside as needed.

Meeting physical needs

- Observe the patient for pallor, diaphoresis and decreased LOC. Remember it is not always necessary to take and record vital signs for this patient—he is dying.
- Reposition the patient in bed as per the nursing assessment dictates, because sensation, reflexes and mobility diminish first in

the legs and gradually in the arms. Make sure the bed sheets cover him loosely to reduce discomfort caused by pressure on arms and legs. Good use of the Waterlow Score (see *Waterlow scoring* earlier in the chapter) and NICE guidelines on pressure ulcer risk assessment and prevention prior to the patient reaching this stage of illness should mean that all risk assessments and care planning have been performed and the patient is being nursed according to these guidelines.

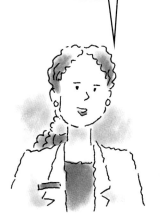

Make your patient's last days as comfortable as possible.

Watch what you say

- When the patient's vision and hearing start to fail, speak to him from near the head of the bed. Because hearing may be acute despite loss of consciousness, avoid speaking inappropriately in his presence.
- Change the bed linens and the patient's gown as needed. Provide skin care during gown changes and adjust the room temperature for patient comfort, if necessary.
- Observe the patient for incontinence or anuria, which can result from diminished neuromuscular control or decreased renal function. If necessary, assess the need for continence aids to prevent skin deterioration or obtain advice from the Continence Advisory Service regarding catheterization. Put on gloves, and wash the perineal area with soap and water as discussed in *Perineal care*. Dry thoroughly to prevent irritation.
- As his condition deteriorates, the patient may breathe mostly through his mouth, causing dryness. Administer mouth care as discussed previously. Elevate the head of the bed to assist with draining of respiratory secretions and aid breathing. Offer fluids frequently, and lubricate the patient's lips and mouth with water to counteract dryness.
- If the unconscious patient's eyes are open, provide appropriate eye care to prevent corneal ulceration, which can cause blindness.
- Administer prescribed analgesia as required and assess effect; if the patient is not pain free, seek advice from the Pain Service in your locality. Keep in mind that, as circulation diminishes, medications given I.M. will be poorly absorbed. Medications should be given I.V., transdermally or subcutaneously, for optimum results.

Meeting emotional needs

- Fully explain all care and treatments to the patient even if he's unconscious because he may still be able to hear. Answer any questions as candidly as possible without sounding callous.

• Allow the patient to express his feelings, which may range from anger to loneliness. Take time to talk with him. Sit near the head of his bed, and avoid looking rushed or unconcerned. Touch him often in neutral areas, such as on his arm or his hand, and allow him to hold your hand if desired.

• Notify family members, if absent, when the patient wishes to see them. Let the patient and family discuss death at their own pace.

• Offer contact with the hospital chaplain for his faith, if appropriate.

Practice pointers

• Overall responsibility for cardiopulmonary resuscitation (CPR) status and decisions for in-patients in the UK rests with consultants. However, the most senior admitting doctor should consider resuscitation status in all patients. Not making a Do Not Attempt Resuscitation (DNAR) decision amounts to the patient being 'for resuscitation' in the event of an arrest occurring. If the patient has a DNAR decision, then ensure that all members of the multidisciplinary team are aware.

• ESCs specific to standard numbers 1–9 (Care, compassion and communication), 21–26 (Infection prevention and control) plus in accordance with 10–20 (Organizational aspects of care), 33–42 (Medicines management) and 27–32 (Nutrition and fluid management).

Write it down

Document-ing care of the dying patient

Record changes in the patient's fluid intake and output and level of consciousness. Note the times of cardiac arrest and the end of respiration, and notify the doctor when these occur.

Family matters

• If family members remain with the patient, show them where the bathrooms, lounges and restaurants are located.

• Explain the patient's needs, treatments and plan of care to them.

• If appropriate, offer to teach them specific skills so they can take part in nursing care. Emphasize that their efforts are important and effective.

• As the patient's death approaches, give them emotional support. (See *Documenting care of the dying patient.*)

Post-mortem care

After the patient dies, care continues and includes preparing him for family viewing, arranging transportation to the morgue and determining the disposition of the

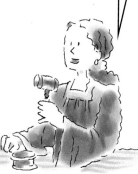

Know the national and local policy on DNAR.

patient's belongings. Post-mortem care also entails comforting and supporting the patient's family and friends, providing for their privacy and informing and supporting the family through the process of registration of death.

Post-mortem care usually begins after a doctor or appropriately trained allied health professional certifies the patient's death. The body of the patient should be cared for and attended to according to both local policy and the patient's cultural and religious beliefs; this may include a family member being involved in the washing and dressing of the patient.

What you need

Basin * soap * blankets * bath towel * washcloths * prescribed lotions * gloves, if the patient has open lesions or has been incontinent * apron * fresh linen * shroud * ID tags (3) * tape * gauze * string.

How you do it

- Give 'Total care' as previously described in this chapter and dress in a shroud, as well as the following.

Preparing for family viewing

- Place the body in the supine position, arms at sides and head on a pillow. Then elevate the head of the bed slightly to prevent discoloration from blood settling in the face.
- If the patient wore dentures and your local policy permits, gently insert them; then close his mouth. Close his eyes by gently pressing on his lids with your fingertips. If they don't stay closed, place moist cotton balls on the eyelids for a few minutes, and then try again to close them. If his jaw is dropping and looking unsightly, place a folded towel under his chin to keep his jaw closed.
- Remove indwelling urinary catheters, tubes and tape, and apply adhesive bandages to puncture sites. Replace soiled dressings.
- Collect all the patient's valuables to prevent loss. If you're unable to remove a ring, cover it with tape to prevent slippage and subsequent loss.
- Cover the body up to the chin with a clean sheet.
- Offer comfort and emotional support to the family and intimate friends. If they wish to see the body, let them do so in private.
- Support the family's needs for spiritual or religious rituals.

• After the family leaves, remove the towel from under the chin of the deceased patient. Pad the wrists and ankles to prevent bruises, and tie them together with gauze or soft string ties.

Preparing for transport

• Fill out the identification tags. Each tag should include the deceased patient's name, hospital number, date of birth, date and time of death, and doctor's name. Tie one tag to the deceased patient's hand or foot, but don't remove his identification bracelet to ensure correct identification.
• Wrap the patient's body in a clean sheet and secure it with tape, secure the second ID tag on the outside of the wrapped body, usually on the chest area.
• If the patient died of an infectious disease, label and dress the body according to local policy.
• Call for portering service or morgue attendant to collect the body. When they arrive to remove the body, close the doors of adjoining rooms if possible.

Handling personal belongings

• Using relevant local policy documents, make a list with a colleague of the deceased patient's personal belongings, including valuables, place them in a plastic bag and attach the third identification tag to it. Store in a secure place until the family or next of kin collect them.

Practice pointers

• If the patient died under suspicious circumstances or within 24 hours of hospital admission, care may be postponed until the medical examiner completes an investigative post-mortem, in this case leave all drips, drains, etc., *in situ*.
• Sign over the deceased patient's personal belongings to his family; make sure a colleague is present as a witness. Obtain the signature of an adult family member to verify receipt of valuables or to state their preference that jewellery remained on the patient.
• Offer emotional support to the deceased patient's family and friends and to other ward patients if appropriate. (See *Documenting post-mortem care*.)
• ESCs specific to standard numbers 1–9 (Care, compassion and communication) and numbers 10–20 (Organizational aspects of care).

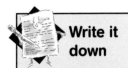

Write it down

Document-ing post-mortem care

Although documentation varies among hospitals, always record the collection or location of storage of the patient's possessions, especially jewellery and money. Also, note the date and time the patient was transported to the morgue. Remember to collate all nursing and medical notes back together.

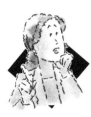

Quick quiz

1. At which anatomical point should clothing be worn above to minimize infection?

    A.   Above the wrist
    B.   Above the elbow
    C.   Above the hand

Answer: B. Above the elbow, to prevent contamination of clothing.

2. Theoretically, between how many care episodes can you use alcohol hand gel before washing?

    A.   1
    B.   0
    C.   3

Answer: C. Three, as long as there has been no physical contamination of body fluids or build-up of residue on your hands from the alcohol hand rub.

3. What PPEs would you require to perform mouth care?

    A.   Gloves and apron only
    B.   Gloves, apron, mask and goggles
    C.   None

Answer: A. Gloves and apron only to prevent contamination of clothing and to safeguard you and your patient from body fluid transfer via the hands.

4. Which group of patients should you ask for consent to perform care?

    A.   All
    B.   None
    C.   Only conscious patients

Answer: A. All, patients must give permission/consent for care to be given; they have every right to refuse.

5. How many ID tags will you require for post-mortem care?

    A.   3
    B.   4
    C.   1

Answer: A. One for the hand or foot, one for the outside of the sheet, and one for the patient's belongings.

Scoring

☆☆☆ If you answered all five items correctly, Wowwee! You know your infection control and hygiene care!

☆☆ If you answered three or four items correctly, Yowzer! Your knowledge is impressive!

☆ If you answered fewer than three correctly, relax, review, and give it another go!

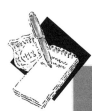

Just the facts

In this chapter, you'll learn:

♦ the A–G of patient assessment

♦ how to perform vital signs, both manually and using electronic equipment

♦ how to clinically monitor your patient using clinical assessment skills and procedures

♦ when and how to escalate your findings using track and trigger systems

♦ about the essential documentation for each procedure.

A–G of assessment

The ABC acronym has been used for many years for assessing the unconscious patient and is widely known. This acronym has been further enhanced, particularly by Dr Gary Smith of Portsmouth University Hospital, and is taught on ALERT courses. It can be used at any time to assess a patient. You should find it helpful whether at the beginning or end of a shift, to give a verbal and written handover; taking or giving a handover to a department nurse during patient transfer; during a shift of duty to physically assess your patient; or during an emergency situation. By using each letter to represent headings you will be able to assess each area of your patient's condition, then in order to act quickly and effectively upon your findings a 'physiological track and trigger system' (see *Early warning system*) can be used, as advised by the National Institute for Health and Clinical Excellence (NICE). The following is a list of questions and prompts that you can use under each heading to guide you through the process:

Airway

Is the patient maintaining his own airway? Does he have an airway adjunct *in situ*, i.e. oropharyngeal airway, nasopharyngeal airway, tracheostomy, laryngectomy? Are they working and clear? Does the patient need suction manoeuvres?

Breathing

How is the patient breathing? Can he talk in full sentences, or does his breathing restrict speech? Is the breathing fast and shallow or slow and deep? (See *Respiration*.) Is he using accessory muscles? Is he gasping for breath? What is the rate? How is his colour, any signs of cyanosis? Any clubbing of the fingers? Is he on oxygen or air therapy; is the prescription correct? If so how much, via which type of delivery device, and what are his oxygen saturations? (See *Pulse oximetry*.) What is his peak flow rate? Does he have a cough? Is it productive or dry? Does he have a wheeze, stridor, crackles or creps? Does he have a chest drain? What type and why? Is it working?

Circulation

What are the heart and/or pulse rates? (See *Pulse*.) What is the rhythm and strength? (regular or irregular, weak, thready or strong). Which anatomical location did you take the pulse from: radial, brachial, femoral, carotid artery? What is the blood pressure? (See *Blood pressure*.) What is the capillary refill time? What are the skin colour, temperature and general condition? Has an electrocardiograph (ECG) been taken; what was the result? Is the patient on intravenous therapy; if so, which fluid is prescribed, over how long, is it running to time? What is the patient's fluid balance? How much urine has he produced? What was the colour? What was the test strip result?

Dysfunction/disability

What is the patient's level of consciousness? (See *Neurological assessment*.) What is his capillary blood glucose level (CBG)? (See Chapter 3.) Does he have any pain? Can he tell you about his pain using a score of 1–3 or can you tell from his facial expressions? Has he had any analgesia?

Exposure

What is the patient's temperature? From which anatomical location was it taken? What was the result? Was the result normal? Are there any lacerations, bruises, reddening or rashes on the skin? Are there any wounds? Describe them: oozing, odour, colour depth, length, signs of healing? What are they being treated with? Is there any oedema? Where? Description, i.e. pitting or non-pitting, fluid loss? What actions have been taken?

Family and friends

Who is the next of kin? Do we have contact details for them? Does the patient wish family and friends to be informed of his condition; if not, who is to be informed? What is the medical history of the immediate family? Do the friends and family know where the patient is, especially after transfer between departments? (If appropriate and the patient wishes them to be informed.)

Goals

What are the expected and planned goals for the patient at this time? Remember these goals must be SMART: specific, measurable, achievable, realistic and timed. What is the estimated date of discharge? How can you help the patient achieve these goals? Do you need to refer the patient to any other multidisciplinary service, i.e. home care, speech and language therapy, pharmacy prescriptions, to prepare for discharge?

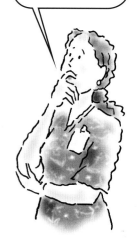

Did I tell Mr Brown where Mrs Brown was transferred to?

Practice pointers

• Use the A–G of patient assessment to give you the entire medical picture of the patient's physiological, psychological and social history.
• Ensure you document all of your findings in the nursing or medical notes as per local policy.
• ESCs specific to standard numbers 1–8 (Care, compassion and communication), 9–20 (Organizational aspects of care), 21–26 (Infection prevention and control), 27–32 (Nutrition and fluid management) and 34–36, 37, 39–42 (Medicines management).

Physiological track and trigger systems

The publication in July 2007 of the NICE *Guidelines for acutely ill patients in hospital* was responded to by most UK hospitals with the introduction of track and trigger systems of various designs. The concept is to ensure patient safety and promote early recognition of acute illness, and the system should used to monitor all adult patients in acute hospitals.

Track

Look at the *Early warning system*, a risk band is identified for each of the vital signs used for patient assessment. Now look horizontally

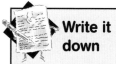

Write it down

Documenting patient assessment

Remember to document your findings for each section of Airway to Goals in the patient's nursing records.

Early warning system

Risk band	Urgent	Warning	Observe-At risk	Normal range	Observe-At risk	Warning	Urgent
Temp (core)		<35.0	<36.0	36.0–37.5		>38.0	>39.0
Pulse	<45	45–49	50–59	60–89	90–114	115–129	>= 130
Systolic blood pressure	<80	80–89 or >40 mmHg drop from normal	90–99 or >20 mmHg drop from normal	100–159	160–179	180–199	>= 200
Respiratory rate	<8			10–19	20–24	25–30	>30
SpO$_2$	<85	85–89	90–93	>= 94			
CNS response (AVPU)		New confusion		Alert	Voice	Pain	Unresponsive
GCS	<10	11–12	13–14	15			
Urine output (Catheterized)		<0.5ml/kg/hr for 2 hours	<0.5ml/kg/hr for 1 hour	0.5–3 ml/kg/hr	>3 ml/kg/hr		
Urine output	<500 ml/24 hours	<750 ml/24 hours	1,000–750 ml/24 hours				

* The most ABNORMAL reading places patient in the associated RISK band
* Interpret physiological data with reference to what is acceptable at the time of assessment and chronic disease state

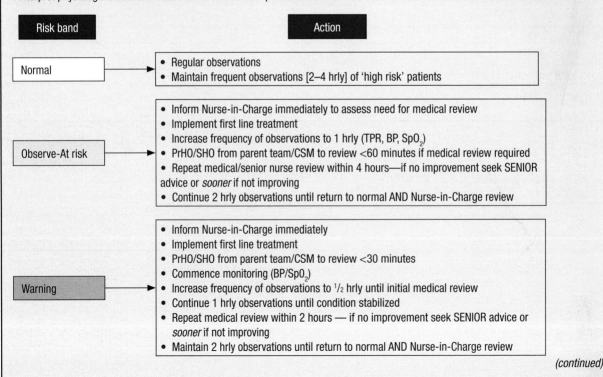

Risk band	Action
Normal	• Regular observations • Maintain frequent observations [2–4 hrly] of 'high risk' patients
Observe-At risk	• Inform Nurse-in-Charge immediately to assess need for medical review • Implement first line treatment • Increase frequency of observations to 1 hrly (TPR, BP, SpO$_2$) • PrHO/SHO from parent team/CSM to review <60 minutes if medical review required • Repeat medical/senior nurse review within 4 hours—if no improvement seek SENIOR advice or *sooner* if not improving • Continue 2 hrly observations until return to normal AND Nurse-in-Charge review
Warning	• Inform Nurse-in-Charge immediately • Implement first line treatment • PrHO/SHO from parent team/CSM to review <30 minutes • Commence monitoring (BP/SpO$_2$) • Increase frequency of observations to $^1/_2$ hrly until initial medical review • Continue 1 hrly observations until condition stabilized • Repeat medical review within 2 hours — if no improvement seek SENIOR advice or *sooner* if not improving • Maintain 2 hrly observations until return to normal AND Nurse-in-Charge review

(continued)

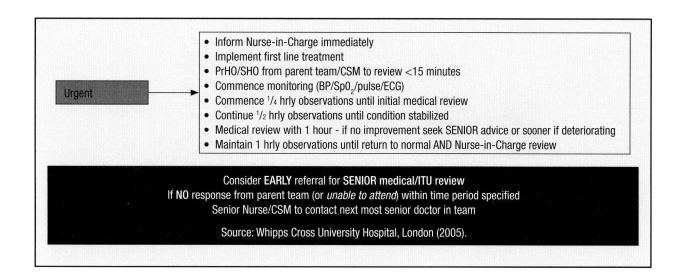

Urgent →

- Inform Nurse-in-Charge immediately
- Implement first line treatment
- PrHO/SHO from parent team/CSM to review <15 minutes
- Commence monitoring (BP/SpO$_2$/pulse/ECG)
- Commence ¼ hrly observations until initial medical review
- Continue ½ hrly observations until condition stabilized
- Medical review with 1 hour - if no improvement seek SENIOR advice or sooner if deteriorating
- Maintain 1 hrly observations until return to normal AND Nurse-in-Charge review

Consider **EARLY** referral for **SENIOR medical/ITU review**
If **NO** response from parent team (or *unable to attend*) within time period specified
Senior Nurse/CSM to contact next most senior doctor in team

Source: Whipps Cross University Hospital, London (2005).

across the table and see how there are ranges for each vital sign. When you have taken a complete set of vital signs for your patient you can easily and quickly interpret these data using this scoring system. This is the 'tracking' part of the system.

Trigger

Each vital sign you take must be interpreted and the instruction/action you follow will be from the most abnormal vital sign. For example, if your patient has the following vital signs:

Blood pressure, 96/64; Core temperature, 36.5; Pulse, 58; Respiratory rate, 6; SpO$_2$, 86%

This would put the blood pressure into the Observe – at risk range (☐); the core temperature would be in the Normal range (☐); the pulse rate would be in the Observe – at risk range (☐); the respiratory rate would be in the Urgent range (■); and the SpO$_2$ would be in the Warning range (■). Therefore the most abnormal vital sign would be the respiratory rate. The colour coding system then tells you what to do. In other words, it allows you to pull the starting pistol 'trigger' and ensure that you have escalated information appropriately and that all the medical professionals that the patient requires to improve his condition are off the starting blocks and ready to run.

I'm on the track and ready for the trigger.

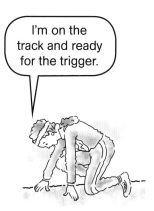

Practice pointers

• Be aware of your local track and trigger system; gain knowledge of how to use it if you are unsure.
• Ensure you escalate your findings; otherwise there is no point in taking vital signs.
• ESCs specific to standard numbers 9–20 (Organizational aspects of care) and 1–8 (Care, compassion and communication).

Temperature

Body temperature represents the balance between heat that metabolism, muscular activity and other factors produce, and heat that is lost through the skin, lungs and body wastes. A stable temperature pattern promotes proper function of cells, tissues and organs; a change in this pattern usually signals the onset of illness.

Choose one of two

Temperature can be measured with one of two types of thermometers: electronic digital or chemical-dot. Oral temperature in adults normally ranges from 36.1° to 37.5°C. Rectal temperature, the most accurate reading, is usually 0.6°C higher; however, this is rarely used due to the higher number of complications and risk. Axillary temperature, the least accurate reading, is usually 0.6–1.1°C lower and tympanic temperature reads 0.5–1°C higher. (See *Types of thermometers.*)

Normal ups and downs

Temperature normally fluctuates with rest and activity. Lowest readings typically occur between 4 and 5 a.m.; the highest readings, between 4 and 8 p.m. Other factors also influence temperature. (See *Differences in temperature.*)

What you need

Electronic thermometer, chemical-dot thermometer or tympanic thermometer ✳ disposable thermometer sheath or probe cover (except for chemical-dot thermometer) ✳ tissue ✳ medical device wipes ✳ if required, gloves and apron.

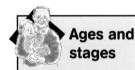

Ages and stages

Differences in temperature

Besides activity level, other factors that influence temperature include sex, age, emotional conditions and environment. Keep these principles in mind:
• Women normally have higher temperatures than men, especially during ovulation.
• Normal temperature is highest in neonates and lowest in elderly persons.
• A hot external environment can raise temperature; a cold environment lowers it.

Types of thermometers

You can take a patient's oral, rectal or axillary temperature with a chemical-dot device or an electronic digital thermometer. You can take tympanic temperature with a tympanic thermometer.

For adults who are awake, alert, oriented and cooperative, use of the tympanic route has become the most frequently used as it is non-invasive and has very few contraindications.

Tympanic thermometer

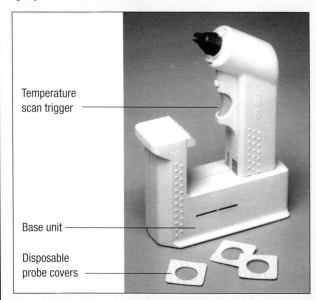

Temperature scan trigger

Base unit

Disposable probe covers

Chemical-dot thermometer

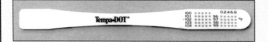

Individual electronic digital thermometer

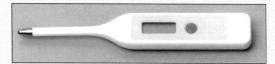

Institutional electronic digital thermometer

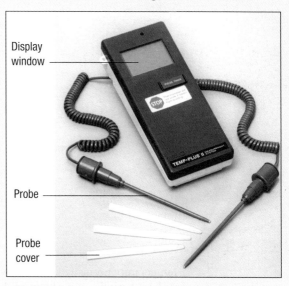

Display window

Probe

Probe cover

How you do it

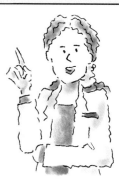

• Explain the procedure to the patient and gain consent. Wash your hands, put on gloves and apron if appropriate. If you're taking an oral temperature and he has had hot or cold liquids, chewed gum or smoked, wait 15 minutes before getting started.

With an electronic thermometer

• Ensure that the equipment is clean. Insert the probe into a disposable probe cover. Ask the patient to keep the probe under the tongue and to the side of the frenulum. Leave the probe in place until the maximum temperature appears on the digital display. Then remove the probe and note the temperature. Clean the equipment before putting away.

With a chemical-dot thermometer

• Remove the thermometer from its protective case by grasping the handle end with your thumb and forefinger, moving the handle up and down to break the seal, and pulling the handle straight out. Leave the chemical-dot thermometer in place for 45 seconds.
• Read the temperature as the last dye dot that has changed colour, or fired; then discard the thermometer and its dispenser case.

With a tympanic thermometer

• Make sure the lens under the probe is clean and shiny. Attach a disposable probe cover.
• Stabilize the patient's head and, if instructed by the manufacturer, gently pull his ear straight back (for children up to age 1) or up and back (for children aged 1 and older to adults).
• Insert the thermometer until the entire ear canal is sealed. The thermometer should be inserted toward the tympanic membrane in the same way that an otoscope is inserted. It should not be painful.
• Press the activation button, and hold it for 1 second. The temperature will appear on the display.
• Record the temperature in the patient's notes and clean the equipment.

Taking an oral temperature

• Put on gloves and position the tip of the thermometer under the patient's tongue on either side of the frenulum, as far back as possible. Placing the tip in this area promotes contact with superficial blood vessels and ensures a more accurate reading.
• Instruct the patient to close his lips but to not bite down with his teeth to avoid breaking the thermometer in his mouth.
• Leave the thermometer in place for the appropriate length of time, depending on which thermometer is used. Record findings and clean equipment.

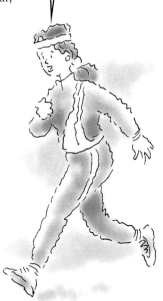

Lowest body temperature typically occurs in the early morning, after a night of rest. Highest occurs in the late afternoon or early evening, after a day of activity. Phew!

Taking an axillary temperature

- Position the patient with the axilla exposed.
- Put on gloves, and gently pat the axilla dry with a facial tissue, because moisture conducts heat. Avoid harsh rubbing, which generates heat.
- Ask the patient to reach across his chest and grasp his opposite shoulder, lifting his elbow.
- Position the thermometer in the centre of the axilla, with the tip pointing toward the patient's head.
- Tell him to keep grasping his shoulder and to lower his elbow and hold it against his chest, to promote skin contact with the thermometer.
- Leave the thermometer in place for the appropriate length of time, depending on which thermometer you're using. Axillary temperature takes longer to register than oral or rectal temperature because the thermometer isn't enclosed in a body cavity.
- Grasp the end of the thermometer, and remove it from the axilla. Remove your gloves and wash your hands.

Practice pointers

- Oral measurement is contraindicated in young children and infants, and in patients who are unconscious or disoriented, or who must breathe through their mouth or are prone to seizures.
- Use the same type of thermometer and method for repeat temperature taking, to ensure more consistent results.
- Store chemical-dot thermometers in a cool area—not in your pocket—because exposure to heat activates the dye dots.
- If your patient is receiving nasal oxygen, know that you can still measure his temperature orally because oxygen administration raises oral temperature by only about 0.27°C. (See *Documenting temperature*.)
- Assess the patient prior to using a tympanic temperature to ensure that: your patient has not been lying on his ear, as it will be warmer; there is no hearing aid *in situ*; he has no ear pain; and that jewellery is not going to obstruct entry to the ear canal.
- ESCs specific to standard numbers 1–8 (Care, compassion and communication), 9–20 (Organizational aspects of care) and 21–26 (Infection prevention and control).

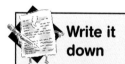

Write it down

Documenting temperature

Record the time, route and temperature on the patient's chart.

Pulse

Blood pumped into an already-full aorta during ventricular contraction creates a fluid wave that travels from the heart to the peripheral arteries. This recurring wave—called a pulse—can be palpated at locations on the body where an artery crosses over bone or firm tissue. (See *Pinpointing pulse sites*.)

Rate, rhythm and volume

Taking a patient's pulse involves determining the number of beats per minute (the pulse rate), the pattern or regularity of the beats (the rhythm), and the volume of blood pumped with each beat. (See *Alternative site for taking a pulse*.) If the pulse is faint or weak, consider using a Doppler ultrasound blood flow detector. (See *Using a Doppler device*.)

What you need

Watch with a second hand ✳ stethoscope (for auscultating apical pulse) ✳ Doppler ultrasound blood flow detector if necessary.

How you do it

• Wash your hands, and ask the patient if you may check his pulse.
• Make sure the patient is comfortable and relaxed because an awkward, uncomfortable position may affect his heart rate.
• Make sure the patient has been resting for at least 10 minutes, as exercise will increase the heart rate.
• Ensure that the patient has not had a cup of tea or coffee (with caffeine content), or a cigarette within the past 10 minutes as this also will increase the heart rate.

Taking a radial pulse

• Place the patient in a sitting or supine position, with his arm supported at his side or across his chest.

Keep the thumb out of it

• Gently press your index, middle and ring fingers on the radial artery, inside the patient's wrist. You should feel a pulse with only moderate pressure; excessive pressure may obstruct blood flow distal to the pulse site. Don't use your thumb to take the patient's pulse; the thumb has a strong pulse of its own and may easily be confused with the patient's pulse.

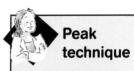

Peak technique

Pinpointing pulse sites

You can assess your patient's pulse rate at several sites, including those shown in the illustration below.

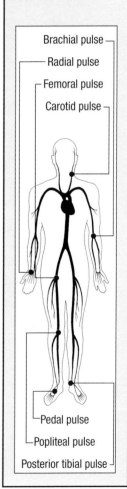

Brachial pulse

Radial pulse

Femoral pulse

Carotid pulse

Pedal pulse

Popliteal pulse

Posterior tibial pulse

One, two, three . . . sixty

• After locating the pulse, count the beats for 60 seconds if the pulse is irregular, or count for 30 seconds and multiply by 2 if the pulse is regular. Counting for a full minute provides a more accurate picture of irregularities.

• While counting the rate, assess the pulse rhythm and volume by noting the pattern and strength of the beats. If you detect an irregularity, repeat the count, and note whether the irregularity

Using a Doppler device

More sensitive than palpation for determining pulse rate, the Doppler ultrasound blood flow detector is especially useful when a pulse is faint or weak. Unlike palpation, which detects arterial wall expansion and retraction, this instrument detects the movement of red blood cells. Here's how you use it.

• Apply a small amount of lubricating gel to the ultrasound probe.
• Position the probe on the skin directly over the selected artery. In the illustration below, the probe is over the posterior tibial artery.
• When using a Doppler probe with an amplifier (as shown below), turn the instrument on and, moving counter-clockwise, set the volume control to the lowest setting. If your model doesn't have a speaker, plug in the earphones, and slowly raise the volume.
• To obtain the best signals, put gel between the skin and the probe, and

tilt the probe 45 degrees from the artery. Slowly move the probe in a circular motion to locate the centre of the artery and the Doppler signal— a hissing noise at the heartbeat. Avoid moving the probe rapidly because this distorts the signal.
• Count the signals for 60 seconds to determine the pulse rate.
• After you have measured the pulse rate, clean the probe with a soft cloth soaked in antiseptic solution, soapy water or as in the manufacturer's instructions. Don't immerse the probe.

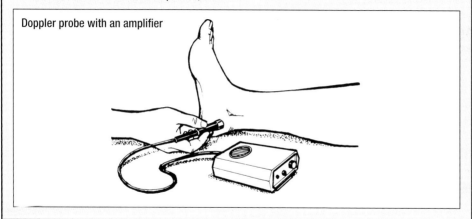

Doppler probe with an amplifier

Ages and stages

Alternative site for taking a pulse

The most common site for taking a pulse is the radial artery in the wrist. This holds true for adults and children older than age 3.

For infants and children younger than age 3, however, it's better to listen to the heart with a stethoscope, rather than palpate a pulse. Because auscultation is done at the apex of the heart, the pulse measured is the *apical pulse*; you will occasionally be asked to measure this in adults too.

Identifying pulse patterns

Type	Rate	Rhythm	Causes and incidence
Normal	60 to 80 beats/minute	● ● ● ●	• Varies with such factors as age, physical activity and gender (infants and children have higher pulse rates than adults and older adults, who have lower pulse rates)
Tachycardia	More than 100 beats/minute	●●●●●●●●	• Accompanies stimulation of the sympathetic nervous system resulting from emotional stress (such as anger, fear or anxiety) or the use of certain drugs and substances (such as caffeine) • May result from exercise or such health conditions as heart failure, anaemia and fever, which increase oxygen requirements and thus pulse rate
Bradycardia	Less than 60 beats/minute	● ● ●	• Accompanies stimulation of the parasympathetic nervous system resulting from drug use, especially cardiac glycosides, and such conditions as cerebral haemorrhage and heart block • May also be present in fit athletes and persons with hypothyroidism
Irregular	Uneven time intervals between beats (for example, periods of regular rhythm interrupted by pauses or premature beats)	●●●● ●●●	• May indicate cardiac irritability, hypoxia, digoxin toxicity, potassium imbalance, or a more serious arrhythmia if premature beats occur frequently (occasional premature beats are normal)

occurs in a pattern or randomly. If you're still in doubt, take an apical pulse. (See *Identifying pulse patterns*.)
• Record your findings on the temperature, pulse, respiration and blood pressure chart (TPR&BP); interpret using the local track and trigger system and escalate appropriately.

Taking an apical pulse
• Help the patient to a supine position, and cover with a blanket/sheet if necessary.

Warm the 'scope first, please
• Keeping in mind that the bell of the stethoscope transmits low-pitched sounds more effectively than the diaphragm, warm the bell

or diaphragm in your hand. Placing a cold stethoscope against the patient's skin may startle him and momentarily increase his heart rate.
- Place the warmed bell or diaphragm over the apex of the heart (normally located at the fifth intercostal space, left of the midclavicular line), and insert the earpieces into your ears.
- Count the beats for 60 seconds, and note their rhythm, volume and strength.
- Remove the stethoscope, and make the patient comfortable.
- Record your findings on the TPR&BP chart.
- Interpret your findings using the local track and trigger system and escalate your findings appropriately.

Taking an apical–radial pulse
- Find another nurse to work with you when taking a patient's apical–radial pulse so that she can palpate the radial pulse while you auscultate the apical pulse with a stethoscope, or vice versa.
- Help the patient to a supine position, and cover with a blanket or sheet as necessary.
- Locate the apical and radial pulses, and then determine a time to begin counting. You should both count beats for 60 seconds.
- Record your findings on the TPR&BP chart.
- Interpret your findings using the local track and trigger system and escalate your findings appropriately.

Practice pointers
- Remember to gain permission after explaining the procedure to your patient.
- Interpret your findings using the local track and trigger system and escalate your findings appropriately.
- When the patient's peripheral pulse is irregular, take an apical pulse to measure the heartbeat more directly.
- Always record your findings on the TPR&BP chart.
- Always act upon your findings.

Working it alone
- First, auscultate at the apex of the heart, holding the stethoscope in place with the hand that holds the watch, and then palpate at the radial artery with the other hand. You can then feel any discrepancies between the apical and radial pulses.
- Some heartbeats detected at the apex can't be detected at peripheral sites. When this occurs, the apical pulse rate is higher than the radial pulse rate; the difference is the pulse deficit. (See *Documenting pulse*.)

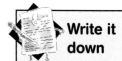

Write it down

Documenting pulse

Record pulse rate, rhythm and strength as well as the time of measurement. 'Full' or 'bounding' describes a pulse of increased strength; 'weak' or 'thready', a pulse of decreased strength. When recording apical pulse, include the intensity of heart sounds. When recording apical–radial pulse, chart the rate according to the pulse site—for example, A/R pulse = 80/76.

Respiration

Respiration is the exchange of oxygen and carbon dioxide between the atmosphere and the body. External respiration, or breathing, occurs through the work of the diaphragm and chest muscles, and delivers oxygen to the lower respiratory tract and alveoli.

Rate, rhythm, depth and sound

Respiration can be measured according to rate, rhythm, depth and sound. These measurements reflect the body's metabolic state, diaphragm and chest-muscle condition, and airway patency.

Respiratory rate is recorded as the number of cycles per minute, with inspiration and expiration making up one cycle; rhythm, as the regularity of these cycles. Depth is recorded as the volume of air inhaled and exhaled with each respiration; sound, as the audible digression from normal, effortless breathing.

Respiration is the first of the vial signs to change during physiological, psychological and pathophysiological changes. It is extremely important that every patient who is being monitored has manual respiratory rate taken regularly.

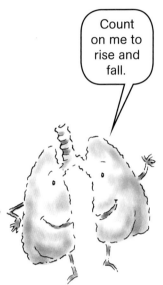

Count on me to rise and fall.

What you need

A watch with a second hand.

How you do it

• The best time to assess your patient's respirations is immediately after taking his pulse rate. Keep your fingertips over his radial artery, and don't tell him that you're counting respirations; otherwise, he'll become conscious of them, and the rate may change.

Watch the movement

• Count respirations by observing the rise and fall of the patient's chest as he breathes. Alternatively, position the patient's opposite arm across his chest, and count respirations by feeling its rise and fall. Consider one rise and one fall to be one respiration.
• Count respirations for 60 seconds, to account for variations in respiratory rate and pattern.
• Observe chest movements for depth of respirations. If the patient inhales a small volume of air, record the depth as shallow; if he inhales a large volume, deep.
• Observe the patient for use of accessory muscles, such as the scalene, sternocleidomastoid, trapezius and latissimus dorsi. Such

Ages and stages

How age affects respiration

When assessing respirations in older patients, keep these points in mind:

- When listening for stridor, check for sternal, substernal and intercostal retractions.
- In infants, an expiratory grunt indicates imminent respiratory distress.
- In older patients, an expiratory grunt indicates partial airway obstruction.

- A child's and adult's respiratory rate may double in response to exercise, illness or emotion.
- Normally, the rate for newborns is 30 to 80 breaths/minute; for toddlers, 20 to 40 breaths/ minute; and for children of school age and older, 15 to 25 breaths/minute.
- Children usually reach the adult rate (12 to 18 breaths/minute) at about age 15.

use indicates weakness of the diaphragm and the external intercostal muscles—the major muscles of respiration.
- Observe the patient for bilateral or unilateral chest movement.

Listen to the sounds

- As you count respirations, watch for and record such breath sounds as stertor, stridor, wheezing and expiratory grunting.
- Stertor is a snoring sound resulting from secretions in the trachea and large bronchi. Listen for it in comatose patients and in patients with a neurological disorder.
- Stridor is an inspiratory crowing sound that occurs in patients with laryngitis, croup or upper respiratory tract obstruction with a foreign body. (See *How age affects respiration*.)
- Wheezing is caused by partial obstruction in the smaller bronchi and bronchioles. This high-pitched, musical sound is common in patients with emphysema or asthma.
- To detect other breath sounds—such as crackles and rhonchi—or the lack of them, you'll need a stethoscope.
- Watch the patient's chest movements and listen to breathing to determine the rhythm and sound of respirations. (See *Identifying respiratory patterns*.)

Practice pointers

- Respiratory rates of less than 10 breaths/minute or more than 18 breaths/minute are usually considered abnormal and should be reported promptly.

Identifying respiratory patterns

Type	Characteristics	Pattern	Possible causes
Apnoea	Periodic absence of breathing	————————	• Mechanical airway obstruction • Conditions affecting the brain's respiratory centre in lateral medulla oblongata
Apnoeustic	Prolonged, gasping inspiration followed by extremely short, inefficient expiration	/\/\/\/\/\/\/\/\/\	• Lesions of respiratory centre
Bradypnoea	Slow, regular respirations of equal depth	∿∿∿∿	• Normal pattern during sleep • Conditions affecting respiratory centre: tumours, metabolic disorders, respiratory decompensation, and use of opiates or alcohol
Cheyne–Stokes	Fast, deep respirations lasting 30 to 170 seconds punctuated by periods of apnoea lasting 20 to 60 seconds	∿∿——∿∿∿——∿∿	• Increased intracranial pressure, severe heart failure, renal failure, meningitis, drug overdose, and cerebral anoxia
Eupnoea	Normal rate and rhythm	∿∿∿∿∿	• Normal respiration
Kussmaul's	Fast (over 20 breaths/minute), deep (resembling sighs), laboured respirations without pause	/\/\/\/\/\/\/\/\/\/\	• Renal failure and metabolic acidosis, particularly diabetic ketoacidosis
Tachypnoea	Rapid respirations, rate rises with body temperature	∿∿∿∿∿∿∿∿∿	• Pneumonia, compensatory respiratory alkalosis, respiratory insufficiency, lesions of the respiratory centre, and salicylate poisoning

• Observe the patient for signs of dyspnoea, such as an anxious facial expression, flaring nostrils, a heaving chest wall and cyanosis. To detect cyanosis, look for the characteristic bluish discoloration of the nail beds and lips, under the tongue, in the buccal mucosa and in the conjunctiva.

• When assessing a patient's respiratory status use A and B from the A–G system, but particularly consider personal and family history. Ask if he smokes and, if he does, the number of years and the number of packs per day. (See *Documenting respirations*.)

• Interpret your findings using the local track and trigger system and escalate your findings appropriately.

• ESCs specific to standard numbers 1–8 (Care, compassion and communication), 9–20 (Organizational aspects of care) and 21–23 (Infection prevention and control), but also in accordance with number 36 (Medicines management).

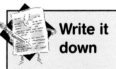

Write it down

Documenting respirations

Record the rate, depth, rhythm and sound of the patient's respirations. Document any actions you have taken due to your findings.

Blood pressure

The force of ventricular contractions, arterial wall elasticity, peripheral vascular resistance, and blood volume and viscosity affect blood pressure, which is the lateral force that blood exerts on arterial walls. Blood pressure measurements consist of systolic pressure and diastolic pressure readings.

Systolic (contract) vs. diastolic (relax)

Systolic pressure occurs when the left ventricle contracts. It reflects the integrity of the heart, arteries and arterioles. Diastolic pressure occurs when the left ventricle relaxes. It indicates blood vessel resistance. Both pressures are measured in millimetres of mercury with a sphygmomanometer and a stethoscope, usually at the brachial artery.

Systolic pressure – diastolic pressure = pulse pressure

Pulse pressure, or the difference between systolic and diastolic pressures, varies inversely with arterial elasticity. Normally, systolic pressure exceeds diastolic pressure by about 40 mmHg. Narrowed pulse pressure, or a difference of less than 30 mmHg, occurs when systolic pressure falls and diastolic pressure rises. These changes reflect reduced stroke volume, increased peripheral resistance or both.

Widened pulse pressure, or a difference of more than 50 mmHg between systolic and diastolic pressures, occurs when systolic pressure rises and diastolic pressure remains constant, or when systolic pressure rises and diastolic pressure falls. These changes reflect increased stroke volume, decreased peripheral resistance or both.

Goin' up

Blood pressure rises with age, weight gain, prolonged stress and anxiety. (See *Effects of age on blood pressure*.)

What you need

Sphygmomanometer ✳ stethoscope ✳ automated vital signs monitor (if you are competent and confident to use it).

Cuffs come in six standard sizes, ranging from newborn to extra-large adult. Disposable cuffs are available.

The automated vital signs monitor is a non-invasive device that measures pulse rate, systolic and diastolic pressures, and mean arterial pressure at preset intervals. However, as these devices cannot give you the required information regarding the pulse (rate, rhythm and strength) they should not be used for measuring the pulse. (See *Using an electronic vital signs monitor*.)

Ages and stages

Effects of age on blood pressure

Blood pressure changes with age. Below are normal blood pressure values, measured in millimetres of mercury (mmHg) at different ages.

Neonate

- Systolic: 50 to 52
- Diastolic: 25 to 30
- Mean: 35 to 40

3 years

- Systolic: 78 to 114
- Diastolic: 46 to 78

10 years

- Systolic: 90 to 132
- Diastolic: 56 to 86

16 years

- Systolic: 104 to 108
- Diastolic: 60 to 92

Adult

- Systolic: 90 to 139
- Diastolic: 60 to 89

- Don't take a blood pressure measurement on the same arm as an arteriovenous fistula or haemodialysis shunt, because blood flow through the device may be compromised. Don't take a blood pressure measurement on the affected side of a mastectomy because it may compromise lymphatic circulation, worsen oedema and damage the arm. Also, don't take blood pressure on the same arm as a peripherally inserted central catheter because it may damage the device.
- Wrap the deflated cuff snugly around the patient's upper arm, 2.5 cm above the brachial artery in the antecubital fossa. The artery mark on the cuff should be in line with the brachial artery, this would indicate that the cuff tubing points down the patient's arm.
- If necessary, connect the appropriate tube to the rubber bulb of the air pump and the other tube to the manometer.

Palpate the systolic

- Palpate the brachial artery as if you were taking the pulse.
- Using the thumb and index finger of your other hand, turn the thumbscrew on the rubber bulb of the air pump clockwise to close the valve.
- Pump air into the cuff while palpating the brachial artery and looking at the anaeroid dial. Continue pumping air until you cannot feel the brachial pulse. Remember the pressure at which you felt the last beat of the pulse; this is the estimate of the systolic pressure.
- Carefully open the valve of the air pump. Then deflate the cuff until the needle points back to zero.

Go with the bell

- Again palpate the brachial artery. This time centre the bell of the stethoscope over the brachial artery where you detect the strongest beats, and hold it in place with one hand. The bell of the stethoscope transmits low-pitched arterial blood sounds more effectively than does the diaphragm. (See *Positioning the blood pressure cuff.*)
- Using the thumb and index finger of your other hand, turn the thumbscrew on the rubber bulb of the air pump clockwise to close the valve.
- Pump air into the cuff while auscultating for the sound over the brachial artery to compress and, eventually, occlude arterial blood flow. Continue pumping air until the anaeroid gauge registers the pressure reading that you obtained through your estimated reading, then slowly increase the pressure by 30 mmHg. For example, estimated reading 100 mmHg then inflate during auscultation to 130 mmHg.
- Carefully open the valve of the air pump. Then deflate the cuff no faster than 2–3 mmHg/second, while watching the mercury column or anaeroid gauge and auscultating for the sound over the artery; each marking on the anaeroid dial represents 2 mmHg.

Positioning the blood pressure cuff

Wrap the cuff snugly around the upper arm above the antecubital fossa (the inner aspect of the elbow).

Proper placement

When measuring an adult's blood pressure, place the lower border of the cuff about 2.5 cm (two fingerwidths) above the antecubital space. The centre of the cuff bladder should rest directly over the medial aspect of the arm. Most cuffs have an arrow for you to position above the brachial artery. You should notice that the tubing is now not occluding the space that your require.

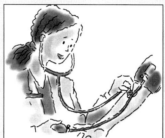

Get a good beat

Place the bell of the stethoscope on the brachial artery at the point where you hear the strongest beats—do not tuck the stethoscope under the BP cuff, *as you will hear noise artefact.*

Tune in to the five sounds

- When you hear the first beat or a clear tapping sound, note the pressure on the gauge—that is, the systolic pressure. (The beat or tapping sound is the first of five Korotkoff sounds. The second sound resembles a murmur or swish; the third, crisp tapping; the fourth, a soft, muffled tone; and the fifth, the last sound heard.)
- Continue to release air gradually while auscultating for the sound over the artery.
- Note the diastolic pressure—the last sound heard to within 2 mmHg.

One mo' time

- Rapidly deflate the cuff. Record the pressure, wait 30 seconds, and then repeat the procedure and record the pressures to confirm your original findings. After doing so, remove and clean the cuff, wash your hands and return equipment to storage.

Practice pointers

- Escalate your findings, don't just sit back thinking job done! Inform your mentor or the nurse in charge if the readings are abnormal according to the track and trigger system.

• For further information on hypertension and acquiring blood pressure measurements, visit the British Hypertension Society website: www.bhsoc.org
• If you cannot palpate the brachial pulse adequately to take an estimated systolic reading, use the radial pulse.
• Use an appropriately sized cuff to prevent associated false readings. (See *Correcting problems of blood pressure measurement*.)
• On admission of a patient to acute care, record the blood pressure in both arms; continue to use the arm (if no contraindications present) which gave the highest reading. Ensure you note the arm used on the TPR&BP chart.
• Palpation of systolic blood pressure may also be important to avoid underestimating results in patients with an auscultatory gap. This gap is a loss of sound between the first and second Korotkoff sounds and may be as great as 40 mmHg. You may find this in patients with venous congestion or hypertension.

Correcting problems of blood pressure measurement

Causes	Nursing actions
False-high reading	
• Cuff too small	• Make sure the cuff bladder encircles 80% of the arm or leg being used for measurement
• Cuff wrapped too loosely, reducing its effective width	• Tighten the cuff
• Cuff deflated too slowly, causing venous congestion in the arm or leg	• Never deflate the cuff more slowly than 2 mmHg per second
• Anaeroid dial tilted	• Read pressures with the anaeroid dial in an upright position
• Measurement poorly timed (for example, after the patient has eaten, ambulated, appeared anxious or flexed his arm muscles)	• Postpone the blood pressure measurement or help the patient relax before measuring his blood pressure
False-low reading	
• Arm or leg positioned incorrectly	• Make sure the patient's arm or leg is level with his heart and supported
• Anaeroid dial below eye level	• Read the anaeroid dial at eye level
• Auscultatory gap (sound fades out for 10 to 15 mmHg, and then returns) unnoticed	• Estimate systolic pressure by palpation before measuring it. Then check this pressure against measured pressure
• Low-volume sounds inaudible	• Before reinflating the cuff, instruct the patient to raise his arm or leg to decrease venous pressure and amplify low-volume sounds. After inflating the cuff, tell him to lower his arm or leg. Then deflate the cuff and listen. If you still fail to detect low-volume sounds, chart palpated systolic pressure

- Interpret your findings using the local track and trigger system and escalate your findings appropriately.
- ESCs specific to standard numbers 1–8 (Care, compassion and Communication), 9–20 (Organizational aspects of care) and 21–23 (Infection prevention and control), and in accordance with 28–29 (Nutrition and fluid management) and 36 (Medicines management).

Make adjustments for special circumstances

- If your patient is crying or anxious, delay measuring his blood pressure, if possible, until he calms down, to avoid falsely elevated readings.
- If your patient is taking antihypertensive medication, measure his blood pressure while he's in a sitting position to ensure accurate results.
- When hypertension is suspected, or you are monitoring an acutely unwell patient, single readings of blood pressure aren't as significant as are patterns of blood pressure over a period of time. (See *Documenting blood pressure*.)

Pulse oximetry

Pulse oximetry is a relatively simple, non-invasive procedure used to monitor arterial oxygen saturation. It can be performed continuously or intermittently.

Light reading

In this procedure, two diodes send red and infrared light through a pulsating arterial vascular bed such as the one in the fingertip. A photo detector slipped over the finger measures the transmitted light as it passes through the vascular bed, detects the relative amount of colour absorbed by arterial blood, and calculates the exact mixed venous oxygen saturation without interference from surrounding venous blood, skin, connective tissue or bone.

Another method, ear oximetry, works by monitoring the transmission of light waves through the vascular bed of a patient's earlobe. Results will be inaccurate if the patient's earlobe is poorly perfused, as from a low cardiac output.

Symbolically speaking

Pulse oximeters usually denote arterial oxygen saturation values with the symbol SpO_2. Invasively measured arterial oxygen saturation values, on the other hand, are denoted by the symbol SaO_2.

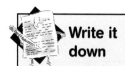

Write it down

Documenting blood pressure

On the patient's chart, record systolic pressure over diastolic pressure (for example, 120/78 mmHg); if necessary, record systolic pressure over two diastolic pressures (for example, 120/78/20 mmHg). Chart an auscultatory gap, if present. If local policy or procedure requires you to chart blood pressures on a graph, use dots or checkmarks and use the correct colour of pen as per policy. Also, document the regularity with which the blood pressure is to be assessed, the extremity used and the size of cuff used.

What you need

Oximeter ✳ finger or ear probe ✳ medical device wipes ✳ nail polish remover, if necessary.

Getting ready

Review the manufacturer's instructions for assembling and cleaning the oximeter.

How you do it

Wash your hands. Explain the procedure to the patient and gain permission.

For pulse oximetry

• Select a finger for the test. Although the index finger is commonly used, a smaller finger may be selected if the patient's fingers are too large for the equipment. Make sure the patient isn't wearing false fingernails, and remove any nail polish from the test finger as these stop the infrared light from passing. Place the transducer (photo detector) probe over the patient's finger so that light beams and sensors oppose each other. If the patient has long fingernails, position the probe perpendicular to the finger, if possible, or clip the fingernail. Always position the patient's hand at heart level to eliminate venous pulsations and to promote accurate readings.
• Turn on the power switch. If the device is working properly, a beep will sound, a display will light momentarily, and the pulse searchlight will flash. The SpO_2 and pulse rate displays will show stationary zeros. After 4–6 heartbeats, the SpO_2 and pulse rate displays will supply information with each beat, and the pulse amplitude indicator will begin tracking the pulse.

For ear oximetry

• Using an alcohol pad, massage the patient's earlobe for 10–20 seconds. Mild erythema indicates adequate vascularization. Following the manufacturer's instructions, attach the ear probe to the patient's earlobe or pinna. Use the ear probe stabilizer for prolonged or exercise testing. Be sure to establish good contact on the ear; an unstable probe may set off the low-perfusion alarm. After the probe has been attached for a few seconds, a saturation reading and pulse waveform will appear on the oximeter's screen.
• Leave the ear probe in place for three or more minutes until readings stabilize at the highest point, or take three separate

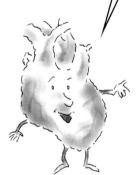

For best pulse oximetry results, keep the patient's hand at my level.

readings and average them. Make sure you revascularize the patient's earlobe each time.
- Remove the probe, turn off and unplug the unit, and clean the probe by gently rubbing it with a medical device wipe.

Practice pointers

- If oximetry has been performed properly, readings are typically accurate. However, certain factors (such as hypothermia or hypotension) may interfere with accuracy. Always set the low saturation and high saturation alarm perimeters on the basis of the saturation aim for each individual patient and never, ever, turn the sound off.
- ESCs specific to standard numbers 1–8 (Care, compassion and communication), 9–20 (Organizational aspects of care) and 21–23 (Infection prevention and control), but also in accordance with number 36 (Medicines management).

Detour over the bridge

- If the patient has compromised circulation in his extremities, you can place a photo detector across the bridge of his nose. Devices are available for this method, never adapt medical equipment for any other purpose than intended.
- If SpO_2 is used to guide weaning the patient from mechanical ventilation, then arterial blood gas analysis should be taken to correlate SpO_2 readings with SaO_2 levels.
- If an automatic blood pressure cuff is used on the same extremity that's used for measuring SpO_2, the cuff will interfere with SpO_2 readings during inflation, causing false readings and the sounding of low perfusion alarms.

Problem solving

Normal SpO_2 levels for ear and pulse oximetry are 95–100% for adults. Lower levels may indicate hypoxaemia, which warrants intervention. Always use the local track and trigger system to interpret your findings and determine your action. However, always know what the saturation aim is for each patient, as clear medical goals should be indicated on an individual patient basis. For example, a patient with a diagnosed respiratory disorder may normally have a SpO_2 of 90%, but during exacerbation of illness this may have fallen to 85%; it would be unachievable and unrealistic to say that we were aiming to achieve oxygen saturations of 95% minimum. For such patients, follow your Trust or employer's policy, notify the doctor, or resuscitate the patient immediately, if necessary. (See *Documenting pulse oximetry*.)

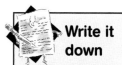 **Write it down**

Document-ing pulse oximetry

In your notes, document the procedure, including the date, time, your name, the procedure type, oximetry measurement, 'track and trigger system' score and actions taken. Record the readings on appropriate flowcharts, if indicated, i.e. TPR&BP.

Neurological assessment

As described in 'A–G of assessment' (above), it is essential to assess and document your patient's level of consciousness and comprehension. As well as using your observation skills to do this, there are many other scoring systems you can use. The Glasgow coma scale (GCS) is the most widely used of these scoring systems and should be the minimal tool used to assess the level of consciousness following a suspected brain injury. Learning to use this assessment scale will enable you and the multidisciplinary team not only to plan and implement care accordingly for your patient, but also to assess its effectiveness and track your patient's progress.

Glasgow coma scale

The Glasgow coma scale (GCS) is so-called as it was developed at the University of Glasgow by Professor Graham M. Teasdale and Professor Bryan Jennett in 1974. The scale uses a point system based on three areas of assessment: eye opening (maximum score of 4), best verbal response (maximum score of 5) and best motor response (maximum score of 6), giving a possible maximum score of 15. The lowest score for each category is 1; thus, the lowest score = 3 (no response to pain, no verbal communication and no eye opening). A GCS of 13–15 therefore would be obtained when a minor injury had occurred; 9–12, a moderate injury; and 8 or less, a severe injury. (See *Glasgow coma scale*.)

Keep your motor running

The best motor response is graded using the following pointers:
• Give the patient a simple command to obey; if he obeys the command, then he would score the maximum 6 points.
• If he does not obey the command correctly, or not at all, then move on to see if he responds to local pain. To assess his response to pain squeeze the trapezium muscle. If he responds immediately and localizes the pain, this would equate to a score of 5 being given.
• Should he not localize pain, observe for him doing one of the following: pulling away from the pain (this indicates withdrawal to pain and would score 4 points); flexing his limbs to pain (this indicates a flexor response and a decorticate posture, score of 3), extension of limbs (indicates an extensor response, where the stimulus causes limb extension or decerebrate posture, a score of 2) and finally a score of 1 for not responding at all to pain.

Glasgow coma scale

	Score	1st Jan 2008																					
Date		1st Jan 2008																						
Time		06.00	07.00																					
Motor response	Score																							
Obeys commands	6																							
Localizes to pain stimuli	5	•	•																					
Withdrawal from pain stimuli	4																							
Extension to pain stimuli	3																							
Flexion to pain stimuli	2																							
No response to pain stimuli	1																							
Verbal response																								
Orientated	5																							
Confusion	4	•	•																					
Inappropriate words	3																							
Incomprehensible speech	2																							
No verbal response	1																							
Eye opening																								
Spontaneous eye opening	4	•	•																					
Open to speech	3																							
Open to pain stimuli	2																							
No response	1																							
Total GCS score		13	13																					
Track and trigger score		Y	Y																					
Initials of nurse		MH	MH																					

Keep talking

The best verbal response is graded using the following pointers:
• He is aware of who he is, where he is, the year, the month and thus is orientated, obtaining a score of 5.
• If he does not meet these criteria, then observe and assess for the following pointers. He responds in a conversational manner but is disorientated and some confusion is noted, then a score of 4 would be given. Inappropriate words would be indicated by him using random words with no conversation being exchanged, and a score of 3 given. Should he respond to you verbally by moaning and not forming words, then incomprehensible speech would be the pointer chosen and a score of 2 given. No verbal response at all indicates a score of 1.

Look into my eyes

Eye opening is graded using the following pointers:
• His eyes open when he is aware you are present, even if you have not spoken; this is spontaneous eye opening and scores 4 points.
• If he does not meet these criteria, then observe and assess for the following pointers. He opens his eyes when you speak or shout, in other words in response to speech, 3 points. Eyes open in response to pain (you should be able to assess this at the same time as assessing motor response, if pain stimuli required; the more practised you are, the more skilled you will become), 2 points. One point for no eye opening. (See *Documenting GCS*.)

Practice pointers

Ensure you are supervised carrying out all of the vital signs until you and your mentor feel you are competent and confident to practise the skill independently.

Friends and relatives

If any relative or friend of the patient communicates to you that they think the patient is behaving abnormally—take action immediately. No one knows the patient better than his friends and family. They are best at assessing neurological function, without a tool.
• ESCs specific to standard numbers 1–8 (Care, compassion and communication), 9–20 (Organizational aspects of care) and 21–23 (Infection prevention and control), but also in accordance with number 36 (Medicines management).

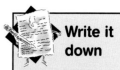

Write it down

Document-ing GCS

Use dots, not ticks, of lines to fill out the GCS chart. Indicate the track and trigger score on the GCS chart. Take, assess and document all other vital signs at the same time as assessing the GCS. Add up the points awarded and document actions taken. Date, time and sign the record.

Height and weight

Height and weight are routinely measured when a patient is admitted due to an acute or chronic illness. An accurate record of the patient's height and weight is essential for calculating dosages of drugs and contrast agents, assessing the patient's nutritional status, and determining the height-to-weight ratio.

What weight tells you

Because body weight is the best overall indicator of fluid status, daily monitoring is important for patients receiving a diuretic or a medication that causes sodium retention. Rapid weight gain may signal fluid retention; rapid weight loss, diuresis.

Scales for every position

Weight can be measured with a standing scale, chair scale or bed scale. Height can be measured with the measuring bar on a standing scale or with a tape measure for a patient confined to a supine position.

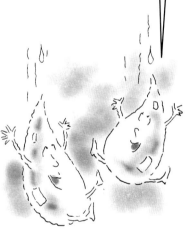

Body weight is the best indicator of fluid status.

What you need

Standing scale with measuring bar or chair or bed scale ✳ wheelchair if needed (to transport patient) ✳ tape measure if needed.

Getting ready

Select the appropriate scale—usually, a standing scale for an ambulatory patient or a chair or bed scale for an acutely ill or debilitated patient. Then make sure the scale is balanced. Standing scales and, to a lesser extent, bed scales may become unbalanced when transported.

How you do it

• Tell the patient that you would like to measure his height and weight and explain the rationale.
• Explain the procedure to him, depending on which type of scale you'll use: standing, chair, or bed, in order to gain informed permission.
• Be aware of the terminology you use with the patient, you do not want to offend; words such as fat should not be used, overweight may be more appropriate. Treat your patient with respect, maintain his privacy and dignity.

Using a standing scale
- Clean the scale's platform with a medical device wipe.
- Tell the patient to remove his robe and slippers or shoes. If the scale has wheels, lock them before the patient steps on. Assist the patient on to the scale and remain close to him to prevent falls.

That's upright balance

- If you're using an upright balance scale, slide the lower rider to the groove representing the largest increment below the patient's estimated weight. Grooves usually represent 10 kg increments, i.e. 10, 20, 30, 40, 50, 60, 70, 80, 90, 100.
- Slide the small upper rider until the beam balances, the small rider usually represents 1 kg increments. Add the upper and lower rider figures to determine the weight.
- Assist the patient off the scale and remain close to him to prevent falls.
- Document and act upon your findings.
- Clean the scale's platform with a medical device wipe.

That's digital

- When using a digital scale, make sure the display reads 0 before use.
- Read the display with the patient standing as still as possible.
- Assist the patient off the scale and remain close to him to prevent falls.
- Document and act upon your findings.
- Clean the scale's platform with a medical device wipe or as per manufacturer's instructions.
- Ensure the scale has been checked and calibrated regularly by your employer's Medical Engineering Department.

Raising the bar

- If you're measuring height, ask the patient to stand erect on the scale's platform, once you have cleaned it with a medical device wipe. Raise the measuring bar above the patient's head, extend the horizontal arm, and lower the bar until it touches the top of the patient's head. Then read the patient's height and document it immediately.
- Help the patient off the scale, and give him his robe and slippers or shoes. Then return the measuring bar to its initial position.

Using a chair scale
- Transport the patient to the weighing area or the scale to the patient's bedside.
- Lock the scale in place to prevent it from moving accidentally and clean it with a medical device wipe or as per local policy.
- Assist the patient into the chair scale using moving and handling standards set for this individual patient.

• Ensure the patient is comfortable and as still as possible, slide the lower rider to the groove representing the largest increment below the patient's estimated weight. Grooves usually represent 10 kg increments, i.e. 10, 20, 30, 40, 50, 60, 70, 80, 90, 100.

• Slide the small upper rider until the beam balances, the small rider usually represents 1 kg increments. Add the upper and lower rider figures to determine the weight.

• Assist the patient out of the chair and back into bed or into their bedside chair, using appropriate moving and handling techniques.

• Document the patient's weight and act upon findings as necessary.

• Then clean the chair scale as per pre procedure, unlock the wheels and remove the scale from the patient's bedside.

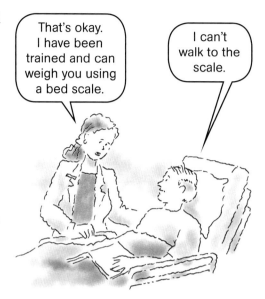

Using a bed scale

There are many makes and models of bed scales available in the UK, both digital and manual. Before using any mechanical aid that hoists, lifts or transports patients, you must be trained by the local moving and handling team or by the manufacturer's trainer, and agree with them that you are confident and competent to use the equipment independently. Therefore this method cannot be described in this book.

Practice pointers

• Reassure and steady patients who are at risk for losing their balance on a scale.

• Weigh the patient at the same time each day (usually before breakfast), in similar clothing, and using the same scale. If the patient uses crutches, weigh him with the crutches. Then weigh the crutches and any heavy clothing and subtract their weight from the total to determine the patient's weight.

• When moving and assisting the patient on to scales, be careful not to dislodge I.V. lines, indwelling catheters and other supportive equipment. (See *Documenting height and weight*.)

Central venous pressure monitoring

Central venous pressure (CVP) monitoring can be used to measure the pressure of the fluid in the central venous system. This, when performed and interpreted in conjunction with TPR&BP, can assist in providing direct correlation to the volume of fluid in the central

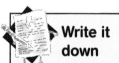

Write it down

Document-ing height and weight

Record the patient's height and weight on the nursing documentation as per local policy; this may be more than one document, i.e. Medicines administration record, Fluid chart, Weight chart.

venous system; is the patient dehydrated or is there fluid overload? (See *Measuring CVP using a water manometer*.) Normal CVP is between 5 and 10 cmH$_2$O. A reading of above 10 cmH$_2$O in relation to fluid volume and status can indicate fluid overload, and a reading below 5 cmH$_2$O may indicate dehydration. There are other reasons for high and low CVP readings, including and not exhaustive of: mechanical error, a blocked catheter, medication, cardiac pathology. It is therefore essential that you are fully aware of the medical aim of CVP readings for the individual patient and of the patient's full plan of care; including past medical history, recent medical and surgical history, and prescribed medications.

The fluids used

Two types of crystalloid fluid can be used for CVP monitoring: 0.9% sodium chloride for the majority of patients and 5% dextrose for patients with liver disease or damage. If the solution is only to be used for measurement and will not be left to infuse between measurements, then a maximum volume of 250 ml per bag will assist in decreasing the risk of accidental fluid overload.

Common factors

To limit discrepancies in measurements between nurses, it is essential that the patient is in the same position and that the same anatomical point is used for every reading. Therefore the patient should have a marked dressing *in situ* as a guide. This and the patient's position and/or the angle of the bed should be communicated to all staff taking readings, via the nursing and medical notes.

Be trendy

As with TPR&BP, a single reading would not be enough to determine treatment. It is essential that regular measurements are taken and recorded, allowing a trend to be seen and acted upon using the track and trigger system in use locally.

What you need

Manometer ✳ I.V. fluid ✳ CVP-giving set ✳ I.V. fluid-giving set ✳ I.V. stand for the manometer ✳ gloves and an apron.

How you do it

- Tell the patient that you would like to measure his central venous pressure and explain the rationale. Explain the procedure to him and gain permission.
- See *Measuring CVP using a water manometer* for procedure guidelines and diagram.

Measuring CVP using a water manometer

- Use the distal lumen of a central venous catheter (CVC). If the patient has a CVC with multiple lumens, the distal lumen may be dedicated to continuous CVP monitoring and the other lumens used for fluid administration. The distal lumen lies in the superior vena cava and is the lumen closest to the right atria.
- To obtain values, position the patient at 30–45 degrees. Zero the transducer, levelling the transducer air–fluid interface stopcock with the right atrium. Read the CVP value from the digital display on the monitor, and note the waveform. Make sure the patient is still when the reading is taken to prevent artefact. Be sure to use this position for all subsequent readings.
- Locate the level of the right atrium by identifying the phlebostatic axis: fifth intercostal space, midaxillary line.
- Mark this point using a pen, but not directly on the patient's skin, use a dressing and then mark the dressing.
- Make sure the manometer base is aligned with the patient's right atrium (the zero reference point). The manometer set usually contains a spirit level on a rod to allow you to determine this quickly.

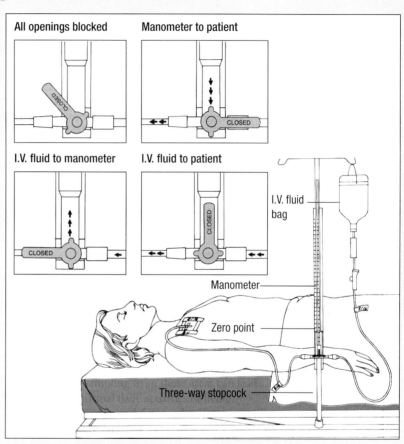

All openings blocked

Manometer to patient

I.V. fluid to manometer

I.V. fluid to patient

I.V. fluid bag

Manometer

Zero point

Three-way stopcock

- After adjusting the manometer's position, examine the typical three-way stopcock. By turning it to any position as shown, you can control the direction of fluid flow.
- Turn the stopcock off to the patient, and slowly fill the manometer with I.V. fluid until the fluid level is 10 to 20 cmH$_2$O higher than the patient's expected CVP value.

Don't overfill the tube because fluid that spills over the top can become a source of contamination.

- Turn the stopcock off to the I.V. fluid and open to the patient. The fluid level in the manometer will drop. When the fluid level comes to rest, it will fluctuate slightly with respirations. Expect it to drop during inspiration and to

(continued)

Measuring CVP using a water manometer *(continued)*

rise during expiration, *due to changes of pressure in the thoracic cavity.*
- Allow the fluid to fluctuate in the same position five times, then record CVP at the end of expiration. Depending on the type of water manometer used, note the value either at the bottom of the meniscus or at the midline of the small floating ball.
- After you have obtained the CVP value, turn the stopcock off to the patient. Recommence any other fluids that you previously stopped and adjust the I.V. drip rate as required.
- Place the patient in a comfortable position.

Practice pointers

- Pre-registration nurses cannot administer medication unsupervised. I.V. fluids are prescribed medications, therefore a competent and confident registered nurse MUST supervise all pre-registration nurses.
- Ensure a closed system of the central venous catheter is maintained, to prevent infection.
- Always use standard infection control procedures when performing CVP manometry.
- Remember to zero the manometer.
- ESCs specific to standard numbers 1–8 (Care, compassion and communication), 9–20 (Organizational aspects of care) and 21–26 (Infection prevention and control), and in accordance with number 29 (Nutrition and fluid management) and 36–42 (Medicines management).

Electrocardiography

Electrocardiography (ECG), which measures the heart's electrical activity as waveforms, is one of the most valuable and commonly used diagnostic tools. An ECG uses electrodes attached to the skin to detect electrical currents moving through the heart. It then transmits these signals to an instrument that produces a record (the electrocardiogram) of cardiac activity.

ECG can be used to identify myocardial ischaemia and infarction, rhythm and conduction disturbances, chamber enlargement, electrolyte imbalances and drug toxicity.

It's like 12 cameras in 10 leads

The standard 12-lead ECG uses a series of electrodes placed on the extremities and the chest wall to assess the heart from 12 different views (leads). The 12-lead ECG should consist of three standard bipolar limb leads (designated I, II, III), three unipolar augmented leads (aVR, aVL, aVF), and six unipolar precordial leads (V1 to V6). The limb leads and augmented leads show the heart from the frontal plane. The precordial leads show the heart from the horizontal plane. However, as the augmented and bipolar leads can do two jobs at once, there are actually only 10 leads.

Using these leads, the ECG device measures and averages the differences between the electrical potential of the electrode sites for each lead, and graphs them over time. This creates the standard ECG complex, called P–QRS–T. The P wave represents atrial depolarization; the QRS complex, ventricular depolarization; and the T wave, ventricular repolarization. The U wave, sometimes present, represents the recovery period of ventricular conduction fibres. (See *Reviewing ECG components*.)

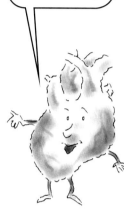

That ECG is a smash hit! It's one of the best ways to see how I'm doing.

Where's the remote?

An ECG is typically accomplished using a multichannel method. All electrodes are attached to the patient at once, and the machine prints a simultaneous view of all leads.

What you need

ECG machine ✳ recording paper ✳ disposable pre-gelled electrodes ✳ 70% alcohol pads, if required ✳ shaving supplies, if required.

Getting ready

Place the ECG machine close to the patient's bed, and plug the power cord into the wall electrical socket.

How you do it

• Before you set up the machine to record a 12-lead ECG, explain the procedure to the patient and gain consent. Tell him that the test records the heart's electrical activity and typically takes about 5 minutes.
• If the patient is not in a single room, close the bed curtains to maintain his privacy.

Reviewing ECG components

This strip shows the components of a normal ECG waveform.

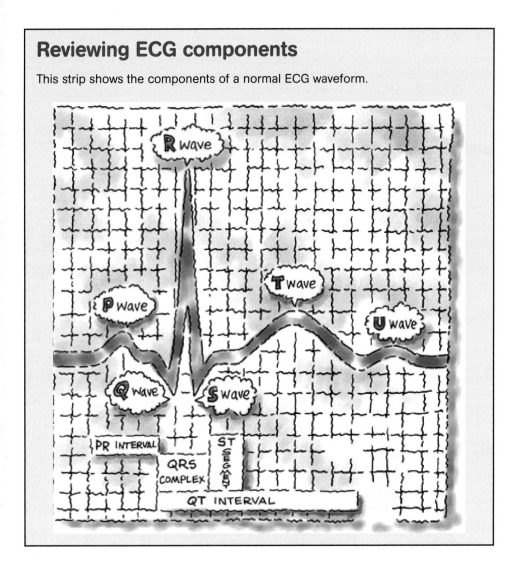

- Have the patient lie in a supine position in the centre of the bed with his arms at his sides. You may raise the head of the bed to promote comfort or if the patient is experiencing breathing difficulties. Expose his arms and legs, and cover him appropriately, to maintain dignity. His arms and legs should be relaxed to minimize muscle trembling, which can cause electrical interference.
- Select flat, fleshy areas to place the electrodes. (See *Positioning chest electrodes*.)

Need an appointment at the salon?

- If an area is excessively hairy, clip it. Clean excess oil or other substances from the skin with 70% alcohol pad to enhance electrode contact.
- Apply the disposable pre-gelled electrodes to the patient's wrists and to the medial aspects of his ankles.

Colour-coded for clarity

- Connect the limb leads to the electrodes.
- You'll see that the tip of each lead is lettered and colour-coded for easy identification. The red or RA lead goes to the right arm; the black or RL lead, to the right leg; the green or LL lead, to the left leg; the yellow or LA lead, to the left arm; and the V1 to V6 leads, to the chest. In other words working clockwise from the right arm, remember this acronym **R**ide **Y**our **G**reen **B**ike—**R**ed, **Y**ellow, **G**reen, **B**lack.

No time to be shy

- Now, expose the patient's chest. Place a disposable electrode at each electrode position. (See *Positioning chest electrodes*.)
- If your patient is a woman, be sure to place the chest electrodes below the breast tissue. In a large-breasted woman, you may need to displace the breast tissue laterally.
- Make sure that the paper speed selector is set to the standard 25 mm/second (2.5 cm/second) and 10 mm (or 1 cm) height. If local policy permits, enter the appropriate patient identification data; otherwise hand write the patient's identification when the ECG is printed.

Ready to roll

- Now you're ready to begin the recording. Ask the patient to relax and breathe normally. Tell him to lie still and not to talk, just for the acquisition process. Then press the auto button. The machine will indicate the acquisition of data to you. The machine will record all 12 leads automatically, recording three consecutive leads simultaneously. Some machines have a display screen so you can preview waveforms before the machine records them.
- When the machine finishes acquiring the data, inform the patient that he may now communicate and move freely again.
- Once the machine has printed the ECG, observe the data for clarity, smudges, etc. If there is no artefact present, remove the electrodes, and clean the patient's skin. After disconnecting the leads from the electrodes, dispose of the electrodes. Clean the machine and return it to storage.
- Inform the doctor that the ECG has been acquired and is ready for interpretation. (See *Documenting ECG*.)

Positioning chest electrodes

To ensure accurate test results, position chest electrodes as follows:

- V_1: Fourth intercostal space at right sternal border
- V_2: Fourth intercostal space at left sternal border
- V_3: Halfway between V_2 and V_4
- V_4: Fifth intercostal space at midclavicular line
- V_5: Fifth intercostal space at anterior axillary line (halfway between V_4 and V_6)
- V_6: Fifth intercostal space at midaxillary line, level with V_4

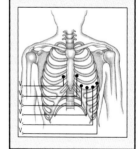

Practice pointers

• If the patient's skin is exceptionally oily, scaly or diaphoretic, rub the electrode site with 70% alcohol swab before applying the electrode to help reduce interference in the tracing.
• After carrying out an ECG it is the technician's responsibility to ensure that it is seen by a doctor and interpreted.
• ESCs specific to standard numbers 1–8 (Care, compassion and communication), 9–20 (Organizational aspects of care) and 21–26 (Infection prevention and control).

Cardiac monitoring

Because it allows continuous observation of the heart's electrical activity, cardiac monitoring is used in patients at risk with, and who are at high risk of developing, life-threatening arrhythmias. Like other forms of electrocardiography (ECG), cardiac monitoring uses electrodes placed on the patient's chest to transmit electrical signals that are converted into a cardiac rhythm tracing on an oscilloscope.

Hardwire vs. wireless

Two types of monitoring may be performed: hardwire or telemetry. In hardwire monitoring, the patient is connected to a monitor at the bedside. The rhythm display appears at the bedside or it may be transmitted to a console at a remote location. Telemetry uses a small transmitter connected to the ambulatory patient to send electrical signals to another location, where they're displayed on a monitor screen.

Regardless of the type, cardiac monitors can display the patient's heart rate and rhythm, produce a printed record of cardiac rhythm, and sound an alarm if the heart rate exceeds or falls below specified limits. Monitors also recognize and count abnormal heartbeats as well as changes.

What you need

Cardiac monitor ✳ monitoring leads ✳ patient cable ✳ disposable pre-gelled electrodes (number of electrodes varies from three to five, depending on the patient's needs) ✳ 70% alcohol pads ✳ optional: shaving supplies, washcloth.

For telemetry
Transmitter ✳ transmitter pouch ✳ telemetry battery pack, leads and electrodes.

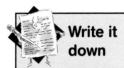

Write it down

Document-ing ECG

If storing the data on the ECG machine, ensure you label the ECG recording with the patient's name, date of birth and hospital identification number. On the ECG itself, record the date, time, patient's name, hospital number and date of birth and appropriate clinical information. In your notes, record that the data have been acquired and the actions you have taken.

Getting ready

Turn on the cardiac monitor to warm up the unit while you prepare the equipment and the patient. Insert the cable into the appropriate monitor socket. Connect the monitoring leads to the cable. In some systems, the monitoring leads are permanently secured to the cable. Each lead should indicate the attachment location: red or RA lead goes to the right arm; the black or RL lead, to the right leg; the green or LL lead, to the left leg; the yellow or LA lead, to the left arm, and ground (C or V). This should appear on the lead—if it's permanently connected—or at the connection of the leads and cable to the patient. Then connect an electrode to each of the leads, carefully checking that each lead is in its correct outlet.

Don't lick it

For telemetry monitoring, insert a new battery into the transmitter. Be sure to match the poles on the battery with the polar markings on the transmitter case. By pressing the button at the top of the unit, test the battery's charge and test the unit to ensure that the battery is operational. If the monitoring leads aren't permanently affixed to the telemetry unit, attach them securely.

How you do it

Explain the procedure to the patient, gain permission, and maintain privacy and dignity. Wash your hands.

For hardwire monitoring
• Expose the patient's chest and determine electrode placement, based on which system and lead you're using. (See *Positioning monitoring leads*.)
• If an area is excessively hairy, clip it or shave it.
• Remove the backing from the pre-gelled electrode. Check the gel for moisture. If the gel is dry, discard the electrode and replace it with a fresh one.

Press firmly

• Apply the electrode to the site and press firmly to ensure a tight seal. Repeat with the remaining electrodes.
• When all the electrodes are in place, check for a tracing on the cardiac monitor. Assess the quality of the ECG. (See *Identifying cardiac monitor problems*.)
• To verify that each beat is being detected by the monitor, compare the digital heart rate display with your count of the patient's heart rate.

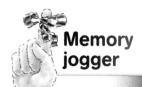

Memory jogger

To help you remember where to place electrodes in a five-electrode configuration, think of the phrase 'white to the upper right'. Then think of snow over trees (white electrode over green electrode) and smoke over fire (black electrode above red electrode). And of course, chocolate (brown electrode) lies close to the heart.

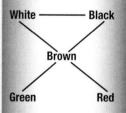

White ———— Black

Brown

Green ———— Red

Positioning monitoring leads

These illustrations show correct electrode positions for some of the monitoring leads you'll use most often. For each lead, you'll see electrode placement for a five-leadwire system and a telemetry system.

In the hardwire system, the electrode position for one lead may be identical to the electrode positions for another lead. In this case, simply change the lead selector switch to the setting that corresponds to the lead you want. In some cases, you'll need to reposition the electrodes.

In the telemetry system, you can create the same lead with two electrodes that you do with three, simply by eliminating the ground electrode.

These illustrations use these abbreviations: RA, right arm; LA, left arm; RL, right leg; LL, Left leg; C, chest; and G, ground.

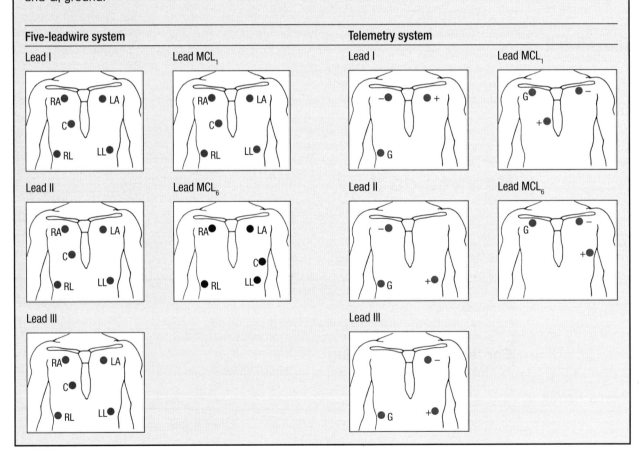

Five-leadwire system

Lead I Lead MCL₁

Lead II Lead MCL₆

Lead III

Telemetry system

Lead I Lead MCL₁

Lead II Lead MCL₆

Lead III

Warning!

Identifying cardiac monitor problems

Problem	Possible causes	Solutions
False–high-rate alarm	• Monitor interpreting large T waves as QRS complexes, which doubles the rate • Skeletal muscle activity	• Reposition electrodes to lead where QRS complexes are taller than T waves. • Place electrodes away from major muscle masses.
False–low-rate alarm	• Shift in electrical axis from patient movement, making QRS complexes too small to register • Low amplitude of QRS • Poor contact between electrode and skin	• Reapply electrodes. Set gain so height of complex is greater than 1 mV. • Increase gain. • Reapply electrodes.
Artefact (waveform interference)	• Patient having seizures, chills, or anxiety • Patient movement • Electrodes applied improperly • Static electricity • Electrical short circuit in leadwires or cable • Interference from decreased room humidity	• Notify doctor and treat patient as ordered. Keep patient warm and reassure him. • Help patient relax. • Check electrodes and reapply, if necessary. • Make sure cables don't have exposed connectors. Change static-causing bedclothes. • Replace broken equipment. Use stress loops when applying leadwires. • Regulate humidity to 40%.

• If necessary, use the gain control to adjust the size of the rhythm tracing, and use the position control to adjust the waveform position on the recording paper.

• Set the upper and lower limits of the heart rate alarm, based on medical aims for the individual patient. Turn the alarm on.

For telemetry monitoring

• Prepare yourself and the patient as for hardwire monitoring.

• Expose the patient's chest, and select the lead arrangement. Remove the backing from one of the pre-gelled electrodes. Check the gel for moistness. If it's dry, discard the electrode and obtain a new one.

• Apply the electrode to the appropriate site. Press your fingers in a circular motion around the electrode to fix the gel and stabilize the electrode. Repeat for each electrode.

• Attach an electrode to the end of each lead.

Walkie-talkie for the heart

• Place the transmitter in the pouch. Tie the pouch strings around the patient's neck and waist, making sure that the pouch fits snugly without causing him discomfort.
• Check the patient's waveform for clarity, position and size. Adjust the gain and baseline as needed.
• To obtain a rhythm strip, press the record key at the central station. Label the strip with the patient's name, date of birth and hospital number, also record the date and time of acquisition. If required, inform the doctor that the rhythm strip has been acquired and place it in the patient's notes, ready for interpretation.

Practice pointers

• Make sure that all electrical equipment and outlets are grounded to avoid electric shock and interference (artefacts). Also ensure that the patient is clean and dry to prevent electric shock.
• If the patient's skin is very oily, scaly or diaphoretic, rub the electrode site with 70% alcohol pad before applying the electrode to help reduce interference in the tracing.
• Assess skin integrity, and reposition the electrodes every 24 hours or as necessary.

Treat the patient, not the rhythm

If the patient is being monitored by telemetry, tell him to remove the transmitter if he takes a shower or bath, but stress that he should let you know before he removes the unit. (See *Documenting cardiac monitoring*.)

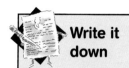

Write it down

Document-ing cardiac monitoring

In your notes, record the date and time monitoring began and the monitoring lead used. Document a rhythm strip at least every 8 hours and with changes in the patient's condition (or as specified by local policy). Label the rhythm strip with the patient's name, date of birth and hospital number, the monitored lead, date and time.

Pain assessment

Several interventions can be used to manage pain. These include analgesic administration, emotional support, comfort measures and cognitive techniques to distract the patient. Severe pain usually requires an opiate analgesic. Invasive measures, such as epidural analgesia or patient-controlled analgesia, may also be required. However, before you can administer treatment for pain you need first to assess the patient's pain, allowing you to plan his care.

What you need

Pain assessment tool or scale.

How you do it

- Explain to the patient how pain medications work together with other pain management therapies to provide relief. Also explain that management aims to keep pain at a low level to permit optimal bodily function. In order to keep his pain at a minimal level you need to ask him a few questions, encourage him to answer honestly.
- To assess pain properly, you must consider both the patient's description and your observations of his physical and behavioural responses. Start by asking him to rank his pain on a scale of 1–3, with 0 denoting no pain and 3 demoting the worst pain imaginable. Besides establishing a baseline, this will help him evaluate pain therapies verbally.

Key questions

Next ask the patient the following questions:
- Where is the pain located?
- How long does the pain last?
- How often does it occur?
- Can you describe the pain?
- What relieves the pain?
- What makes the pain worse?
    Bear in mind that his experiences, self-image and beliefs about his condition will influence his answers to these questions.

Other clues

Observe the patient's behavioural responses to pain. Also note physiological responses, which may be sympathetic or parasympathetic.
- Behavioural responses include altered body position, moaning, sighing, grimacing, withdrawal, crying, restlessness, muscle twitching and immobility.
- Sympathetic responses—commonly associated with mild to moderate pain—include pallor, elevated blood pressure, dilated pupils, skeletal muscle tension, dyspnoea, tachycardia and diaphoresis.
- Parasympathetic responses—commonly associated with severe, deep pain—include pallor, decreased blood pressure, bradycardia, nausea and vomiting, weakness, dizziness and loss of consciousness.

Partners in pain management

Work with the patient, the doctors and the pain team to develop a plan of care that uses interventions that fit the patient's lifestyle. These may include prescribed medications, emotional support, comfort measures, cognitive techniques and education about pain

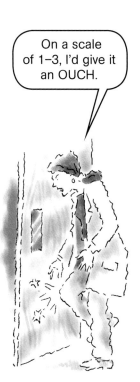

On a scale of 1–3, I'd give it an OUCH.

and its management. Emphasize the importance of maintaining good bowel habits, respiratory function and mobility because pain increases problems in these areas.

Implement your plan of care

Because individuals respond to pain differently, you'll find that what works for one person may not work for another. However, the following care aspects should always be provided:
• Administer medication and adjunctive medication as prescribed and required. Remember that a pre-registration nurse cannot administer medications without supervision by a registered nurse.
• Provide emotional support by spending time with the patient. His inability to manage the pain may cause him to be anxious and frustrated, such feelings can worsen pain.
• Perform comfort measures such as encouraging or assisting with repositioning, as this will reduce muscle spasms.
• Provide oral hygiene as required, because a common side-effect of pain medications (analgesia) is drying of the mucous membranes of the mouth.
• Use cognitive therapies such as distraction, guided imagery, deep breathing and relaxation to help the patient enhance the effect of analgesics. You can easily use these 'mind-over-pain' techniques at the bedside. Choose the method the patient prefers. If possible, start these techniques when the patient feels little or no pain. If he feels persistent pain, begin with short, simple exercises. Before beginning, dim the lights, remove the patient's restrictive clothing, and eliminate noise from the environment.

A brief get-away

For distraction, have the patient recall a pleasant experience or focus his attention on an enjoyable activity. For instance, he can use music as a distraction by turning on the radio when the pain begins. Have him close his eyes and concentrate on listening, raising or lowering the volume as his pain increases or subsides. Note, however, that distraction is usually effective only against brief pain episodes lasting less than 5 minutes.

Without ever leaving the house

• For guided imagery, help the patient concentrate on a peaceful, pleasant image such as a walk on the beach. Encourage him to concentrate on the details of the image he has selected by asking about its sight, sound, smell, taste and touch. If available, use

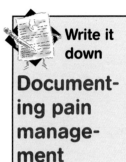

Write it down

Document-ing pain manage-ment

Document pain as a fifth vital sign, recording it as frequently as other vital signs. In your notes, record:

• each step of the nursing process
• subjective information elicited from the patient, using his own words
• location, quality and duration of pain
• precipitating factors
• pain relief method used
• nursing interventions and patient's responses
• alternative treatments to consider the next time pain occurs (if pain wasn't relieved)
• complications of drug therapy.

audiotapes of sounds to help with guided imagery. The positive emotions evoked by this exercise minimize pain.

• For deep breathing, have the patient stare at an object and then slowly inhale and exhale as he counts aloud to maintain a comfortable rate and rhythm. Have him concentrate on the rise and fall of his abdomen. Encourage him to feel more and more weightless with each breath while he concentrates on the rhythm of his breathing or on any restful image.

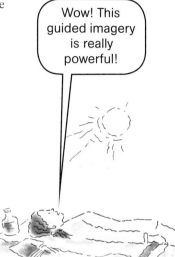

Wow! This guided imagery is really powerful!

Focus, tense, relax

For muscle relaxation, have the patient focus on a particular muscle group. Then ask him to tense the muscles and note the sensation. After 5–7 seconds, tell him to relax the muscles and concentrate on the relaxed state. Have him note the difference between the tense and relaxed states. After he tenses and relaxes one muscle group, have him proceed to another and another until he has covered his entire body.

Practice pointers

• Evaluate your patient's response to pain management. If he's still in pain, reassess him and alter your plan of care after discussion with the multidisciplinary team.
• The most common adverse effects of analgesics include respiratory depression (the most serious), sedation, constipation, nausea and vomiting. (See *Documenting pain management*.)
• ESCs specific to standard numbers 1–8 (Care, compassion and communication) and 33–42 (Medicines management).

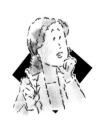

Quick quiz

1. Which heart rate in an adult would be considered normal using the early warning system?
    A. 60 to 89 beats/minute
    B. 90 to 114 beats/minute
    C. >130 beats/minute

Answer: A. A heart rate of between 60 and 89 beats/minute in an adult who is hospitalized is within the normal range.

2. What is the normal range for CVP?
    A. 15–20 cmH$_2$O
    B. 5–10 cmH$_2$O
    C. 0–10 cmH$_2$O

Answer: B. 5–10 cm of water is the normal range for CVP.

3. Why do you estimate systolic blood pressure?
    A. When you can't find a stethoscope
    B. When your patient is restless
    C. Because it makes the procedure more comfortable and less painful for the patient.

Answer: C. Estimation of systolic pressure prior to auscultation means that you have already established a pressure to inflate to, minimizing the need to increase to pressures such as 300 mmHg before deflating.

Scoring

☆☆☆ If you answered all three items correctly, congratulations! You are an assessment pro!

☆☆ If you answered two items correctly, great! You are prepared for assessing patients!

☆ If you answered fewer than two correctly, don't despair. Just review the chapter and try again!

3 Specimen collection

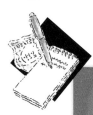

Just the facts

In this chapter, you'll learn:

♦ about procedures for collecting specimens and how to perform them (see Chapter 8, for enhanced skills, i.e. venepuncture, Papanicolaou test, etc.)

♦ what patient care, complications and patient teaching are associated with each procedure

♦ about essential documentation for each procedure.

Practice pointers

Follow the code

Important information is obtained from specimens you collect, not only as a guide to treatment and care of patients but also for definitive diagnosis. The information can only be obtained if you follow the correct process when collecting the specimen and give specific and detailed information with it; this is your responsibility if you are collecting the specimen. Specimens should only be taken when there are clinical signs of infection, clinical indications present or following agreement with an Infection Control Advisor or Health Protection Unit as part of a screening programme.

Before the procedure you must always communicate to your patient the reason, process and side effects of the procedure in order to obtain permission. When collecting, handling or processing specimens you must wear appropriate personal protective clothing to avoid exposure to body fluids and potentially pathogenic organisms, and, of course, perform good hand hygiene before and after the procedure. Always ensure that you are transporting specimens safely too; use specifically designed containers and never overfill them, ensure lids are sealed tightly and seal the container in a two-compartment specimen bag with the container in one compartment and the laboratory request form in the second. Label both the container and the laboratory request form.

- ESCs specific to standards: Infection prevention and control, all; Medicines management, 36, 41 and 42. Care, compassion and communication, 1–9; and in accordance with standard Organizational aspects of care, 10–20.

Capillary blood glucose (CBG)

Reagent strip tests (such as Glucostix, Chemstrip bG and Multistix) are a quick, easy way to test a patient's blood glucose level. A drop of capillary blood—obtained by fingerstick, heelstick, or earlobe puncture—provides the blood sample.

These tests can detect or monitor elevated blood glucose levels in patients with diabetes. They can also screen for diabetes mellitus and help distinguish diabetic coma from non-diabetic coma. What's more, they can be performed in the hospital, doctor's surgery or patient's home.

Match the colour to the chart

In blood glucose tests, a reagent patch on the tip of a hand-held plastic strip changes colour in response to the amount of glucose in the blood sample. Comparing the colour change after 60 seconds with a standardized colour chart provides a semi-quantitative measurement of blood glucose levels, but this method is less commonly used due to the lowering cost of portable devices meters (such as Glucometer II, Accu-Chek II or One Touch), which provide quantitative measurements and are just as accurate as other laboratory tests, and therefore are the preferred method. Some meters store successive test results electronically to help determine glucose patterns, so are ideal for the patient at home.

What you need

Reagent strips ✳ soap, water and handtowels ✳ clinical waste bag ✳ sharps bin ✳ gloves and apron ✳ portable blood glucose meter ✳ gauze pads ✳ disposable mechanical blood-letting device ✳ watch or clock with a second hand.

How you do it

- Calibrate the device, using control agents for both high and low calibration, to prevent false positive/negative readings. Follow manufacturers' instructions and local policy as to when, how often and who can perform this procedure.
- Explain the procedure to the patient and gain permission.

- Next, select the puncture site—usually the fingertip for an adult or a child. (See *Not appropriate for all*.)
- Wash your hands, put on gloves and an apron.
- Ask or assist the patient to wash and dry their hands using warm water and soap, to prevent cross-infection and help dilate the capillaries.

Prep the meter

- Switch on the meter.
- Check that the reagent strip lot number matches the number that appears on screen; if it does not, insert the batch strip from the reagent strip container into the device. This will change the lot number and configure the device to work with the reagent strips you have. You must perform this step whenever you acquire or change to a new container of reagent strips.
- Insert a reagent strip into the device without touching the reagent patch on the end, to prevent contamination and inaccurate readings.
- The device will now indicate via pictures (usually a flashing drop of blood) that it is ready for a sample of blood.

At the fingertip

- To collect a sample from the fingertip using the preferred method (a disposable mechanical blood-letting device, such as an Autolet, which uses a spring-loaded lancet), position the lancet on the side of the patient's third, fourth or small finger, perpendicular to the lines of the fingerprints. The thumb, second finger or the pad of the fingertip should not be used as these are used for the pincer movement of the hand and also to feel. Continuous sampling from these areas can lead to nerve damage, thus inhibiting normal daily activities of living.
- Depress the lever or button quickly and firmly; this, in turn, will pierce the skin sharply and quickly to minimize the patient's anxiety and pain and to increase blood flow.
- Discard the lancet immediately in a sharps bin!
- After puncturing the fingertip, wipe away the first drop of blood as this assists in preventing cross-contamination from the skin and also from serous fluid being acquired, leading to a less than accurate result.
- Touch the second drop of formed blood to the reagent patch on the strip, covering the entire patch; the meter will begin to process the blood and acquire the data.

Under pressure

- After collecting the blood sample, briefly apply pressure to the puncture site to prevent painful extravasation of blood into subcutaneous tissues. Ask the adult patient to hold a gauze pad firmly over the puncture site until bleeding stops.
- Make sure you leave the blood on the strip and the strip in the device until the reading appears digitally on the screen.

Ages and stages

Not appropriate for all

The fingertip or earlobe of an adult or a child is typically chosen as the site for capillary blood glucose testing. However, these sites are not appropriate for infants. The heel or great toe is commonly the preferred site for an infant.

• Once the reading has been acquired and noted, remove the reagent strip from the meter, and dispose of it in the clinical waste. Check the puncture site and ask the patient if he would like a dressing. Clean the meter, as per manufacturer's instructions.

Document and act

• Document capillary blood glucose (CBG). (See *Documenting CBG*.)
• Act upon your findings; remember a normal CBG is between 4 and 7 mmol/l, but check for specific instructions and aims for individual patients.

Practice pointers

• Ensure you are confident and competent to perform this skill by accessing local teaching sessions and working with your mentor until you are both satisfied competency has been achieved. Check local policy as students may not always be allowed to perform this procedure. This will maintain patient safety.
• Before using reagent strips, check the expiration date on the package and replace outdated strips. Check for special instructions related to the specific reagent strip. Protect the strips from light, heat and moisture.
• Before using a blood glucose meter, calibrate it and run it with a control sample to ensure accurate test results, document these findings. Follow the manufacturer's instructions for calibration.

Stay away from the cold

• Avoid selecting cold, cyanotic or swollen puncture sites, to ensure an adequate blood sample. (See *Checking capillary blood glucose*.)
• To help detect abnormal glucose metabolism and diagnose diabetes mellitus, the doctor may order other blood glucose tests. (See *Documenting CBG*.)

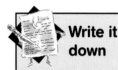

Write it down

Document-ing CBG

Record the reading from the portable blood glucose meter or a colour chart in your notes or on a special flowchart, if available. Also record the time and date of the test. Note interventions/actions you took, and sign.

Home care connection

Checking capillary blood glucose

If the patient will be using the portable blood glucose meter system at home, teach him the proper use and disposal of the lancet or Autolet, as well as maintenance and cleaning of the portable blood glucose meter, as necessary. Also, provide written guidelines to reinforce your teaching.

Collecting a random urine specimen for urinalysis

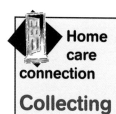

A random urine specimen is collected for urinalysis as part of the patient assessment process or at various times during hospitalization. It permits screening for urinary and systemic disorders and prevents unnecessary laboratory testing. (See *Collecting urine*.) Urinalysis can give information regarding the following factors in relation to urine: colour, pH, specific gravity, glucose, ketones, blood, nitrates, protein and leucocytes. It is essential that you are aware of why you are testing for these factors as they are only indicators of possible disease presence; further urine and fasting blood tests should always be performed if positive presence of the following is found, before diagnosis is made.

Colour

- In its normal state, urine should be clear and the colour of straw. Remember though that some medications and food can alter the colour of urine, such as amitryptiline (blue to green), indomethacin (green), tetracyclines (yellow to orange), beetroot (pink–red), rhubarb (brown–black).
- Debris may indicate the presence of disease.
- Cloudiness is not normal and may indicate the present of infection, dehydration and/or disease process.

Acid or alkali

- The pH test relates to acidity. Normal range for pH is between 5 and 6.
- A pH of above 7 indicates stale urine, which can be an indication of infection.
- A pH below 4 indicates acidic urine; with this level of pH, patients are at risk of forming uric acid calculi.

Specific gravity

- Monitors the ability of the kidney to concentrate or dilute urine. It is determined by comparing the weight of urine with that of an equivalent volume of distilled water, which has a specific gravity of 1.000. Because urine contains dissolved salts and other substances, its specific gravity is greater than 1.000. Urine specific gravity ranges from 1.003 (very dilute) to 1.035 (highly concentrated); normal values range from 1.010 to 1.025.
- High concentration can indicate dehydration.
- Low concentration can indicate increased kidney function or fluid overload.

Home care connection

Collecting urine

If your patient will be collecting a random urine specimen at home, instruct him to collect the specimen in a clean container with a tight-fitting lid and to keep it on ice or in the refrigerator (separate from food items) for up to 24 hours.

Low urine specific gravity indicates that the patient is failing to reabsorb water…

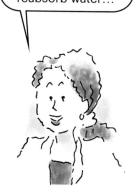

Glucose

- Presence of glucose in urine found during urinalysis can be an indicator of diabetes mellitus.
- Glucose may also be present if renal absorption is abnormal.

Ketones

- Ketones are produced by the breakdown of fatty acids. So when the patient has not eaten and is using stored fat as the main source of energy, ketones will be present; for example, in a patient with anorexia, diabetes mellitus, or a patient on a low or zero carbohydrate diet.
- The smell of ketones is often described as having a distinctive 'pear drop' or 'nail polish remover' type smell.

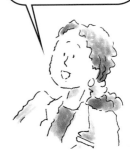

...which may indicate acute renal failure, diabetes insipidus, or several other conditions.

Protein

- Often present during the course of a urinary tract infection (UTI), or in renal or urological disease processes.
- Can indicate hypertension, pyrexia, congestive cardiac failure, pre-eclampsia, infection or, again, diabetes.

Blood

- The presence of blood can be as a result of contamination from menstrual fluid, post-catheterization or post-operative trauma (especially urological surgery).
- Can also indicate renal tract infection, kidney stones, tumour or malignancy, kidney trauma or reflux syndrome in patients with recurring UTIs.

Leucocytes

- You should also know leucocytes as white blood cells; you will then remember that white blood cells are present in higher numbers when the body is trying to fight infection or foreign bodies. Therefore, high leucocyte presence can indicate rejection of a new kidney or organ, inflammation, disease or infection.

Nitrate

- Nitrates should not normally be present at all, there is no high or low figure to observe—just check for their presence. Many, but not all, bacterial strains produce nitrates, so their presence can be an indicator of infection. But remember some bacteria do not produce nitrates (i.e. staphylococci, enterococci and *Pseudomonas*) so a negative result does not always mean no infection present.

What you need

Clean or disposable container, bedpan or urinal with cover ✳ gloves and apron ✳ label ✳ reagent strips and associated colour chart ✳ medical device or surface wipes ✳ measuring jug, if necessary.

How you do it

- Inform the patient that you need a urine specimen for analysis. Explain the procedure to him and his family, if necessary, to promote cooperation and prevent accidental disposal of specimens, and to gain permission.
- Provide privacy. Instruct the patient on bed rest to void into a clean bedpan or urinal, with the bed curtains drawn. Ask the ambulatory patient to void into a specific container in the bathroom. Label the container *before use*, with his name, date of birth and hospital number (*thus preventing contamination of your pen when the specimen pot has been used*) and ask him to return the specimen to you for testing, *this will prevent data being correlated with the wrong patient*.

Test, record, discard

- Put on gloves and apron.
- Pour some urine into a sterile specimen pot in case you need to send a specimen to the laboratory. *By doing this now you have prevented contamination of the specimen with the reagent strip.*
- Take one reagent strip and dip into urine sample, follow manufacturer's guidelines for how long to leave strip in the sample, as this varies between manufacturers.
- Use the manufacturer's colour chart to cross-reference each individual colour change on the reagent strip, do not allow the strip to come into contact with the chart; if you inadvertently spill urine on the outside of the container, clean with a surface or medical device wipe and allow it to dry to prevent cross-contamination. Follow the manufacturer's guidelines for how long to wait before cross-referencing to the colour chart.
- If the patient's urine output must be measured and recorded, pour the urine into the measuring jug, measure and record. Otherwise, discard the urine and disposable container (if used) as per local policy.
- Remove and discard gloves and apron in clinical waste, wash your hands.
- Document your findings, *to enable communication with all multidisciplinary team members as required*. (See *Documenting urine specimen collection*.)
- Take appropriate actions as required and as local policy states, i.e. send the previously decanted urine specimen to the laboratory for testing; document this in the patient's records.

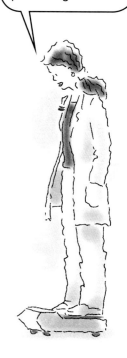

I've used up my recent food intake as energy, now I'm burning fat and producing ketones.

Clean and return

• Put on gloves. Clean the measuring container and urinal or bedpan, and return them to their proper storage area. Discard disposable items.
• Wash your hands thoroughly to prevent cross-contamination. Offer the patient a washcloth, soap, water and hand towels to wash and dry his hands.

Collecting a catheter specimen of urine (CSU)

Obtain a catheter specimen of urine (CSU) by aspirating a specimen with a catheter tip syringe via the needle-free collection port, thus maintaining a closed system. It requires a non-touch sterile collection technique to prevent catheter contamination, specimen contamination and urinary tract infection. Clamping the drainage tube and emptying the urine into a container are contraindicated, as this opens the system to infection. (See *Possible portals of infection*.)

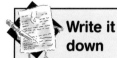

Write it down

Document- ing urine specimen collection

Record the time and date of specimen collection and analysis. Specify the test results as well as the appearance, odour, and colour and unusual characteristics of the specimen. If necessary, record the urine volume on the fluid balance chart. Sign the documentation.

Possible portals of infection

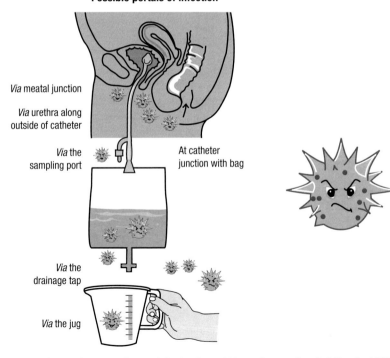

Via meatal junction

Via urethra along outside of catheter

Via the sampling port

At catheter junction with bag

Via the drainage tap

Via the jug

Source: Corrine Cameron-Watson, Infection Control Nurse, Queens Hospital, Romford, UK

What you need

Non-sterile gloves ✳ apron ✳ 70% alcohol swab ✳ 10 ml syringe ✳ tube clamp ✳ sterile specimen container with lid ✳ label ✳ laboratory request form and sample bag.

How you do it

• Check the identification details on the laboratory request form with the patient, to ensure the correct patient is identified.
• Explain the procedure to the patient and gain permission.
• Label the sterile container with the patient's name, hospital number and date of birth prior to use to prevent cross-contamination of your pen.
• Wash your hands and put on gloves and an apron.
• The drainage tube will have a built-in sampling port, wipe the port with an alcohol pad for 10–30 seconds and allow the alcohol to dry, it is only when alcohol has dried that bacteria are eliminated.
• Check the expiry date and remove the syringe from its packaging using a non-touch technique, to prevent cross-infection.
• Insert the tip of the syringe into the clean, dry sampling port at a 90-degree angle to the tubing. Aspirate the specimen into the syringe. Remove the syringe with sample content.
• Clean the port again using a 70% alcohol swab.
• Transfer the specimen to the pre-labelled sterile container.
• Place the labelled sample and laboratory request form in a sample bag and send it to the laboratory immediately (ideally urine should be examined in the laboratory within 2 hours), or place it in a dedicated medical fridge (for no longer that 48 hours), as bacteria will multiply at room temperature, giving misleading results.
• Remove your gloves and apron and dispose of in clinical waste and wash your hands.
• Document procedure (see *Documenting CSU collection*).

Practice pointers

• If a urine culture is to be performed, list current antibiotic therapy on the laboratory request form.
• Never take a CSU from the drainage bag, this urine may have been stagnant for many hours.
• Do not use a needle to aspirate the sample through a needle-free port, you are at higher risk of contaminated sharps injury.

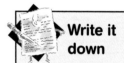

Write it down

Documenting CSU collection

In your notes, record:

• time of specimen collection and method of aspiration
• what you have done with the specimen, i.e. transported to the laboratory, waiting in fridge for collection, etc.
• specific test requested
• appearance, odour, and colour and unusual characteristics of the specimen
• the fact that it came from an indwelling catheter. If necessary, record the urine volume on the fluid balance chart.

Timed urine collection

Because hormones, proteins and electrolytes are excreted in small, variable amounts in urine, specimens for measuring these substances must typically be collected over an extended period to yield quantities of diagnostic value.

A 24-hour specimen is used most commonly because it provides an average excretion rate for substances eliminated during this period. Timed specimens may also be collected for shorter periods, such as 2 or 12 hours, depending on the information needed.

After the challenge

A timed urine specimen may also be collected after administering a challenge dose of a chemical—inulin, for example—to detect various renal disorders.

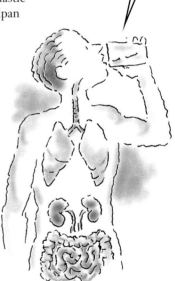

This test is sure to quench the patient's thirst.

What you need

Large collection bottle with a cap or stopper, or a commercial plastic container ✳ preservative, if necessary ✳ gloves and apron ✳ bedpan or urinal if patient doesn't have an indwelling catheter ✳ measuring jug if patient's intake and output must be measured ✳ refrigerator ✳ label ✳ laboratory request form.

Obtain large collection bottles from the laboratory and check that preservatives have already been added.

How you do it

• Explain the procedure to the patient, to gain permission and his cooperation plus to prevent accidental disposal of urine during the collection period. Emphasize that failure to collect all urine during the collection period invalidates the test and requires that it begin again—even missing one!
• Follow standard infection control procedures and instruction as in CSU collection when handling urine, completing documentation and ensuring safe arrival at the laboratory.

Don't forget

• Communicate to all multidisciplinary team (MDT) members at handover and via the patient's notes that the collection is in progress. This will eliminate the need for patient-care reminders over the patient's bed, etc., which he may find offensive and does not preserve his privacy and dignity.

• Instruct the patient to save all urine during the collection period, to notify you after each voiding, and to avoid contaminating the urine with stool or toilet tissue, as far as possible. Explain any dietary or drug restrictions, and make sure he understands and is willing to comply with them.

For 2-hour collection

• If possible, encourage the patient to drink 500–1,000 ml of water up to 30 minutes before collection begins. After 30 minutes, ask him to void. Put on gloves and discard this specimen so the patient starts the collection period with an empty bladder.
• If prescribed and not contraindicated, administer a challenge dose of medication (such as glucose solution), and record the time.
• If possible, offer the patient a glass of water at least every hour during the collection period to stimulate urine production. After each voiding, put on gloves and an apron and add the specimen to the collection bottle, using a non-touch technique.

15-minute warning

• Instruct the patient to void about 15 minutes before the end of the collection period, if possible, and add this specimen to the collection bottle.
• At the end of the collection period, send the appropriately labelled collection bottle to the laboratory immediately, along with a properly completed laboratory request form.

For 12-hour and 24-hour collection

• Put on gloves, and ask the patient to void. Then discard this urine so the patient starts the collection period with an empty bladder. Record the time.
• After putting on gloves and an apron, pour the first urine specimen into the collection bottle.
• Remove and discard your gloves and wash your hands.
• Then refrigerate the bottle until the next voiding, or send each full bottle individually to the laboratory (ensure correct labelling) for adequate storage if not available at ward level.

One more time

• After putting on gloves, collect all urine voided during the prescribed period. Just before the collection period ends, ask the patient to void again, if possible. Add this last specimen to the collection bottle, refrigerate to inhibit deterioration of the specimen, and remove and discard your gloves in the clinical waste.
• Wash your hands, then label the collection bottle, and send it to the laboratory with a properly completed laboratory request form.

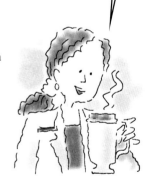

Be sure to tell your patient that exercise and ingestion of coffee, tea, or drugs can alter test results.

Practice pointers

- Keep the patient well hydrated before and during the test to ensure adequate urine flow.
- Before collection of a timed specimen, make sure the laboratory will be open when the collection period ends to help ensure prompt, accurate results. To avoid contamination, never store a specimen in a refrigerator that contains food or medication.
- If the patient has an indwelling catheter in place, put the collection bag in an ice-filled container at his bedside.
- Inform the patient that exercise and ingestion of coffee, tea or drugs can alter test results.
- If you accidentally discard a specimen during the collection period, you'll need to restart the collection. This may result in an additional day of hospitalization, which may cause the patient unnecessary personal and financial stress. Therefore, emphasize to everyone involved in his care, as well as to family and other visitors, the need to save all the patient's urine during the collection period. (See *Documenting timed urine collection*.)

Write it down

Documenting timed urine collection

Record the date and intervals of specimen collection and when the collection bottle(s) was sent to the laboratory.

Straining urine for calculi

Renal calculi, or kidney stones, may develop anywhere in the urinary tract. They may be excreted with the urine or become lodged in the urinary tract, causing haematuria, urine retention, renal colic and, possibly, hydronephrosis.

Sizes vary

Ranging in size from microscopic to several centimetres, calculi form in the kidneys when mineral salts—principally calcium oxalate or calcium phosphate—collect around a nucleus of bacterial cells, blood clots or other particles. Other substances involved in calculus formation include uric acid, xanthine and ammonia.

Strain carefully

Testing for calculi requires careful straining of all of the patient's urine through a gauze pad or fine-mesh sieve and, at times, quantitative laboratory analysis of questionable specimens. Such testing typically continues until the patient passes the calculi or until surgery.

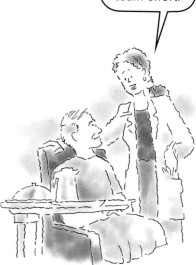

Straining urine for stones is a team effort.

What you need

Strainer or gauze pad ✷ measuring jug ✷ rubber band ✷ urinal or bedpan ✷ gloves and apron ✷ laboratory request form ✷ specimen container (for use if calculi are found).

How you do it

• Explain the procedure to the patient and his family, if possible, to ensure cooperation, to gain permission and to stress the importance of straining all the patient's urine.
• Communicate to all MDT members at handover and via the patient's notes that collection and straining is in progress. This will eliminate the need for patient-care reminders over the patient's bed, etc., which he may find offensive and does not preserve his privacy and dignity.
• Tell the patient to notify you after each voiding.

Improvise!

• If a commercial strainer isn't available, unfold a gauze pad, place it over the top of a graduated measuring jug, and secure it with a rubber band.
• Put on gloves and an apron. With the gauze secured over the mouth of the collection container, pour the specimen from the urinal or bedpan into the container. If the patient has an indwelling catheter in place, strain all urine from the collection bag before discarding it.

Detective work

• Examine the strainer for calculi. If you detect calculi or if the filter looks questionable, place the filtrate in a specimen container, and send it to the laboratory with a laboratory request form.
• Remove and discard your gloves and apron, wash your hands.
• Document, sign and date your findings and actions.

Practice pointers

• Save and send to the laboratory small or suspicious-looking residue in the specimen container, because even tiny calculi can cause haematuria and extreme pain.
• Be aware that calculi may appear in various colours, each of which has diagnostic value.
• If the patient will be straining his urine at home, teach him how to use a strainer, and tell him how important it is to strain all his urine for the prescribed period. (See *Documenting straining urine for calculi*.)

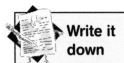 **Write it down**

Document-ing strain-ing urine for calculi

Chart the time of the specimen collection and transport to the laboratory, if necessary. Describe the filtrate passed, and note whether pain or haematuria occurred during the voiding, sign and date.

Stool collection

Stool is collected to determine if blood, ova and parasites, bile, fat, pathogens, or such substances as ingested drugs are present. Visual examination of stool characteristics—such as colour, consistency and odour—can reveal such conditions as gastrointestinal (GI) bleeding and steatorrhoea.

Random or specific

Stool specimens are collected randomly or for specific periods, such as 72 hours. Because stool specimens can't be obtained on demand, proper collection requires careful instructions to the patient to ensure an uncontaminated specimen.

What you need

Specimen container with lid ✳ gloves and apron ✳ tongue blade ✳ paper towel or paper bag ✳ bedpan or portable commode ✳ laboratory request form.

How you do it

• Explain the procedure to the patient, to ensure permission and cooperation is granted and to prevent inadvertent disposal of timed stool specimens.

Collecting a random specimen

• Tell the patient to notify you when he has the urge to defecate. Have him defecate into a clean, dry bedpan or portable commode. Instruct him not to contaminate the specimen with urine or toilet tissue because urine inhibits faecal bacterial growth and toilet tissue contains bismuth, which interferes with test results.
• Put on gloves and apron.

Specimen representative

• Using the spoon cap of the specimen container or a tongue blade, transfer the most representative stool specimen from the bedpan to the specimen container, and cap the container. If the patient passes blood, mucus or pus with the stool, be sure to include this with the specimen.
• If a tongue blade was used to collect the specimen, wrap it in a paper towel or place it in a paper bag and discard it in the clinical waste. Remove and discard your gloves, and wash your hands thoroughly to prevent cross-contamination.

It's a fact—stool specimens can't be obtained on demand. You'll have to work carefully with the patient to ensure proper collection.

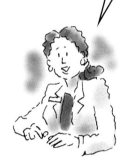

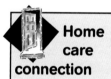

Home care connection

Collecting a stool specimen

If the patient is to collect a stool specimen at home, instruct him to collect it in a clean container with a tight-fitting lid, to wrap the container in an opaque plastic bag or paper bag if available, and to keep it in the refrigerator (separate from food items) until it can be transported.

Collecting a timed specimen

• Communicate to all MDT members at handover and via the patient's notes that timed stool collection is in progress. This will eliminate the need for patient-care reminders over the patient's bed, such as 'save all stool', which he may find offensive and, of course, does not preserve his privacy and dignity.
• After putting on gloves, collect the first specimen, and include this in the total specimen.

Complete transfer

• Obtain the timed specimen as you would a random specimen, but remember to transfer all stool to the specimen container.
• If stool must be obtained with an enema, use only tap water or normal saline solution.
• As per local policy, send each specimen to the laboratory immediately with a laboratory request form, or if permitted, refrigerate the specimens collected during the test period, and send them when collection is complete. Remove and discard gloves and apron in clinical waste and decontaminate hands thoroughly.
• Make sure the patient is comfortable after the procedure and that he has the opportunity to thoroughly clean his hands and perianal area. Perineal care may be necessary for some patients (see Perineal care, Chapter 1).

Practice pointers

• To prevent contamination, never place a stool specimen in a refrigerator that contains food or medication. (See *Collecting a stool specimen*.)
• Notify the doctor if the stool specimen looks unusual. (See *Documenting stool collection*.)

Write it down

Documenting stool collection

In your notes, record:

• time and date of specimen collection
• colour, odour and consistency of the stool
• unusual characteristics
• whether the patient had difficulty passing the stool
• signature.

Faecal occult blood test

Faecal occult blood tests are valuable for detecting occult blood (hidden GI bleeding), which may be present with colorectal cancer and GI ulcers such as duodenal ulcers. They are also useful for distinguishing between true melena and melena-like stools. Certain medications, such as iron supplements and bismuth compounds, can darken stools so that they resemble melena.

Look for blue

Two common occult blood screening tests are Haematest (an orthotolidin reagent tablet) and the Haemoccult slide (filter paper impregnated with guaiac). Both tests produce a blue reaction in a faecal smear if occult blood loss exceeds 5 ml in 24 hours. A newer test, Colocare, requires no faecal smear. In the UK, these tests are usually performed in the laboratory; however, they can be performed in the clinical area if the testing kit is available.

Repeat three times

To confirm a positive result, the test must be repeated at least three times while the patient follows a meatless, high-residue diet. Even then, a confirmed positive result doesn't necessarily indicate colorectal cancer. It does indicate the need for further diagnostic studies because GI bleeding can result from many causes other than cancer, such as ulcers and diverticula. These tests are easily performed on collected specimens or smears from a digital rectal examination (DRE).

What you need

Test kit ✳ gloves and apron ✳ glass or porcelain plate ✳ tongue blade or other wooden applicator.

How you do it

- Put on gloves and apron and collect a stool specimen.

Haematest reagent tablet test

- Use a tongue blade or other wooden applicator to smear a bit of the stool specimen on the filter paper supplied with the test kit. Or, after performing a digital rectal examination, wipe the finger you used for the examination on a square of the filter paper.
- Place the filter paper with the stool smear on a glass plate.
- Remove a reagent tablet from the bottle, and immediately replace the cap tightly. Then place the tablet in the centre of the stool smear on the filter paper.
- Add one drop of water to the tablet, and allow it to soak in for 5–10 seconds. Add a second drop, letting it run from the tablet onto the specimen and filter paper. If necessary, tap the plate gently to dislodge water from the top of the tablet.

2-minute read

- After 2 minutes, the filter paper will turn blue if the test is positive. Don't read the colour that appears on the tablet itself or that develops on the filter paper after the 2-minute period.
- Note the results and discard the filter paper.
- Remove and discard your gloves and apron, and wash your hands thoroughly.

Haemoccult slide test

• Open the flap on the slide packet, and use a tongue blade or other wooden applicator to apply a thin smear of the stool specimen to the guaiac-impregnated filter paper exposed in box A. Or, after performing a digital rectal examination, wipe the finger you used for the examination on a square of the filter paper.
• Apply a second smear from another part of the specimen to the filter paper exposed in box B because some parts of the specimen may not contain blood.
• Allow the specimens to dry for 3–5 minutes.

Positive result

• Open the flap on the reverse side of the slide package, and place 2 drops of Haemoccult developing solution on the paper over each smear. A blue reaction will appear in 30–60 seconds if the test result is positive.
• Record the results, and discard the slide package.
• Remove and discard your gloves, and wash your hands thoroughly.

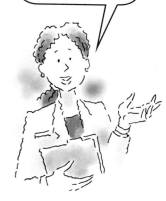

You'll get the best results if the patient maintains a high-fibre, meatless diet during the test period.

Practice pointers

• Use of the Bristol Stool Chart to describe and guide on type of faeces is commonly used in the UK. (See Lewis, S.J. and Heaton, K.W. (1997) Stool form scale as a useful guide to intestinal transit time. *Scandinavian Journal of Gastroenterology* 32(9): 920–924.)
• Make sure stool specimens aren't contaminated with urine, soap solution, lubricating jelly or toilet tissue, and test them as soon as possible after collection.
• Test samples from several portions of the same specimen because occult blood from the upper GI tract isn't always evenly dispersed throughout the formed stool; likewise, blood from colorectal bleeding may occur mostly on the outer stool surface.
• Discard outdated tablets. Protect Haematest tablets from moisture, heat and light.
• If no test kit is available in the clinical setting, then the test should be undertaken by the laboratory. Use stool specimen containers to send three consecutive specimens to the laboratory with a request form.

Repeat if positive

• If repeat testing is necessary after a positive result, explain the test to the patient. Instruct him to maintain a high-fibre diet and to refrain from eating red meat, poultry, fish, turnips and horseradish for 48–72 hours before the test, as well as throughout the collection period, because these substances may alter test results.
• As prescribed, have the patient discontinue use of iron preparations, bromides, iodides, *Rauwolfia* derivatives,

Home care connection

Home tests for faecal occult blood

Most faecal occult blood tests require the patient to collect a specimen of his stool and smear some of it on a slide. In contrast, some new tests don't require the patient to handle stool, making the procedure safer and simpler. One example is a test called Colocare. If your patient will be performing the Colocare test at home, include these instructions in your patient teaching:

• Tell him to avoid red meat and vitamin C supplements for 2 days before the test.
• Advise him to check with his doctor about the need for discontinuing medications before the test. Drugs that can interfere with test results include aspirin, indomethacin, corticosteroids, phenylbutazone, reserpine, dietary supplements, anticancer drugs and anticoagulants.
• Tell him to flush the toilet twice just before performing the test to remove any toilet-cleaning chemicals from the bowl.
• Instruct him to defecate into the toilet—but to throw no toilet paper into the bowl— and, within 5 minutes, to remove the test pad from its pouch and float it printed side up on the surface of the water.
• Tell him to watch the pad for 15 to 30 seconds for evidence of blue or green colour changes, and have him record the result on the reply card.
• Emphasize that he should perform this test with three consecutive bowel movements and then send the completed card to his doctor. However, he should call his doctor immediately if he notes a positive colour change in the first test.

Write it down

Document- ing a faecal occult blood test

Record the time and date of the test, the result, and unusual characteristics of the stool tested. Sign and date the entry and report positive results to the doctor.

indomethacin, colchicine, salicylates, potassium, phenylbutazone, oxyphenbutazone, bismuth compounds, steroids and ascorbic acid for 48–72 hours before the test and during it, to ensure accurate test results and avoid possible bleeding, which some of these compounds can cause. (See *Home tests for faecal occult blood* and *Documenting a faecal occult blood test*.)
• If the first test was undertaken using a kit in the clinical area then the repeat testing should be undertaken by the laboratory. Use a stool specimen container and lab form to send the specimen to the laboratory.

Sputum collection

Sputum, which is secreted by mucous membranes lining the bronchioles, bronchi and trachea, helps protect the respiratory tract from infection. When expelled from the respiratory tract, sputum carries saliva, nasal and sinus secretions, dead cells and bacteria from the respiratory tract. Sputum specimens may be cultured to identify respiratory pathogens.

Three methods

Expectoration is the usual method of sputum specimen collection. It may require ultrasonic nebulization, hydration or chest percussion and postural drainage. Less common methods for sputum specimen collection include tracheal suctioning and nasopharyngeal suctioning.

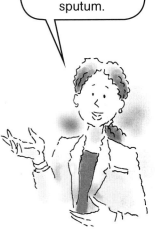

Expectoration is the most common method for collecting sputum.

What you need

Expectoration method
Sterile specimen container with tight-fitting cap ✳ gloves and apron ✳ tissues ✳ label ✳ laboratory request form.

For tracheal suctioning
12–14 French sterile suction catheter ✳ laboratory request form ✳ sterile gloves ✳ apron ✳ mask or goggles ✳ sterile in-line specimen trap (Lukens trap) ✳ portable suction machine, if wall unit is unavailable ✳ oxygen therapy ✳ label ✳ lubricating jelly.

Commercial suction kits contain all the equipment except the suction machine and an in-line specimen container.

Getting ready

Equipment and preparation depend on the method of collection. Gather the appropriate equipment for the task.

How you do it

• Ask the patient if you may collect a specimen of sputum (not saliva), and explain the procedure to promote cooperation and gain permission. If possible, collect the specimen early in the morning, before breakfast, to obtain an overnight accumulation of secretions.

Collection by expectoration
• Ask the patient to sit in a chair or at the edge of the bed.
• Ask the patient to rinse his mouth with normal tap water to reduce specimen contamination. (Avoid mouthwash or toothpaste because they may affect the mobility of organisms in the sputum sample.) Encourage him to take 3 or 4 deep breaths, then ask him to cough deeply and expectorate directly into the specimen container. To obtain enough sputum for testing purposes (approximately 15 ml) this may need to be repeated two or three times. Encourage the patient to take deep breaths, to prevent hypoxia, between each attempt.
• Put on gloves and apron.

Label and send

- Cap the container and, if necessary, clean its exterior. Remove and discard your gloves, and wash your hands thoroughly. Label the container with the patient's name and date of birth, hospital number, doctor's name, and date and time of collection. Also, include on the laboratory request form whether the patient was febrile or taking antibiotics and whether sputum was induced (because such specimens commonly appear watery and may resemble saliva). Send the specimen to the laboratory immediately.

Collection by tracheal suctioning

- If the patient can't produce an adequate specimen by coughing, prepare to suction him to obtain the specimen. Explain the suctioning procedure to him and inform him that he may cough, gag or feel short of breath during the procedure. Offer reassurance and agree a hand signal the patient can use to indicate he requires you to interrupt the procedure.

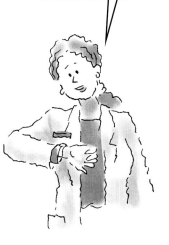

Sputum should be collected early in the morning.

Testing . . . testing . . .

- Check the suction machine to make sure it's functioning properly. Then place the patient in an upright position.
- Administer oxygen to the patient before beginning the procedure. If the patient is already receiving oxygen, increase the flow rate or percentage being delivered, to oxygenate the patient and prevent hypoxia. (See *Suctioning can be dangerous*.)
- Wash your hands thoroughly.
- Put on non-sterile gloves, gloves and goggles.
- Connect the suction tubing to the male adapter of the in-line specimen trap. Attach the sterile suction catheter to the rubber tubing of the trap. (See *Attaching a specimen trap to a suction catheter*.)

Warning!

Suctioning can be dangerous

Tracheal suctioning can be dangerous because it deprives your patient of oxygen. Remember to administer oxygen as prescribed both pre and post procedure. If your patient becomes hypoxic or cyanotic during suctioning, remove the catheter immediately and administer high-flow oxygen using a non-rebreathe mask and 15 litres of oxygen.

Patients with cardiac disease may develop arrhythmias during the procedure as a result of suctioning. Other potential complications include tracheal trauma or bleeding, vomiting, aspiration and hypoxaemia.

Attaching a specimen trap to a suction catheter

When collecting a sputum specimen using tracheal suctioning, you'll need to attach the specimen trap to the suctioning catheter. Follow the steps below for connecting and disconnecting the trap.

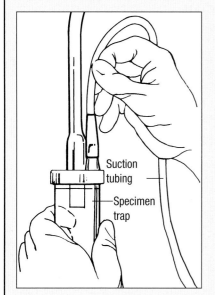

Suction tubing
Specimen trap

With gloves on, push the suction tubing onto the male adapter of the in-line trap.

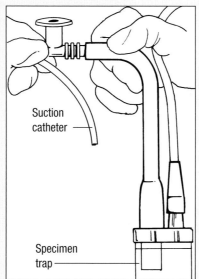

Suction catheter

Specimen trap

Insert the suction catheter into the rubber tubing of the trap.

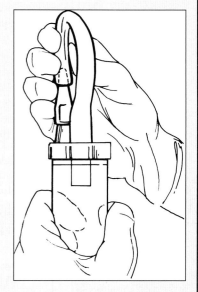

After suctioning, disconnect the in-line trap from the suction tubing and catheter. To seal the container, connect the rubber tubing to the male adapter of the trap.

• Tell the patient to tilt his head back slightly. Insert a nasopharyngeal airway if indicated. Then lubricate the catheter with jelly, and gently pass it through the patient's nostril.
• When the catheter reaches the larynx, the patient will cough. As he does, quickly advance the catheter into the trachea. Tell him to take several deep breaths through his mouth to ease insertion.
• To obtain the specimen, apply suction for 5–10 seconds but never longer than 15 seconds because prolonged suction can cause hypoxia. If the procedure must be repeated, let the patient rest for 4–6 breaths. When collection is completed, discontinue the suction, gently remove the catheter, and administer oxygen, or recommence prescribed oxygen therapy.

Careful clean-up

- Detach the catheter from the in-line trap, gather it up in your dominant hand, and pull the glove cuff inside out and down around the used catheter to enclose it for disposal. Remove and discard the other glove and your goggles.
- Apply a clean pair of non-sterile gloves. Detach the trap from the tubing connected to the suction machine. Seal the trap tightly by connecting the rubber tubing to the male adapter of the trap. Examine the specimen to make sure it's actually sputum, not saliva. Label the trap's container as an expectorated specimen, and send it to the laboratory immediately with a completed laboratory request form.
- Offer the patient a glass of water or mouthwash.

Practice pointers

- If you do not have a specimen trap for obtaining a sample, suction the patient as above, but use a sterile receiver bottle on the suction machine. Once suctioning has been performed, transfer a sample of sputum from the sterile bottle, using a sterile tongue depressor or spoon, to a specimen container, label and send to the lab. Apply a new catheter and bottle to the suction machine at the end of the procedure.
- If you can't obtain a sputum specimen through tracheal suctioning, refer the patient to physiotherapy for chest percussion to loosen and mobilize secretions, and position the patient for optimal drainage. After 20–30 minutes, repeat the tracheal suctioning procedure.
- Before sending the specimen to the laboratory, examine it to make sure it's actually sputum, not saliva, because saliva will produce inaccurate test results.
- Because expectorated sputum is contaminated by normal mouth flora, tracheal suctioning provides a more reliable specimen for diagnosis. (See *Documenting sputum collection*.)

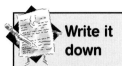

Write it down

Documenting sputum collection

In your notes, record:

- collection method used
- time and date of collection
- patient's response
- colour and consistency of the specimen
- your signature.

Throat specimen collection

Correct collection and handling of a throat specimen helps the laboratory staff identify pathogens accurately with a minimum of contamination from normal bacterial flora. Collection normally involves using a swab to sample inflamed tissues and exudates from the throat.

What you need

Gloves and apron ✳ tongue blade ✳ penlight ✳ sterile cotton-tipped swab ✳ sterile culture tube with or without transport medium as required (or commercial collection kit; swabs for methicillin-resistant *Staphylococcus aureus* (MRSA) should be taken using a dry swab, and swabs for culture should be taken with transport medium) ✳ label ✳ laboratory request form.

How you do it

- Maintain privacy and dignity by drawing bed curtains as necessary and draping patient with a blanket.
- Explain the procedure to the patient to ease his anxiety and ensure cooperation and gain informed permission.
- Tell the patient that he may gag during the swabbing but that the procedure will probably take less than 1 minute.
- Instruct the patient to sit erect at the edge of the bed or in a chair, facing you. Then wash your hands and put on gloves and an apron.

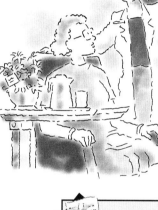

Collecting a throat specimen may cause you to gag, but the procedure will be over quickly.

In the spotlight

- Ask the patient to tilt his head back. Depress his tongue with the tongue blade, and illuminate his throat with the penlight to check for inflamed areas.
- If the patient starts to gag, withdraw the tongue blade and tell him to breathe deeply. After he's relaxed, reinsert the tongue blade but not as deeply as before.

From side to shining side

- Using the cotton-tipped swab, wipe the tonsillar areas from side to side, including any inflamed or purulent sites. Make sure you don't touch the tongue, cheeks or teeth with the swab to avoid contaminating it with oral bacteria.
- Withdraw the swab, and immediately place it in the culture tube. If you're using a commercial kit, push the swab into the medium to keep the swab moist.
- Remove and discard your gloves and apron as per local policy, and wash your hands.
- Label the specimen with the patient's name, date of birth, hospital number, the doctor's name, your initials or signature, and the date, time and site of collection.

Identify your suspect

- On the laboratory request form, indicate whether any organism is strongly suspected.
- Send the specimen to the laboratory immediately to prevent growth or deterioration of microbes.

Practice pointers

- Note recent antibiotic therapy on the laboratory request form. (See *Documenting throat specimen collection*.)

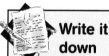

Write it down

Document-ing throat specimen collection

In your notes, record:

- time, date and site of specimen collection
- recent or current antibiotic therapy
- unusual appearance or odour of the specimen
- sign and date the entry.

Nasal specimen collection

Nasopharyngeal specimen collection involves using a sterile cotton-tipped swab to collect a specimen from the nasopharynx, to help identify pathogens. As the nose is usually a dry area, the dry cotton-tipped swab should be dipped in sterile saline solution before the collection. After the specimen has been collected, the swab is immediately placed in a sterile tube without transport medium if the indication is for MRSA. If the request is for culture and sensitivity, then a sterile tube with transport medium should be used.

What you need

Gloves and apron ✳ penlight ✳ sterile, flexible cotton-tipped swab ✳ sterile saline solution ✳ sterile culture tube with/or without transport medium ✳ label ✳ laboratory request form.

How you do it

- Explain the procedure to the patient and gain permission.
- Maintain privacy and dignity by drawing bed curtains as necessary.
- Inform the patient that he may gag or feel the urge to sneeze during the swabbing but that the procedure takes less than 1 minute.
- Have the patient sit erect at the edge of the bed or in a chair, facing you. Then wash your hands and put on gloves and an apron.

Clear passages

- Ask the patient to blow his nose to clear his nasal passages. Then check his nostrils for patency with a penlight.
- Tell the patient to occlude one nostril first and then the other as he exhales. Listen for the more patent nostril because you'll insert the swab into it.
- Ask the patient to cough to bring organisms to the nose for a better specimen.
- While the sterile swab is still in the package, bend it in a curve, and then open the package without contaminating the swab.
- Ask the patient to tilt his head back, and gently pass the swab through the nostril 1–2 cm, keeping the swab near the septum and floor of the nose. Rotate the swab quickly, and remove it.
- Remove the cap from the culture tube, insert the swab, and break off the contaminated end. Then close the tube tightly.
- Remove and discard your gloves and apron and wash your hands.
- Label the specimen for culture or MRSA as appropriate, complete a laboratory request form and send the specimen to the laboratory immediately. If you're collecting a specimen to isolate a possible virus, check with the laboratory for the recommended collection technique. (See *Documenting nasal specimen collection*.)

Write it down

Document-ing nasal specimen collection

In your notes, record:

- time, date and site of specimen collection (right or left)
- recent or current antibiotic therapy
- unusual appearance or odour of the specimen
- sign, date and time of the entry.

Wound specimen collection

Wound specimen collection involves using a sterile cotton-tipped swab to collect a specimen from inflamed tissues or exudate to help identify pathogens. After the specimen is collected, the swab is immediately placed in a sterile tube containing a transport medium and, in the case of sampling for anaerobes, an inert gas.

What you need

Sterile gloves ✳ apron ✳ sterile forceps ✳ alcohol ✳ sterile swabs ✳ sterile 10 ml syringe ✳ sterile 21G needle ✳ sterile culture tube with transport medium (or commercial collection kit for aerobic culture) ✳ labels ✳ special anaerobic culture tube containing carbon dioxide or nitrogen ✳ fresh dressings for the wound ✳ laboratory request form ✳ optional: rubber stopper for needle.

How you do it

- Explain the procedure to the patient and gain permission.
- Maintain privacy and dignity by drawing bed curtains as necessary and draping patient with a blanket.
- Undress the wound and prepare the patient as described in Chapter 4, Aseptic technique.
- Clean the area around the wound with warmed saline solution to reduce the risk of contaminating the specimen with skin bacteria. Then allow the area to dry.

Aerobic culture

- For an aerobic culture, use a sterile cotton-tipped swab to collect as much exudate as possible, or insert the swab deeply into the wound and gently rotate it. Remove the swab from the wound, and immediately place it in the aerobic culture tube. Label the culture tube and send the tube to the laboratory immediately with a completed laboratory request form. Never collect exudate from the skin and then insert the same swab into the wound; this could contaminate the wound with skin bacteria.

Anaerobic culture

- For an anaerobic culture, insert the sterile cotton-tipped swab deeply into the wound, rotate it gently, remove it, and immediately place it in the anaerobic culture tube. (See *Anaerobic specimen collector*.)
- Apply a new dressing to the wound.

> Avoiding contamination with skin bacteria is a key part of wound specimen collection.

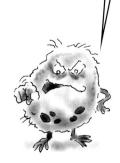

Anaerobic specimen collector

Because most anaerobes die when exposed to oxygen, they must be transported in tubes filled with carbon dioxide or nitrogen. The anaerobic specimen collector shown here includes a tube filled with carbon dioxide, a small inner tube and a swab attached to a plastic plunger.

Before specimen collection, the small inner tube containing the swab is held in place with the rubber stopper (as shown on the left). After collecting the specimen, quickly replace the swab in the inner tube and depress the plunger to separate the inner tube from the stopper (as shown on the right), forcing it into the larger tube and exposing the specimen to a carbon dioxide-rich environment.

Before   **After**

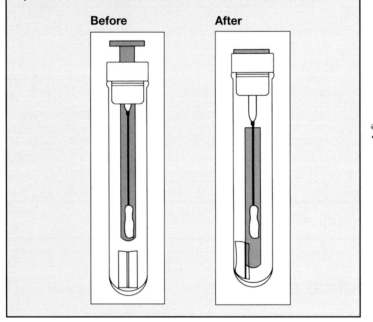

Practice pointers

• Note recent antibiotic therapy on the laboratory request form. (See *Documenting wound specimen collection*.)
• Remember to administer prescribed analgesia at an appropriate time before the procedure.
• If the doctor has requested to view and assess the wound, contact her and inform her of the time that you will be removing the wound dressing, to minimize exposure of the wound to organisms.

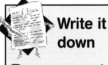

Write it down

Document-ing wound specimen collection

In your notes, record:

• time, date and site of specimen collection
• recent or current antibiotic therapy
• unusual appearance or odour of the specimen
• sign, date and time entry in notes.

Ear specimen collection

Ear specimen collection involves using a sterile swab to collect a specimen from the ear canal to identify pathogens. After the specimen is collected, the swab is immediately placed in a sterile tube containing a transport medium.

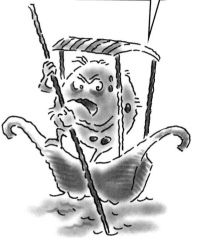

If I'm in the ear canal, ear specimen collection is the way to find out.

What you need

Gloves ✳ apron ✳ normal saline solution ✳ two 5 cm × 5 cm gauze pads ✳ sterile swabs ✳ sterile culture tube with transport medium ✳ label ✳ laboratory request form.

How you do it

* Wash your hands, put on gloves and apron.
* Explain the procedure to the patient and gain permission.
* Maintain privacy and dignity by drawing bed curtains as necessary.
* Gently clean excess debris from the patient's ear with normal saline solution and gauze pads.
* Moisten the sterile swab and insert into the ear canal, and rotate it gently along the walls of the canal to avoid damaging the eardrum.
* Withdraw the swab, being careful not to touch other surfaces to avoid contaminating the specimen.
* Place the swab in the sterile culture tube with transport medium.
* Remove and discard your gloves and apron, and wash your hands.
* Label the specimen for culture and sensitivity (or as instructed), complete a laboratory request form, and send the specimen to the laboratory immediately.

Practice pointers

* Note recent antibiotic therapy on the laboratory request form. (See *Documenting ear specimen collection*.)

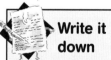 **Write it down**

Document- ing ear specimen collection

In your notes, record:

* time, date and site of specimen collection
* recent or current antibiotic therapy
* unusual appearance or odour of the specimen
* sign, time and date entry in notes.

Eye specimen collection

Eye specimen collection involves using a sterile swab to collect specimen to identify pathogens. After the specimen is collected, the swab is immediately placed in a sterile tube containing a transport medium.

What you need

Sterile gloves ✳ apron ✳ sterile normal saline solution ✳ two 5 cm × 5 cm gauze pads ✳ sterile swabs ✳ sterile wire culture loop (for corneal scraping) ✳ sterile culture tube with transport medium ✳ label ✳ laboratory request form.

How you do it

- Wash your hands, put on apron and then sterile gloves.
- Explain the procedure to the patient and gain permission.
- Maintain privacy and dignity by drawing bed curtains as necessary.
- Gently clean excess debris from the outside of the eye with normal saline solution and gauze pads, wiping from the inner to the outer canthus.

Lowering the lower eyelid

- Retract the lower eyelid to expose the conjunctival sac. Gently rub the sterile swab over the conjunctiva, being careful not to touch other surfaces. Hold the swab parallel to the eye, rather than pointed directly at it, to prevent corneal irritation or trauma due to sudden movement. (If corneal scraping is required, a doctor will perform the procedure using a wire culture loop.)
- Immediately place the swab or wire loop in the culture tube with transport medium.
- Remove and discard your gloves and apron then wash your hands.
- Label the specimen for culture, complete a laboratory request form, and send the specimen to the laboratory immediately.

Practice pointers

- Note recent antibiotic therapy on the laboratory request form.
- Don't use an antiseptic before culturing, to avoid irritating the eye and inhibiting growth of organisms in the culture. If the patient is a child or an uncooperative adult, ask a co-worker to restrain the patient's head to prevent eye trauma resulting from sudden movement. (See *Documenting eye specimen collection*.)

Perineal specimen

Correct perineal specimen collection and handling of the swab specimen helps the laboratory staff identify pathogens accurately with a minimum of contamination from normal bacterial flora. Collection normally involves sampling the tissue posterior to the anus with a sterile swab.

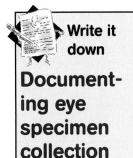

Write it down

Document-ing eye specimen collection

In your notes, record:

- time, date and site of specimen collection
- any recent or current antibiotic therapy
- unusual appearance or odour of the specimen
- sign, time and date entry in notes.

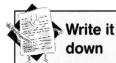

What you need

Gloves ✳ apron ✳ sterile swab ✳ sterile culture tube with transport medium ✳ label ✳ laboratory request form.

How you do it

- Explain the procedure to the patient and gain permission.
- Maintain privacy and dignity by drawing bed curtains as necessary and draping patient with a blanket.
- Wash your hands, and put on gloves and apron.

Not far to go

- Remove the swab from the container and maintain sepsis using a non-touch technique.
- Gently part the patient's buttocks and rotate the swab against the perineum, posterior to the anus.
- Place the swab in a culture tube with transport medium.
- Remove and discard your gloves and apron then wash your hands.
- Label the specimen for culture, complete a laboratory request form, and send the specimen to the laboratory immediately.

Practice pointers

- Note recent antibiotic therapy on the laboratory request form. (See *Documenting perineal specimen collection*.)

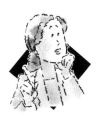

Quick quiz

1. From which fingers should you not obtain a capillary blood glucose sample?
   - A. Third
   - B. Fifth
   - C. Thumb or forefinger

Answer: C. The thumb, 2nd finger or the pad of the fingertip should not be used as these are used for the pincer movement of the hand and also to feel. Continuous sampling from these areas can lead to nerve damage, thus inhibiting normal daily activities of living.

2. How can the normal colour of urine be described?
   - A. Grass
   - B. Straw
   - C. Earth

Answer: B. Normal urine should be straw coloured plus odour and debris free.

> **✎ Write it down**
>
> **Documenting perineal specimen collection**
>
> In your notes, record:
>
> - time, date and site of specimen collection
> - recent or current antibiotic therapy
> - unusual appearance or odour of the specimen
> - sign, time and date the entry.

3. When obtaining a CSU, why is a needle not used on the sampling port?

    A. Increased risk of needlestick injury

    B. It is not sterile

Answer: A. Any unnecessary use of needles will increase your risk of needlestick injuries.

4. When obtaining a sputum specimen using suction what PPEs should you wear?

    A. Face mask

    B. Face mask, apron and gloves

    C. Gloves

Answer: B. It is your responsibility to protect yourself from bacteria and pathogens by wearing personal protective equipment supplied by your employer/host trust.

5. Which food item should the patient avoid for 48 to 72 hours before faecal occult blood testing, as well as throughout the collection period?

    A. Horseradish

    B. Tomatoes

    C. Beets

Answer: A. The patient should maintain a high-fibre diet and refrain from eating red meat, poultry, fish, turnips and horseradish for 48 to 72 hours before the test as well as throughout the collection period.

Scoring

⭐⭐⭐ If you answered all five items correctly, Wowwee! You're quite a specimen!

⭐⭐ If you answered three or four items correctly, Yowzer! Your collection knowledge is impressive!

⭐ If you answered fewer than three correctly, relax, review, and give it another go!

④ Wound and ulcer care

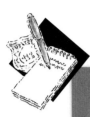

Just the facts

In this chapter, you'll learn:

♦ how to perform aseptic technique

♦ how to perform wound assessment

♦ about wound care and treatments

♦ about performing pressure ulcer assessment

♦ measures to prevent pressure ulcers

♦ patient teaching and documentation associated with each treatment.

Essential skills clusters

Essential skills clusters associated with and specific to wound and ulcer assessment, prevention and care:

• Care, compassion and communication: associated with all numbers, 1–9.

• Organisational aspects of care: associated with numbers 10–15, 17–20 and specific to number 18.

• Infection prevention and control: specific to all numbers, 21–26.

• Nutrition and fluid management: specific to numbers 27–29 (as part of the risk assessment process).

• Medicines management: specific to numbers 34, 36, 38–41 (but only when medication is being used in wound or pressure ulcer care).

Aseptic technique

Absence of sepsis

Aseptic technique is the practice used during clinical procedures on a patient. Its main aim is to prevent or minimize contamination of sterile areas of the body; in other words, prevent the introduction or carriage of microorganisms. These infections come from three main areas: the hands of healthcare staff, the patient's own body and the environment. Therefore poor asepsis can lead to the risk of cross-infection from these areas to the patient. Remember you have a duty of care to safeguard the well-being of your patients.

Indications for use

Aseptic technique should be used during any invasive procedure, for example:
• when dressing wounds that are healing by primary intention
• when removing or manipulating invasive devices such as drains, sutures or clips
• when inserting devices, i.e. catheters (urinary, intravenous, central venous, etc.)
• when taking a catheter specimen of urine (CSU).
Or when a clean technique is insufficient to protect the patient from cross-infection.

SICP reminder

It is essential to remember to use the standard infection control procedures (SICPs) described in Chapter 1. These were effective hand hygiene and use of personal protective equipment (PPE). However, here are a few more to remember: safe use and disposal of sharps, safe disposal of waste (as per local policy), decontamination of medical devices and the environment, disposal of single-use patient and equipment items after one use to minimize the risk of cross-infection.

What you need

Dressing trolley ✳ sterile dressing pack, containing a disposable plastic tray, gauze, sterile gloves, sterile field, disposable clinical waste bag ✳ sterile saline solution for wound cleansing ✳ jug ✳ warm water ✳ detergent, warm water, 70% alcohol or chlorhexidine solution for cleaning trolley surface ✳ sterile 20 ml syringe and 20 ml sterile saline for irrigation ✳ prescribed or appropriate dressings ✳ appropriate local documentation.

May I assess your wound and redress it to prevent infection?

Getting ready

Discuss and explain the procedure with the patient and gain permission. Wash the trolley with detergent and water then allow to dry. Assemble all equipment on the bottom shelf of this clean, dry trolley and prepare the clinical treatment room (preferable) for the patient. Place the sterile saline solution packet for wound cleansing in a jug and add warm water, enough to barely cover the packaging. If you do not have access to a clinical treatment room and will be performing the procedure by or on the patient's bed, either at home or in a hospital ward, ensure the bed linen and surrounding areas are clean and free from clutter and dust, close the bed curtains or bedroom door to maintain privacy and dignity, and take your trolley to the patient.

How you do it

- Wash your hands (see Hand hygiene, Chapter 1) and put on your apron.
- Loosen the dressing, but do not expose to environment and possible contamination risk.
- Wash your hands or use alcohol gel.
- Decontaminate the top and sides of the dressing trolley using the 70% alcohol or chlorhexidine solution and allow it to dry.
- Check the expiry dates and ensure that all packaging is intact to ensure that only sterile products are used.
- Open the sterile pack and allow it to drop on to the top shelf of the dressing trolley, do not allow the outer pack to touch the trolley to prevent contamination.
- Open the inner pack using only the outer corners of the pack, thus any potential contamination is kept to the outer corners only. Open any further sterile equipment and allow it to drop on to the sterile field.
- Remove the warmed saline solution from the water jug, open without touching the inner packaging and pour into a galley pot.
- To arrange the contents of the sterile pack, carefully pick up the clinical waste bag from the top opening, put your hand inside, without touching the outside of the bag to keep it sterile. Use this covering to arrange your contents.
- Keeping your hand inside the clinical waste bag now remove the dressing; fold the bag inside out, the contents should now be secured inside and the bag can be used for further clinical waste.
- Assess the wound and take appropriate actions (see Wound assessment, below).

Applying sterile gloves

1. Open glove packaging using outside edges only and tip out inside packaging onto sterile field, then wash your hands.
2. Open the inner packaging using outer edges of packaging only until gloves are exposed.
3. Pick up the left glove using your right hand; pick it up by the cuff only.
4. Hold the glove at the fold of the cuff, insert your left hand and pull the glove onto your hand.
5. Once pulled onto your hand adjust if necessary but only touch the inside of the glove.
6. Pick up the right glove by tucking your gloved left hand in between the fold of the cuff and pull the glove over your right hand. Readjust fingers once both gloves are *in situ*.

When applying the right glove ensure that the sterile left glove does not touch your skin.

1.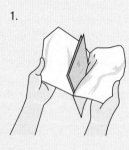

2.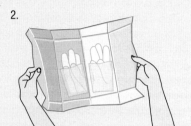

3.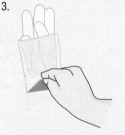

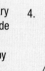

4.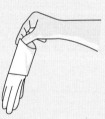

5.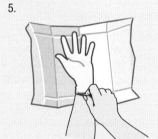

6.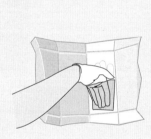

- Decontaminate hands again, using alcohol gel and allow to dry, in case of re-contamination.
- Apply sterile gloves. (See *Applying sterile gloves*.)

Don't touch!

- Clean around the wound, if deemed necessary by wound assessment, using gauze and the warmed saline solution. Do not allow your gloved hand to touch the patient. (See *Non-touch technique*.) Pick up the gauze in your dominant hand (the use of forceps should be minimized to prevent trauma to the area), place the gauze in the warmed saline solution and allow it to absorb some of the warmed

Non-touch technique

When performing aseptic procedures use the non-touch tecnhique. Never allow your sterile gloved hand to touch the patient, this indicates possible contamination and that hand can now NOT be taken back to the sterile field. Only ever allow the sterile equipment you are using to touch the patient, for example, when cleaning with gauze and saline solution only allow the sterile gauze to touch the patient—not your hand. Any equipment that has been in direct contact with the patient must then be placed directly in the clinical waste bag, without your hand touching the bag! Should you accidentally come into contact with the patient or the waste with your gloved hand, remove your gloves (both), decontaminate your hands, open clean sterile gloves on to the sterile field and apply them. In the same light, should you accidentally place contaminated waste on the sterile field, stop the procedure, cover the wound with a sterile dressing towel and start from the beginning.

solution, the warming of the solution aids re-vascularization and minimizes discomfort. Squeeze out the excess over the galley pot.
• Irrigate the wound as required. Irrigation cleans tissues and flushes cell debris and drainage from an open wound. Irrigation helps the wound heal properly from the inside tissue layers outward to the skin surface; it also helps prevent trauma and premature surface healing over an abscess pocket or infected tract. Do not use too much pressure when irrigating *as this can remove granulating tissue as well as necrotic tissue.*
• Apply a new sterile dressing as appropriate.
• Discard contaminated equipment appropriately in clinical or household waste (use local policy). Return the trolley to storage after cleaning with detergent and water.
• Ensure patient comfort.
• Document the procedure. (See *Documenting wound assessment.*)

Practice pointers

• Know your standard infection control procedures.
• Prepare your equipment and double check you have everything you require prior to undertaking the procedure.
• Maintain aseptic technique at all times.
• Practise putting on sterile gloves.

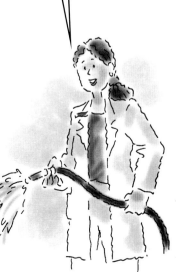

Hose it down! Irrigation cleans tissues and flushes away cell debris from an open wound.

Wound assessment

Most wounds will heal without difficulty; however, some wounds are subject to factors that will prevent them from healing normally, such as diabetes mellitus, peripheral vascular disease, previous ulceration, infection, etc. It is therefore very important to assess the wound and take a detailed clinical history from the patient or relative before you begin to plan the treatment of the wound. In order to assess the wound, you should be looking at a number of factors:

Pain

Pain will always be a factor in wound assessment and should be dealt with before you actually begin to physically assess the wound. Always prepare the patient for the wound assessment by asking them about their pain (use local policy and pain scoring tool) and offering analgesia as required before you begin to remove dressings, change dressings, assess the wound, etc. It is also essential to document the pain assessment as the type of pain the patient is experiencing may be arising from different aetiologies and will be treated in different ways. If pain cannot be controlled in the local area then referral to the pain control team should be made.

Site and surround

Of course it is important to record and describe the site of the wound, you don't want to be searching for it to assess it! The site of the wound can also assist diagnosis, for example a foot ulcer could be indicative of diabetes mellitus, a wound on the calf may well be of a venous aetiology.

Assess the surrounding area of skin; is there cellulites present? Is it red, pale, hot to touch, bleeding, bruised, excoriated? Is there excess exudate? All of these factors will affect how the wound is treated from the onset and also at each follow-on assessment.

Size matters

As with any ongoing patient monitoring technique, a baseline record is required in order for comparison and identification of progress to be made. In order to estimate size and have a direct comparison, photograph the wound at initial inspection using a polaroid camera and grid photo paper. The squares of the photo paper will allow you to estimate the size and assess progress at each further assessment.

Another method is to trace around the wound margins using clean, clear grid acetate. You have recorded the precise size of the wound to aid you in further assessments—but, from this you can also estimate the surface area of the wound, simply multiply the length by

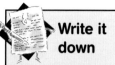

Write it down

Document-ing wound assessment

Make sure you record your findings every time you assess/expose the wound. Include comments on the following:

- colour
- size
- pain
- wound edges
- wound bed
- actions taken, i.e. dressings applied, irrigation, etc.

Date, time and sign the entry in the patient notes.

the width at the widest points of the wounds. Remember this is only an estimate as many factors will affect this technique, such as how the patient is positioned, stretching of the skin and limb placement.

Round the edges

Look at the wound edges, describe and document how they appear. This may have an important impact upon diagnosis, as wounds of different aetiologies present with different wound edges.

Off to bed

If you can remember that healthy, granulating tissue is pink in colour and has no odour, then this will assist you in assessing the wound bed, as anything else is abnormal. (See *Tailoring wound care to wound colour*.) For example, the presence of white or cream tissue

---

Tailoring wound care to wound colour

With any wound, promote healing by keeping it moist, clean and free from debris. For open wounds, use wound colour to guide the specific management approach and to assess how well the wound is healing.

Red or pink wounds

Red or pink, the colour of healthy granulation tissue, indicates normal healing. Cover a red wound, keep it moist and clean, and protect it from trauma. Use a transparent dressing (such as Tegaderm or Opsite), a hydrocolloid dressing (such as DuoDerm), or a gauze dressing moistened with sterile normal saline solution or impregnated with petroleum jelly or an antibiotic.

Yellow wounds

Yellow is the colour of exudate produced by microorganisms in an open wound. Exudate usually appears whitish yellow, creamy yellow, yellowish green or beige. Dry exudate appears darker.

If your patient has a yellow wound, clean it and remove exudate, using irrigation; then cover it with a moist dressing. Use absorptive, alginate products (for example, Kaltostat or Aquacel) or a moist gauze dressing with or without an antibiotic. You may also use high-pressure irrigation.

Black wounds

Black, the least healthy colour, signals necrosis. You should debride a black wound. After removing dead tissue, apply a dressing to keep the wound moist and to guard against external contamination. As prescribed, use hydrocolloid products daily.

Multicoloured wounds

You may note two or even all three colours in a wound. In this case, classify the wound according to the least healthy colour present. For example, if your patient's wound is red and yellow, classify it as a yellow wound.

covering a wound bed (slough): this tissue is dead and is preventing vascularization of the wound and thus wound healing, it needs to be removed. Necrotic tissue, which is dark in colour, is non-viable tissue, as it has a limited to no blood supply and will not heal, and eschar tissue is dry and black and, again, dead. Dark red tissue, or bleeding tissue, can indicate the presence of infection and this needs to be treated after the bacteria have been identified from a wound swab. When describing and documenting this information it should be quantified. Wound documentation in your local policy may already assist you with this; if it doesn't, then use of the following will assist in follow-on assessments: excessive (+++), moderate (++), minimal (+) and absent (−).

Remember that the main signs and symptoms of infection are pain, heat, redness and swelling; however, additional signs of infection can include increased exudate, bleeding, abnormal granulation and odour. Assess and document all of these factors every time you assess the wound. Practice your core values and communication; the wound may be offensively smelling to you, but the patient may be offended if you wrinkle your nose and express this.

Surgical wound management

Two primary methods for managing a draining surgical wound, dressing and pouching, can help prevent infection and promote patient comfort and healing. Pouching also allows you to measure wound drainage.

Lightly seeping wounds with drains or minimal drainage can be managed with packing and gauze dressings. Chronic wounds may require an occlusive dressing, whereas those with copious, excoriating drainage need pouching to protect the surrounding skin. You may use the colour of the wound to help determine which type of dressing to apply. (See *Tailoring wound care to wound colour*.) When handling wound drainage, always follow standard precautions.

What you need

Clinical waste bag ✳ clean gloves ✳ sterile gloves ✳ apron and face shield or goggles, if indicated ✳ sterile gauze pads ✳ large absorbent dressings, if indicated ✳ sterile cotton-tipped applicators ✳ sterile dressing set ✳ topical medication, if ordered ✳ adhesive or other tape ✳ soap and water ✳ optional: forceps, skin protectant, non-adherent pads, collodion spray or acetone-free adhesive remover, warmed sterile normal saline solution and jug.

For a wound with a drain
Sterile scissors ✳ sterile gauze pads ✳ drain ✳ sterile pre-cut pads or drain dressings ✳ adhesive tape (hypoallergenic if the patient is hypersensitive) ✳ surgical mask.

For pouching a wound
Collection pouch with drainage port ✳ sterile gloves ✳ apron ✳ skin protectant ✳ sterile gauze pads.

Getting ready

Ask the patient about allergies to tapes, dressings and solutions you'll be using, such as iodine, and verify this in their nursing or medical notes. Assemble all equipment in the clinical room; check the expiration date on each sterile package and inspect for tears.

Place a clinical waste bag near the patient's bed, but avoid reaching across the sterile field or the wound when disposing of soiled articles. Form a cuff by turning down the top of the waste bag to provide a wide opening and to prevent contamination of instruments or gloves by touching the bag's edge.

How you do it

• Explain the procedure to the patient to allay his fears and gain permission, ensure his cooperation.
• Provide teaching to the patient as well as to responsible family members if the dressing will be changed at home. (See *Caring for surgical wounds*.)

Removing the old dressing
• Check the medical notes, nursing care plan and prescription chart for specific wound care and medication instructions. Note the location of surgical drains to avoid dislodging them during the procedure.
• Assess the patient's condition, provide privacy and position him as necessary, exposing only the wound site.
• Wash your hands and put on an apron, face shield (if necessary) and gloves.
• Loosen the soiled dressing by holding the patient's skin and pulling the tape or dressing toward the wound to prevent stress on the incision.

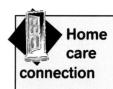

Home care connection

Caring for surgical wounds

If your patient needs wound care after discharge, provide appropriate teaching and refer to the primary care team, i.e. community nurse or GP surgery. If he's caring for the wound himself, stress the importance of using aseptic technique, and teach him how to examine the wound for signs of infection and other complications.

Put on a show

Also show him how to change dressings. Give him written instructions for all procedures to be performed at home.

- Slowly remove the soiled dressing. If the gauze adheres to the wound, loosen the gauze by moistening it with sterile normal saline solution.
- Observe the dressing for the amount, type, colour and odour of drainage, then discard the dressing and gloves in the clinical waste bag.

Caring for the wound

- Wash your hands. Establish a sterile field with all the equipment and supplies you'll need for giving wound care and the dressing change. Squeeze ointment (if prescribed) on to the sterile field. If you're using an antiseptic from an non-sterile bottle, pour the antiseptic cleaning agent into a sterile container so you won't contaminate your gloves. Then put on sterile gloves.
- Saturate the sterile gauze pads with the prescribed cleaning agent.
- If ordered, obtain a wound culture; then proceed to clean the wound.
- Pick up the moistened gauze pad or swab, and squeeze out the excess solution.

Start from the top

- Working from the top of the incision, wipe once to the bottom and then discard the gauze pad. With a second moistened pad, wipe from top to bottom next to the incision, and then continue to work outward from the incision in lines running parallel to it.
- Use sterile, cotton-tipped applicators for efficient cleaning of tight-fitting wire sutures, deep and narrow wounds, and wounds with pockets. Remember to wipe only once with each applicator.
- If the patient has a surgical drain, clean the drain's surface last by wiping in half or full circles from the drain site outward.
- Clean to at least 2.5 cm beyond the end of the new dressing. If you aren't applying a new dressing, clean to at least 5 cm beyond the incision.

Infection detection

- Check to make sure that the edges of the incision are lined up properly, and check for signs of infection (heat, redness, swelling, induration and odour) or separation. If you observe such signs, or if the patient reports pain at the wound site, notify the doctor.
- Irrigate the wound, as necessary.
- Wash the skin surrounding the wound with soap and water and pat dry using a sterile 10 cm × 10 cm gauze pad. Avoid oil-based soap because it may interfere with pouch adherence. Apply any prescribed topical medication and skin protectant, if needed.

- If planned, pack the wound with gauze pads or manufactured pharmaceutical product, using sterile forceps. Pack the wound, but not tightly, using the wet-to-damp method and making sure to wring out the pad so that it's slightly moist.

Applying a fresh gauze dressing

- Gently place sterile gauze pads at the centre of the wound, and move progressively outward to the edges of the wound site. Extend the gauze at least 2.5 cm beyond the incision in each direction, and cover the wound evenly with enough sterile dressings (usually two or three layers) to absorb all drainage until the next dressing change. Place additional dressings at the lower part of the wound to absorb drainage as it collects there. Use large absorbent dressings to form outer layers, if needed, to provide greater absorbency.
- Secure the dressing's edges to the patient's skin with strips of tape or Montgomery straps to prevent skin excoriation, which may occur with repeated dressing changes. (See *How to make Montgomery straps*.)
- Properly dispose of the solutions and waste bag, and clean or discard soiled equipment and supplies according to local policy.

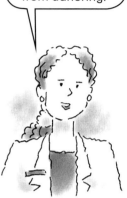

Oil alert! Using an oil-based soap may prevent the pouch from adhering.

How to make Montgomery straps

An abdominal dressing requiring frequent changes can be secured with Montgomery straps to promote the patient's comfort. If ready-made straps aren't available, follow these steps to make your own:

- Cut four to six strips of 5 cm or 7.5 cm wide hypoallergenic tape of sufficient length to allow the tape to extend about 15 cm beyond the wound on each side.
- Fold one of each strip 5 cm to 7.5 cm back on itself (sticky sides together) to form a non-adhesive tab. Then cut a small hole in the folded tab's centre, close to its top edge. Make as many pairs of straps as you'll need to secure the dressing snugly.
- Clean the patient's skin to prevent irritation. After the skin dries, apply a skin protectant. Then apply the sticky side of each tape to a skin barrier sheet composed of opaque hydrocolloidal or non-hydrocolloidal materials, and apply the sheet directly to the skin near the dressing.

Next, thread a separate piece of twill tape (about 30.5 cm) through each pair of holes in the straps, and fasten each tie as you would a shoelace.

Don't secure the ties too tightly.

- Repeat this procedure according to the number of Montgomery straps needed.
- Replace Montgomery straps whenever they become soiled (every 2 to 3 days). If skin maceration occurs, place new tapes about 2.5 cm) away from the irritation.

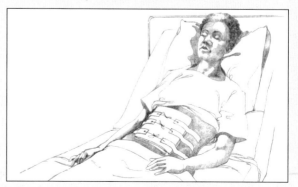

Dressing a wound with a drain

• Prepare a drain dressing by using sterile scissors to cut a slit in a sterile gauze pad or use pre-packaged dressings. Don't use a cotton-lined gauze pad because cutting the gauze opens the lining and releases cotton fibres into the wound.

• Gently press one pad close to the skin around the drain so that the tubing fits into the slit. Press the second pad around the drain from the opposite direction so that the two pads encircle the tubing.

• Layer as many uncut sterile gauze pads or large absorbent dressings around the tubing as needed to absorb expected drainage. Tape the dressing in place.

Pouching a wound

• If your patient's wound is draining heavily or if drainage may damage surrounding skin, you'll need to apply a pouch. First, measure the wound and then cut an opening 1 cm larger than the wound in the facing of the collection pouch.

• Apply a skin protectant as needed. Some protectants are incorporated within the collection pouch and also provide adhesion.

• Make sure that the drainage port at the bottom of the pouch is closed firmly to prevent leaks. Then gently press the contoured pouch opening around the wound, starting at its lower edge, to catch any drainage. The pouch drain may be directed toward the side if the patient is on bed rest, and directed toward the patient's leg if he's ambulatory, to allow ease of emptying.

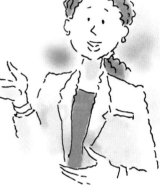

If the wound is draining heavily, you need to apply a pouch.

Gloves and goggles

• To empty the pouch, put on clean gloves and a face shield, or mask and goggles, if necessary to avoid any splashing. Then insert the pouch's bottom half into a measuring container and open the drainage port. Note the colour, consistency, odour and amount of fluid. If necessary or requested, obtain a culture specimen and send it to the laboratory immediately. Remember to follow standard precautions when handling body fluids.

• Wipe the bottom of the pouch and the drainage port with an alcohol wipe to remove drainage and reseal the port. Change the pouch only if it leaks or fails to adhere.

Practice pointers

• If the patient has two wounds in the same area, cover each wound separately with layers of sterile gauze pads. Then cover each site with a large absorbent dressing secured to the patient's skin with tape. Don't use a single, large absorbent dressing to cover both sites because drainage quickly saturates a pad, promoting cross-contamination.

• When packing a wound, don't pack it too tightly because this compresses adjacent capillaries and may prevent the wound

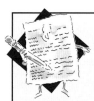

Write it down

Documenting surgical wound management

In your notes, record:

- date, time and type of wound management procedure
- amount of soiled dressing and packing removed
- wound appearance (size, condition of margins, presence of necrotic tissue) and odour
- type, colour, consistency and amount of drainage
- presence and location of drains
- additional procedures such as irrigation
- topical medication application
- type and amount of new dressing or pouch applied
- patient's tolerance of the procedure.

Document special or detailed wound care instructions and pain management steps on the plan of care. Record drainage colour and amount on the intake and output sheet.

edges from contracting. Avoid overlapping damp packing on to surrounding skin because it macerates the intact tissue.

- For the recent post-operative patient or a patient with complications, check the dressing every 15–30 minutes. For the patient with a properly healing wound, check the dressing at least once every 8 hours. (See *Documenting surgical wound management*.)

Be sensitive to sensitivity

- If your patient is sensitive to adhesive tape, use paper or silk tape because it's less likely to cause a skin reaction and peels off more easily than adhesive tape.

Wound dehiscence and evisceration management

Occasionally, the edges of a wound may fail to join or may separate even after they seem to be healing normally. This development, called wound dehiscence, may lead to evisceration, in which a portion of the viscera (usually a bowel loop) protrudes through the incision. Evisceration, in turn, can lead to peritonitis and septic shock. (See *Recognizing dehiscence and evisceration*.) Dehiscence and evisceration are most likely to occur 6–7 days after surgery and may be caused by poor nutrition, chronic pulmonary or cardiac disease, localized wound infection, or stress on the incision (from coughing or vomiting).

What you need

Two sterile towels ✳ 1 litre of sterile normal saline solution ✳ sterile irrigation set, including a basin, solution container, and 50 ml catheter-tip syringe ✳ several large abdominal dressings ✳ sterile, waterproof drape ✳ protective bed pads ✳ sterile gloves ✳ apron.

If the patient will return to theatre, gather the following equipment after the open wound is treated: I.V. administration set and I.V. fluids ✳ equipment for nasogastric (NG) intubation ✳ medication, as prescribed ✳ suction apparatus.

Getting ready

Provide reassurance and ask the patient to stay in bed. If possible, stay with him while someone else notifies the doctor and collects the necessary equipment.

Place a pad under the patient to keep the sheets dry when you moisten the exposed viscera. Using aseptic technique, unfold a sterile towel to create a sterile field. Open the package containing the irrigation set, and place the basin, solution container, and 50 ml syringe on the sterile field.

Open the bottle of normal saline solution and pour 400 ml into the solution container and 200 ml into the sterile basin. Open several large abdominal dressings, and place them on the sterile field.

How you do it

• Wash your hands and put on the sterile gloves and apron, place one or two of the large abdominal dressings into the basin to saturate them with saline solution.
• Place the moistened dressings over the exposed viscera, followed by a sterile, waterproof drape to prevent the sheets from getting wet.
• Moisten the dressings every hour by withdrawing saline solution from the container through the syringe and then gently squirting the solution on the dressings.

Darkness visible

• When you moisten the dressings, inspect the colour of the viscera. If it appears dusky or black, notify the doctor immediately. With its blood supply interrupted, a protruding organ may become ischaemic and necrotic.
• Keep the patient on absolute bed rest at an angle of no more than 20 degrees' elevation, with his knees flexed to prevent injury and reduce stress on the incision.
• Don't allow the patient to have anything by mouth, monitor the patient's vital signs every 15 minutes and take appropriate action according to the track and trigger system in use to detect and prevent shock.

Recognizing dehiscence and evisceration

Dehiscence or evisceration may occur as a surgical intervention.

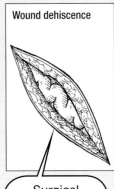

Wound dehiscence

Surgical wound layers separate.

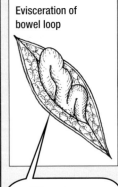

Evisceration of bowel loop

The viscera (in this case, the bowel loop) protrude through the incision.

- Continue to reassure the patient, and if necessary, prepare him to return to theatre.

Practice pointers

- If you're caring for a post-operative patient who is at risk for poor healing, make sure he gets an adequate supply of protein, vitamins and calories. Monitor his dietary deficiencies, and discuss any problems with the doctor and dietician.
- When irrigating the wound, ensure that the fluid runs from the clean to the dirty area, to prevent contamination of the wound.
- You may need to prepare the patient for theatre by initiating an I.V.; inserting an NG tube and connecting to suction, according to medical instruction; and administering pre-operative medication. Because the NG intubation may make the patient gag or vomit, causing further evisceration, the doctor may choose to insert it in theatre or the anaesthetic room. Make sure that the patient has signed a consent form before administering pre-operative medications, and that your documentation in the nursing and medical records is fully completed, thus ensuring that the theatre staff are made fully aware of the patient's recent history. (See *Documenting dehiscence and evisceration management*.)
- Gauze has been used in this text to demonstrate dressing wounds; however, gauze is not always appropriate. Many types of dressings are available that are appropriate for different types of wounds. Have a look at the *British National Formulary* (Appendix: Wound and elastic hosiery) for this underpinning knowledge.

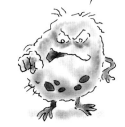

If you aren't careful during irrigation, my pathogenic friends and I will run rampant.

Write it down

Documenting dehiscence and evisceration management

In your notes, document:

- when the problem occurred, date and time
- patient's activity preceding the problem
- patient's condition
- time the doctor was notified
- appearance of the wound or eviscerated organ
- amount, colour, consistency and odour of drainage
- nursing actions taken
- patient's vital signs and response to the incident
- doctor's actions.

Finally, be sure to change the patient's plan of care to reflect nursing actions needed to promote proper healing.

Traumatic wound management

Traumatic wounds include abrasions, lacerations, puncture wounds and amputations. In an abrasion, the skin is scraped, with partial loss of the skin surface. In a laceration, the skin is torn, causing jagged, irregular edges; the severity of a laceration depends on its size, depth and location. A puncture wound occurs when a pointed object, such as a knife or glass fragment, penetrates the skin. Traumatic amputation refers to removal of part of the body, a limb, or part of a limb.

In cases of trauma, first stabilize the patient's airway, breathing and circulation. Then treat the traumatic wound according to the type and cause.

What you need

Sterile basin ✳ normal saline solution ✳ sterile gauze pads ✳ sterile gloves ✳ clean gloves ✳ apron ✳ sterile cotton-tipped applicators ✳ dry sterile dressing, non-adherent pad or petroleum gauze ✳ protective bed pad ✳ optional: scissors, towel, goggles, mask, gown, 50 ml catheter-tip syringe, surgical scrub brush, antibacterial ointment, porous tape, sterile forceps, sutures and suture set, hydrogen peroxide.

Getting ready

Place a protective bed pad under the area to be cleaned. Remove any clothing covering the wound. If necessary, cut hair around the wound with scissors to promote cleaning and treatment. Assemble needed equipment in the treatment room or at the patient's bedside. Fill a sterile basin with normal saline solution. Make sure the treatment area has enough light to allow close observation of the wound.

How you do it

• Check the patient's past medical history for previous tetanus immunization and, if needed and prescribed, arrange for immunization and administration of analgesia.
• Wash your hands and put on an apron and gloves, plus mask and goggles if spraying or splashing of body fluids is possible. Depending on the type and location of the wound, wear sterile or clean gloves.

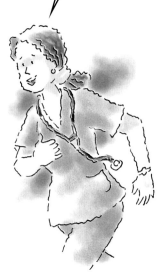

First focus on the ABCs. Then treat the traumatic wound.

For an abrasion

- Flush the scraped skin with normal saline solution.
- Remove dirt or gravel with a sterile gauze pad moistened with normal saline solution and rub in the opposite direction from which the dirt or gravel became embedded. If the wound is extremely dirty, you may use a surgical brush to scrub it.
- With a small wound, allow it to dry and form a scab. With a larger wound, you may need to cover it with a non-adherent pad or petroleum gauze and a light dressing. Apply antibacterial ointment as prescribed.

For a laceration

- Moisten a sterile gauze pad with normal saline solution. Clean the wound gently, working outward from its centre to about 5 cm beyond its edges. Discard the soiled gauze pad and use a fresh one as necessary. Continue until the wound appears clean.
- If the wound is dirty, you may irrigate it with a 50 ml catheter-tip syringe and normal saline solution.
- Assist the doctor in suturing the wound edges using the suture kit, or apply sterile strips of porous tape.
- Apply the prescribed antibacterial ointment and a dry sterile dressing over the wound.

For a puncture wound

- If the wound is minor, allow it to bleed for a few minutes before cleaning it. For a larger puncture wound, you may need to irrigate it before applying a dry dressing.
- Stabilize any embedded foreign object until the doctor can remove it. After he removes the object and bleeding has stabilized, clean the wound as you would clean a laceration or deep puncture wound.

For an amputation

- Apply a gauze pad moistened with normal saline solution to the amputation site. Elevate the affected part, and immobilize it for surgery.
- Recover the amputated part, and prepare it for transport to a hospital where microvascular surgery is performed.

Practice pointers

- Before wound care, assess the patient's need for pain medication or an agent prescribed to promote comfort.
- When irrigating a traumatic wound, avoid using high pressure because higher pressure can seriously interfere with healing, kill cells and allow bacteria to infiltrate the tissue.
- After a wound has been cleaned, the doctor may want to debride it to remove dead tissue and reduce the risk of infection and scarring. If this is necessary, pack the wound lightly with gauze pads soaked in normal saline solution until debridement.
- Observe for signs and symptoms of infection, such as warm, red skin at the site or purulent discharge. Be aware that infection of a traumatic wound can delay healing, increase scar formation, and trigger systemic infection such as septicaemia.
- Observe all dressings. If oedema is present, loosen the dressing to avoid impairing circulation to the area. (See *Documenting traumatic wound management*.)

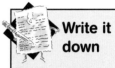

Write it down

Document- ing traumatic wound management

In your notes, document:

- date and time of the procedure
- wound size and condition
- medication administration
- specific wound care measures
- patient teaching.

Suture removal

The goal of suture removal is to remove skin sutures from a healed wound without damaging newly formed tissue. Usually, for a sufficiently healed wound, sutures are removed 7–10 days after insertion, wounds on the peripheries, such as the face, head and hands, may be removed after 5–7 days. Techniques for removal depend on the method of suturing, but all require aseptic technique to prevent contamination. Sutures are usually removed by a nurse on instruction by the doctor or advanced nurse practitioner, this may be in the form of written communication in the medical notes; make sure you know the plan for your patient.

What you need

Clinical waste bag ✳ adjustable light (as necessary) ✳ clean gloves, if the wound is dressed ✳ sterile gloves ✳ apron ✳ sterile forceps ✳ normal saline solution ✳ sterile gauze pads ✳ sterile curve-tipped suture scissors ✳ optional: adhesive butterfly strips or Steri-Strips and skin protectant spray or dressing.

Pre-packaged, sterile suture-removal packs are available.

Getting ready

Assemble all equipment in the treatment room if available, or at the patient's bedside. Check the expiration date on each sterile package and inspect for tears. Follow aseptic technique preparation guide.

How you do it

- Check the medical notes or wound care plan to confirm the details for this procedure.
- Check for patient allergies, especially to adhesive tape and topical solutions or medications.
- Explain the procedure to the patient, obtain permission, provide privacy, maintain dignity and position him so he's comfortable without placing undue tension on the suture line.
- Wash your hands, put on gloves and apron, loosen the dressing as described in aseptic technique.

Consider the visible part of a suture contaminated. After all, I might be there.

All healed up?

- Assess the wound; observing the patient's wound for possible gaping, drainage, inflammation, signs of infection and embedded sutures. Notify the doctor if the wound has failed to heal properly.
- Establish a sterile work area with all the equipment and supplies you'll need for suture removal and wound care. Wash your hands and open the sterile suture-removal tray if you're using one, open all other equipment on to the sterile field, including sterile gloves before you put them on.
- Wipe the incision gently with sterile gauze pads soaked in a normal saline solution to remove surface encrustations.
- Then proceed according to the type of suture you're removing. (See *Methods for removing sutures*.) Because the visible part of a suture is exposed to skin bacteria and considered contaminated, be sure to cut sutures at the skin surface on one side of the visible part of the suture. Remove the suture by lifting and pulling the visible end off the skin to avoid drawing this contaminated portion back through subcutaneous tissue.

Skip over for support

- If requested in the medical plan or wound care plan, remove every other suture to maintain some support for the incision. Then go back and remove the remaining sutures on the requested date.
- After removing sutures apply a light sterile gauze dressing, if needed, then discard your gloves, apron and soiled equipment, and clean the equipment according to local policy.

Methods for removing sutures

Removal techniques depend in large part on the type of sutures to be removed. The illustrations here show removal steps for four common suture types. Keep in mind that for all suture types, it's important to grasp and cut sutures in the correct place to avoid pulling the exposed (thus contaminated) suture material through subcutaneous tissue.

Plain interrupted sutures

Using sterile forceps, grasp the knot of the first suture and raise it off the skin. This will expose a small portion of the suture that was below skin level. Place the rounded tip of sterile curved-tip suture scissors against the skin, and cut through the exposed portion of the suture. Then, still holding the knot with the forceps, pull the cut suture up and out of the skin in a smooth continuous motion to avoid causing the patient pain. Discard the suture. Repeat the process for every other suture, initially; if the wound doesn't gape, you can then remove the remaining sutures as per the plan of care.

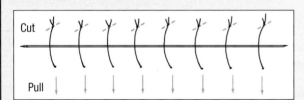

Plain continuous sutures

Cut the first suture on the side opposite the knot. Next, cut the same side of the next suture in line. Then lift the first suture out in the direction of the knot. Proceed along the suture line, grasping each suture where you grasped the knot on the first one.

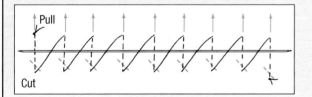

Mattress interrupted sutures

If possible, remove the small, visible portion of the suture opposite the knot by cutting it at each visible end and lifting the small piece away from the skin to prevent pulling it through and contaminating subcutaneous tissue. Then remove the rest of the suture by pulling it out in the direction of the knot. If the visible portion is too small to cut twice, cut it once and pull the entire suture out in the opposite direction. Repeat these steps for the remaining sutures, and monitor the incision carefully for infection.

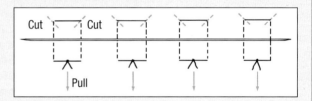

Mattress continuous sutures

Follow the procedure for removing mattress interrupted sutures, first removing the small visible portion of the suture, if possible, to prevent pulling it through and contaminating subcutaneous tissue. Then extract the rest of the suture in the direction of the knot.

Practice pointers

• If the patient has interrupted sutures or an incompletely healed suture line, remove only those sutures specified by the doctor. He may want to leave some sutures in place for an additional day or two to support the suture line.

• If the patient has both tension and regular sutures in place, check the doctor's instruction for the sequence in which they are to be removed. Because tension sutures link underlying fat and muscle tissue and give added support to the obese or slow-healing patient, they usually remain in place for up to 21 days.

• If the wound dehisces during suture removal, apply butterfly adhesive strips or Steri-Strips to support and approximate the edges, and call the doctor immediately to repair the wound. Leave the strips in place for 3–5 days, as ordered. (See *Documenting suture removal*.)

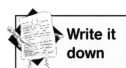

Write it down

Documenting suture removal

In your notes, record:

• date and time of suture removal
• type and number of sutures
• appearance of the suture line
• signs of wound complications
• dressings or butterfly strips applied
• patient's tolerance of the procedure.

Skin staple and clip removal

Skin staples or clips may be used instead of standard sutures to close lacerations or surgical wounds. When properly placed, staples and clips distribute tension evenly along the suture line with minimal tissue trauma and compression, facilitating healing and minimizing scarring.

What you need

Clinical waste bag ✳ sharps bin ✳ adjustable light (if required) ✳ clean gloves ✳ sterile gloves ✳ apron ✳ sterile gauze pads ✳ sterile staple or clip extractor ✳ sterile cotton-tipped applicators ✳ optional: butterfly adhesive strips or Steri-Strips, skin protectant spray or dressing. Pre-packaged, sterile, disposable staple or clip extractors are available.

Getting ready

Assemble all equipment in the treatment room (if available) or at the patient's bedside. Check the expiration date on each sterile package and inspect for tears. Follow aseptic technique preparation guide.

How you do it

• Before you remove skin staples and clips, check the medical notes and wound care plan to confirm the exact timing and details for this procedure.

• Check for patient allergies and verify in medical or nursing records. Explain the procedure to the patient, gain permission, provide privacy, maintain dignity and place him in a comfortable position that doesn't place undue tension on the incision. Adjust the light to shine directly on the incision.

• Wash your hands, put on clean gloves and apron, and carefully loosen the dressing.

• Establish a sterile work area with all the equipment and supplies you'll need for removing staples or clips and for cleaning and dressing the incision. Open the package containing the sterile staple or clip extractor, maintaining asepsis. Put on sterile gloves and using the clinical waste bag remove the dressing.

• Assess the patient's incision and notify the doctor of gaping, drainage, inflammation and other signs of infection.

• Wipe the incision gently with sterile gauze pads soaked in a normal saline solution to remove surface encrustations.

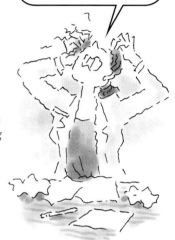

Staples and clips distribute tension evenly along the tissue line. If only I had something to distribute my tension!

1: Extract. 2: Repeat step 1

• Pick up the sterile staple or clip extractor. Then, starting at one end of the incision, remove the staple or clip. (See *Removing a staple*.) Hold the extractor over the sharps bin, and release the handle to discard the staple or clip. Repeat the procedure for each staple or clip until all are removed.

Removing a staple

Follow these steps to remove a staple from a wound using a staple remover.

The staple remover changes the shape of the staple and pulls the prongs out of the intradermal tissue.

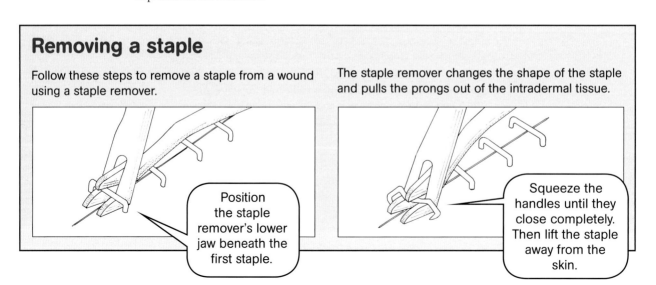

Position the staple remover's lower jaw beneath the first staple.

Squeeze the handles until they close completely. Then lift the staple away from the skin.

• Apply a sterile gauze dressing, if needed, to prevent infection and irritation from clothing. Then discard your gloves and properly dispose of soiled equipment and supplies according to local policy.

Practice pointers

• Carefully check the doctor's instructions or wound care plan for the time and extent of staple or clip removal. The doctor may want you to remove only alternate staples or clips initially and to leave the others in place for an additional day or two to support the incision.
• If extraction is difficult, notify the doctor; staples or clips placed too deeply within the skin or left in place too long may resist removal.

If you need some support

• If the wound dehisces after staples or clips are removed, apply butterfly adhesive strips or Steri-Strips to approximate and support the edges, and call the doctor immediately to repair the wound. While waiting for the doctor's arrival in the clinical area, follow the instructions given in Wound dehiscence and evisceration management, earlier in this chapter. Leave the strips in place for 3–5 days. (See *Documenting skin staple and clip removal.*)

Negative pressure wound therapy

Negative pressure wound therapy, also known as vacuum-assisted closure pressure therapy, is used to enhance delayed or impaired wound healing. The negative pressure closure device applies localized sub-atmospheric pressure to draw the edges of the wound toward the centre. A special dressing is placed in the wound or over a graft or flap, and negative pressure wound therapy is applied. This wound packing removes fluids from the wound and stimulates growth of healthy granulation tissue.

Negative pressure wound therapy is indicated for acute and traumatic wounds, pressure ulcers, and chronic open wounds, such as diabetic ulcers, meshed grafts, and skin flaps. It's contraindicated for fistulas that involve organs or body cavities, necrotic tissue with eschar, untreated osteomyelitis and malignant wounds. This therapy should be used cautiously in patients with active bleeding, in those taking anticoagulants, and when achievement of wound haemostasis has been difficult.

What you need

Clinical waste bag ✳ goggles ✳ gown, if indicated ✳ emesis basin ✳ normal saline solution ✳ clean gloves ✳ sterile gloves ✳ apron

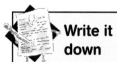

Write it down

Document-ing skin staple and clip removal

In your notes, record:

• date and time of staple or clip removal
• number of staples or clips removed
• appearance of the incision
• dressings or butterfly strips applied
• signs of wound complications
• patient's tolerance of the procedure.

✳ sterile scissors ✳ protective bed pad ✳ 35 ml piston syringe with 19G catheter ✳ reticulated foam ✳ fenestrated tubing ✳ evacuation tubing ✳ skin protectant wipe ✳ transparent occlusive air-permeable drape ✳ evacuation canister ✳ vacuum unit.

Getting ready

Assemble the vacuum-assisted closure device at the bedside according to the manufacturer's instructions. Set negative pressure according to the instructions of the doctor or tissue viability nurse (25 to 200 mmHg).

How you do it

• Check the wound care plan, and assess the patient's condition, including pain assessment. Administer analgesia prior to procedure if required.
• Explain the procedure to the patient, gain permission, provide privacy, maintain dignity and wash your hands. If necessary, put on a gown and goggles to protect yourself from wound drainage and contamination.
• Place a protective bed pad under the patient to catch any spill, avoid linen changes and maintain the patient's comfort. Position him to allow maximum wound exposure. Place the emesis basin under the wound to collect any drainage.
• Put on clean gloves. Remove the soiled dressing and discard it in the waterproof trash bag. Attach the 19G catheter to the 35 ml piston syringe and irrigate the wound thoroughly using normal saline solution.
• Clean the area around the wound with normal saline solution; wipe intact skin with a skin protectant wipe and allow it to dry well. Remove and discard your gloves.

Fun with foam

• Put on sterile gloves. Using sterile scissors cut the foam to the shape and measurement of the wound. More than one piece of foam may be necessary if the first piece is cut too small.
• Carefully place the foam in the wound. Next, place the fenestrated tubing into the centre of the foam. The fenestrated tubing embedded into the foam delivers negative pressure to the wound.
• Place the transparent occlusive air-permeable drape over the foam, enclosing the foam and the tubing together. Remove and discard your gloves.

- Connect the free end of the fenestrated tubing to the tubing that's connected to the evacuation canister.

Flick the switch

- Turn on the vacuum unit.
- Make sure the patient is comfortable.
- Properly dispose of drainage, solution, linen-saver pad, and waste bag, and clean and dispose of soiled equipment and supplies according to local policy.

Practice pointers

- Change the dressing every 48 hours. Try to coordinate the dressing change with the doctor's visit so he can inspect the wound.
- Measure the amount of drainage every shift.
- Audible and visual alarms alert you if the unit is tipped greater than 45 degrees, if the canister is full, if the dressing has an air leak, or if the canister becomes dislodged.
- Cleaning and care of wounds may temporarily increase the patient's pain and increases the risk for infection. (See *Documenting negative pressure therapy*.)

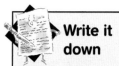

Write it down

Document-ing negative pressure therapy

In your notes, document:

- frequency and duration of therapy
- amount of negative pressure applied
- size and condition of the wound
- patient's response to the procedure.

Closed-wound drain management

A closed-wound drain, such as the Haemovac or Jackson–Pratt system, consists of perforated tubing connected to a portable vacuum unit. It's commonly inserted during surgery with the distal end of the tubing lying within the wound and leaving the body from another site. A closed-wound drain helps reduce the risk of infection, skin breakdown, and the number of dressing changes. It also promotes healing. The drain is usually sutured to the skin and the exit site is often treated as an additional surgical wound.

What you need

Alcohol pads ✳ gloves ✳ apron ✳ clinical waste bag ✳ sterile gauze pads ✳ antiseptic cleaning agent or normal saline solution.

How you do it

- Explain the procedure to the patient, gain permission, provide privacy, maintain dignity and wash your hands.

Using a non-disposable closed-wound drainage system

The portable closed-wound drainage system draws drainage from a wound site, such as the chest wall post-mastectomy (as shown below left), by means of a tube.

To empty the drainage in a non-disposable system, remove the plug and empty it into a jug. To re-establish suction, compress the drainage unit against a firm surface to expel air and, while holding it down, replace the plug with your other hand (as shown below centre).

The same principle is used for the Jackson–Pratt bulb drain (as shown below right).

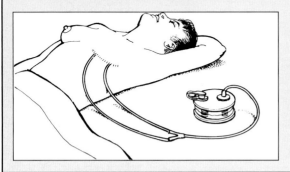 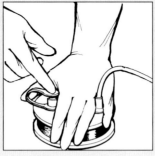 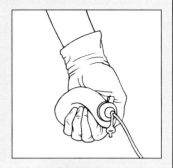

- Wearing gloves and an apron, unclip the vacuum unit from the patient's bed or gown and release the vacuum by removing the spout plug on the collection chamber. The container will expand completely as it draws in air.
- Empty the unit's contents into a graduated cylinder or, if a disposable unit, note the amount and appearance of the drainage. If diagnostic tests will be performed on the fluid specimen, pour the drainage directly into a sterile laboratory container.
- Use a pre-soaked alcohol pad to clean the unit's spout and plug (if non-disposable unit), then re-establish the vacuum by fully compressing the vacuum unit with one hand and apply a new unit or, if a non-disposable unit, by replacing the spout plug with your other hand. (See *Using a non-disposable closed-wound drainage system*.)

(Un)do the twist

- Check the patency of the equipment, making sure the tubing is free from twists and kinks and working properly. (See *Complications of drains*.) If re-inflation occurs, recompress the unit and make sure the spout plug is secure.
- Secure the vacuum unit to the patient's gown below the wound, making sure that there's no tension on the drainage tubing. Remove and discard your gloves, and wash your hands.

Warning!

Complications of drains

With a closed-wound drain, monitor for occlusion of the tubing by fibrin, clots or other particles that can reduce or obstruct drainage.

Bad mistake

Also, be careful not to mistake chest tubes for closed-wound drains. Unlike a closed-wound drain, the vacuum of a chest tube should never be released.

Suture surveillance

- Observe the sutures that secure the drain to the patient's skin; look for signs of pulling, tearing, swelling or infection of surrounding skin. Gently clean the sutures with sterile gauze pads soaked in the normal saline solution
- Properly dispose of drainage, solutions, and the clinical waste bag, and clean or dispose of soiled equipment and supplies according to local policy.

Practice pointers

- Drainage must be emptied and measured frequently to maintain maximum suction and prevent strain on the suture line. Empty the drain and measure its contents once during each shift if drainage has accumulated, and more often if drainage is excessive. If the patient is ambulatory, empty the device before ambulation to remove excess drainage, maintain maximum suction and avoid straining the drain's suture line.
- If the patient has more than one closed drain, number the drains (do not use 'right' and 'left' as this can lead to confusion), so you can record drainage from each site. (See *Documenting closed-wound drain management*.)

Stump and prosthesis care

Patient care immediately after limb amputation includes psychological care as well as the physical care of monitoring drainage from the stump, positioning the affected limb, assisting with exercises prescribed by a physical therapist, and wrapping and conditioning the stump.

Post-operative stump care will vary slightly, depending on the amputation site (arm or leg). After the stump heals, it requires only routine daily care, such as proper hygiene and continued muscle-strengthening exercises.

Clean and lube

The prosthesis, when in use, also requires daily care. Typically, a plastic prosthesis must be cleaned, lubricated and checked for proper fit. As the patient recovers from the physical and psychological trauma of amputation, he will need to learn correct procedures for routine daily care of the stump and the prosthesis.

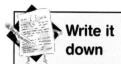

Write it down

Documenting closed-wound drain management

In your notes, record:

- date and time you empty the drain
- appearance of the drain site
- presence of swelling or other signs of infection
- equipment malfunction and nursing action taken
- patient's tolerance of the procedure.

On the intake and output sheet, record drainage colour, consistency, type and amount. If the patient has more than one closed-wound drain, number the drains and record the information above separately for each drainage site.

What you need

For post-operative stump care

Pressure dressing ✳ abdominal pad ✳ suction equipment ✳ overhead trapeze ✳ adhesive tape, bandage clips or safety pins ✳ sandbags or trochanter roll (for a leg) ✳ elastic stump shrinker or 10 cm elastic bandage.

For stump and prosthesis care

Mild soap or alcohol pads ✳ gloves and apron ✳ stump socks or athletic tube socks ✳ two washcloths ✳ two towels ✳ appropriate lubricating oil.

How you do it

• Perform routine post-operative care. Frequently assess the patient's respiratory status and level of consciousness, monitor vital signs and I.V. infusions, check tube patency, and promote patient comfort and safety.

Monitoring stump drainage

• *Because gravity causes fluid to accumulate at the stump*, frequently check the amount of blood and drainage on the dressing. Notify the doctor if drainage or blood accumulations increase rapidly. If excessive bleeding occurs, notify the doctor immediately and apply a pressure dressing and further elevate the limb.
• Tape the abdominal pad over the moist part of the dressing as needed. *Providing a dry area helps prevent bacterial infection.*
• Monitor the suction drainage equipment, and note the amount and type of drainage.

Positioning the extremity

• *To prevent contractures*, position an arm with the patient's elbow extended and the shoulder abducted.
• *To correctly position a leg*, elevate the foot of the bed slightly and place sandbags or a trochanter roll against the patient's hip *to prevent external rotation*. Don't place a pillow under the thigh to flex the hip; *this can cause hip flexion contracture*. For the same reason, tell the patient to avoid prolonged sitting.
• After a below-the-knee amputation, maintain knee extension *to prevent hamstring muscle contractures.*

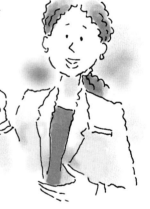

Phantom pain isn't a fantasy. It can be a real complication of an amputation.

Firm basis for care

After leg amputation, place the patient on a firm surface in the prone position for at least 4 hours per day, with his legs close together and without pillows under his stomach, hips, knees or stump (unless this position is contraindicated). *This position helps prevent hip flexion, contractures and abduction; it also stretches the flexor muscles.*

Assisting with prescribed exercises

• After arm amputation, encourage the patient to exercise the remaining arm *to prevent muscle contractures.* Help him perform isometric and range-of-motion (ROM) exercises for both shoulders, as prescribed by the physical therapist, *because prosthesis use requires both shoulders.*

• After leg amputation, stand behind the patient and, if necessary, support him with your hands at his waist during balancing exercises.

• Instruct the patient to exercise the affected and unaffected limbs *to maintain muscle tone and increase muscle strength.* A patient with a leg amputation may perform push-ups, as ordered (in the sitting position, arms at his sides), or pull-ups on the overhead trapeze *to strengthen his arms, shoulders and back in preparation for using crutches.*

Wrapping and conditioning the stump

• Apply an elastic stump shrinker *to prevent oedema and shape the limb in preparation for the prosthesis.* Wrap the stump so that it narrows toward the distal end. *This helps to ensure comfort when the patient wears the prosthesis.*

• Instead of using an elastic stump shrinker, you can wrap the stump in a 10 cm elastic bandage. To do this, stretch the bandage to about two-thirds its maximum length as you wrap it diagonally around the stump, with the greatest pressure distally. (Depending on the size of the patient's leg, you may need to use two 10 cm bandages.) Secure the bandage with clips, safety pins or adhesive tape. Make sure the bandage covers all portions of the stump smoothly *because wrinkles or exposed areas encourage skin breakdown.* (See *Wrapping a stump.*)

• If the patient experiences throbbing after the stump is wrapped, remove the bandage immediately and reapply it less tightly. *Throbbing indicates impaired circulation.*

• Check the bandage regularly. Rewrap it when it begins to bunch up at the end (usually about every 12 hours for a moderately active patient) or every 24 hours.

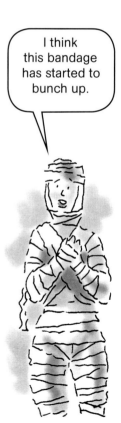

I think this bandage has started to bunch up.

Wrapping a stump

Proper stump care helps protect the limb, reduces swelling, and prepares the limb for a prosthesis. As you perform the procedure, teach it to the patient.

- Obtain two 10 cm elastic bandages.
- Centre the end of the first bandage at the top of the patient's thigh.
- Unroll the bandage downward over the stump and to the back of the leg.

- Make three figure-eight turns to adequately cover the ends of the stump. As you wrap, be sure to include the roll of flesh in the groin area. Use enough pressure to ensure that the stump narrows toward the end so that it fits comfortably into the prosthesis.

- Use the second 10 cm bandage to anchor the first bandage around the waist. For a below-the-knee amputation, use the knee to anchor the bandage in place.
- Secure the bandage with Clipsor adhesive tape.
- Check the stump bandage regularly, and rewrap it if it bunches at the end.

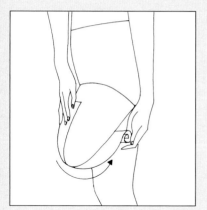 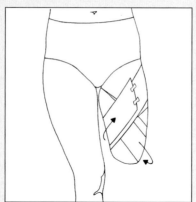 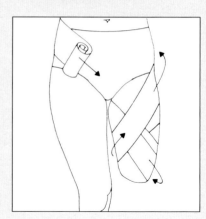

- After removing the bandage to rewrap it, massage the stump gently, always pushing *toward* the suture line rather than away from it. *This stimulates circulation and prevents scar tissue from adhering to the bone.*

Push to heal

- When healing begins, instruct the patient to push the stump against a pillow. Then have him progress gradually to pushing against harder surfaces, such as a padded chair, then a hard chair. *These conditioning exercises help the patient adjust to experiencing pressure and sensation in the stump.*

Caring for the healed stump

- *To prevent a rash*, bathe the stump but never shave it. If possible, bathe the stump at the end of the day *because warm water may cause swelling, making reapplication of the prosthesis difficult.*

Inspection report

- Inspect the stump for redness, swelling, irritation and calluses. Report these findings to the doctor. Tell the patient to avoid putting weight on the stump. (The skin should be firm but not taut over the bony end of the limb.)
- Continue muscle-strengthening exercises *so the patient can build the strength he'll need to control the prosthesis.*
- Change the patient's stump socks as necessary *to avoid exposing the skin to excessive perspiration, which can be irritating.* Wash the socks in warm water and gentle non-detergent soap; lay them flat on a towel to dry. *Machine washing or drying may shrink the socks.*

Caring for the plastic prosthesis

- Wipe the plastic socket of the prosthesis with a damp cloth and mild alcohol *to prevent bacterial accumulation.*
- Wipe the insert (if the prosthesis has one) with a dry cloth.
- Dry the prosthesis thoroughly; if possible, allow it to dry overnight.
- Maintain and lubricate the prosthesis, as instructed by the manufacturer.
- Check for malfunctions and adjust or repair the prosthesis as necessary *to prevent further damage.*
- Check the condition of the shoe on a foot prosthesis frequently, and change it as necessary.

Applying the prosthesis

- Apply a stump sock. Keep the seams away from bony prominences.
- If the prosthesis has an insert, remove it from the socket, place it over the stump, and insert the stump into the prosthesis.
- If it has no insert, merely slide the prosthesis over the stump. Secure the prosthesis on to the stump according to the manufacturer's directions.

Practice pointers

- If a patient arrives at the hospital with a traumatic amputation, the amputated part may be saved for possible re-implantation. (See *Caring for an amputated body part.*)
- Teach the patient how to care for his stump and prosthesis properly. Make sure he knows what signs and symptoms indicate problems in the stump. Explain that a 10 lb (4.5 kg) change in body weight will alter his stump size and require a new prosthesis socket *to ensure a correct fit.* (See *Caring for a stump at home.*)

- Exercise of the remaining muscles in an amputated limb must begin the day after surgery. A physical therapist will direct these exercises. For example, arm exercises progress from isometrics to assisted ROM to active ROM. Leg exercises include rising from a chair, balancing on one leg, and ROM exercises of the knees and hips. (See *Documenting stump and prosthesis care.*)

Caring for an amputated body part

After traumatic amputation, a surgeon may be able to reimplant the severed body part through microsurgery. The chance of successful reimplantation is much greater if the amputated part has received proper care.

If a patient arrives at the hospital with a severed body part, first make sure the bleeding at the amputation site has been controlled. Then follow these guidelines for preserving the body part.

- Put on sterile gloves. Place several sterile gauze pads and an appropriate amount of sterile gauze in a sterile basin, and pour sterile Normasol or 0.9% sodium chloride solution over them. Never use any other solution, and don't try to scrub or debride the part.
- Holding the body part in one gloved hand, carefully pat it dry with sterile gauze. Place saline-soaked gauze pads over the stump; then wrap the whole body part with saline-soaked gauze. Wrap the gauze with a sterile towel, if available. Then put this package in a watertight container or bag and seal it.
- Fill another plastic bag with ice and place the part, still in its watertight container, inside. Seal the outer bag. (Always protect the part from direct contact with ice—and never use dry ice. Otherwise, irreversible tissue damage may occur, making the part unsuitable for reimplantation.) Keep this bag ice-cold until the doctor is ready to do the reimplantation surgery.
- Label the bag with the patient's name, date of birth, hospital number, identification of the amputated part and date and time when cooling began.

Note: The body part must be wrapped and cooled quickly.

Irreversible tissue damage occurs after only 6 hours at ambient temperature. However, hypothermic management seldom preserves tissues for more than 24 hours.

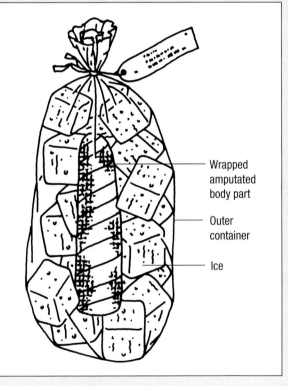

Wrapped amputated body part

Outer container

Ice

Home care connection

Caring for a stump at home

Before your patient returns home after a limb amputation, emphasize that proper care of his stump can speed healing. Tell him to inspect the stump carefully every day, using a mirror, and to continue proper daily stump care. Instruct him to call the doctor if the incision appears to be opening, looks red or swollen, feels warm, is painful to touch, or is seeping drainage.

Tell the patient to massage the stump toward the suture line to mobilize the scar and prevent its adherence to bone. Advise him to avoid exposing the skin around the stump to excessive perspiration, which can be irritating. Tell him to change his elastic bandages or stump socks during the day to avoid this.

Ease the pain

Tell the patient that he may experience twitching, spasms, or phantom limb pain as his stump muscles adjust to amputation. Advise him that he can ease these symptoms not only with prescribed medication but also with heat, massage or gentle pressure. If his stump is sensitive to touch, tell him to rub it with a dry washcloth for 4 minutes three times per day.

Stress the importance of performing prescribed exercises to help minimize complications, maintain muscle strength and tone, prevent contractures and promote independence. Also urge him to maintain proper positioning to prevent contractures and oedema.

Write it down

Documenting stump and prosthesis care

In your notes, record:

- date, time, and specific procedures performed for all postoperative care
- amount and type of drainage
- condition of the dressing
- need for dressing reinforcement
- appearance of the suture line and surrounding tissue
- signs and symptoms of skin irritation or infection
- complications and nursing actions taken

- patient's tolerance of exercise
- patient's psychological reaction to the amputation.

During routine daily care, document:

- date, time, type of care given
- condition of the skin and suture line, including signs and symptoms of irritation (such as redness or tenderness)
- patient's progress in caring for the stump or prosthesis
- your signature.

Anti-embolism stocking application

Elastic anti-embolism stockings are used to help prevent deep vein thrombosis and pulmonary embolism in post-operative, bedridden, elderly or other at-risk patients. They work by squeezing superficial leg veins and increasing venous return to the heart. Anti-embolism stockings can provide equal pressure over the entire leg or a graded pressure that's greatest at the ankle and decreases over the length of the leg.

Measuring for anti-embolism stockings

Measure the patient carefully to ensure that his anti-embolism stockings provide enough compression for adequate venous return.

To choose the correct knee-length stocking, measure the circumference of the calf at its widest point (top left) and the leg length from the bottom of the heel to the back of the knee (bottom left).

To choose a thigh-length stocking, measure the calf as for a knee-length stocking and the thigh at its widest point (top right). Then measure the leg length from the bottom of the heel to the gluteal fold (bottom right).

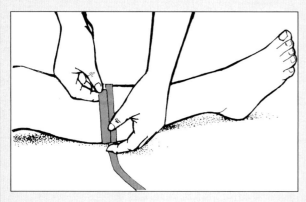

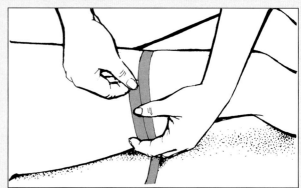

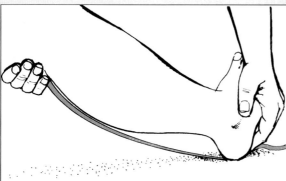

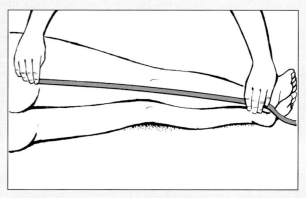

What you need

Tape measure ✳ anti-embolism stockings of correct size and length.

Getting ready

Measure the patient for the correct size stocking, according to the manufacturer's specifications. (See *Measuring for anti-embolism stockings*.)

How you do it

• First, check the prescription and assess the patient's condition. If his legs are cold or cyanotic, notify the doctor before proceeding.
• After explaining the procedure to the patient, provide privacy, and wash your hands thoroughly.
• Have the patient lie down.

Applying a knee-length stocking

• Begin by turning the stocking inside out until the foot part remains inside the stocking.
• Ease the turned-in foot section over the toes, while supporting the ankle, and stretch it until the heel rests in the heel pocket. The toe should be visible through the toe window, if any.
• Gather the loose material at the ankle, and slide the rest of the stocking up over the heel with short pulls, alternating front and back, until it rests 2.5–5 cm below the bottom of the knee. Gently snap the fabric around the ankle to ensure a tight fit and to eliminate gaps, and see that the fabric is smooth over the foot. (See *Applying anti-embolism stockings*.)
• Repeat the procedure for the second stocking.

Applying a thigh-length stocking

• Follow the procedure for applying a knee-length stocking.
• With the patient's leg extended, stretch the rest of the stocking over the knee, then flex the patient's knee and pull the stocking over the thigh until the top is 2.5–7.5 cm below the gluteal fold. Remember to stretch the stocking from the top, front and back, to distribute the fabric evenly. Gently snap the fabric behind the knee to eliminate gaps, which could reduce pressure.

Applying a waist-length stocking

• Follow the procedure for applying knee-length and thigh-length stockings, and extend the stocking top to the gluteal fold.
• Fit the patient with the adjustable belt that accompanies the stockings, making sure that the waistband and the fabric don't interfere with any incision, drainage tube, catheter or other device.

Applying anti-embolism stockings

Gather the loose part of the stocking at the toes, and pull this portion toward the heel.

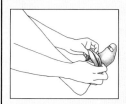

Then gather the loose part of the stocking, and bring it over the heel with short, alternating front and back pulls.

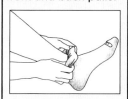

Insert the index and middle fingers into the gathered part of the stocking at the ankle, and ease it upward by rocking it slightly up and down.

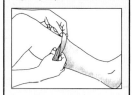

Practice pointers

• Anti-embolism stockings usually aren't used on patients with skin lesions, gangrene, poor circulation, excessive oedema, recent vein ligation or grafts.

• If you find the patient's measurements are outside the range indicated, ask the doctor if she wants to order custom-made stockings.

• Stockings should be applied in the morning, before oedema develops. If the patient has been walking, have him lie down and elevate his legs for 15–30 minutes before applying the stockings to facilitate venous return.

• Don't allow the stockings to roll or turn down at the top or toe because this can cut off circulation.

• Check the patient's toes at least once every 4 hours, noting skin colour and temperature, sensation, swelling and ability to move. If complications occur, remove the stockings and notify the doctor immediately. Remove the stockings once daily to bathe the skin and perform skin assessment, observing for irritation and breakdown.

• Review anti-embolism stocking application with the patient, if necessary. (See *Reviewing anti-embolism stocking care* and *Documenting anti-embolism stocking application.*)

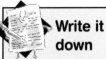

Write it down

Document-ing anti-embolism stocking application

In your notes, record:

• date and time of stocking application and removal
• stocking length and size
• condition of the leg before and after treatment
• condition of the toes during treatment
• complications
• patient's tolerance of the treatment
• sign, date and time the entry.

Home care connection

Reviewing anti-embolism stocking care

If the patient requires anti-embolism stockings after discharge, teach him or a family member how to apply them correctly and explain why he needs to wear them.

Instruct the patient or family member to care for the stockings properly and to replace them when they lose elasticity. Tell the patient that he should wear the stockings at all times (except during bathing) to provide continuous protection against thrombosis. Tell him to keep a second pair handy to wear while the first pair is being laundered.

- Take care of your back. Ensure you position yourself close to the patient by elevating the bed, try to prevent overreaching, stooping or twisting to maintain safe moving and handling practices. You must have attended a university or host trust moving and handling teaching session prior to commencing clinical placement.

Sequential compression therapy

> Sequential compression therapy uses a wave-like motion to massage the legs, which promotes blood flow.

Sequential compression therapy massages the legs in a wave-like, milking motion that promotes blood flow and deters thrombosis. It may be used with other measures to prevent deep vein thrombosis, such as anti-embolism stockings and anticoagulant medications. Anti-embolism stockings and sequential compression sleeves are commonly used pre-operatively and post-operatively because blood clots tend to form during surgery.

What you need

Measuring tape ✳ sizing chart for the brand of sleeves you're using ✳ pair of compression sleeves in correct size ✳ connecting tubing ✳ compression controller.

Getting ready

Wash your hands, explain the procedure to the patient and gain permission, have the patient rest in bed so that you can measure the circumference of the upper thigh at the gluteal fold. Find the patient's thigh measurement on the sizing chart, and locate the corresponding size of the compression sleeve.

Remove the compression sleeves from the package and unfold them, laying them with the cotton lining facing up.

How you do it

- Place the patient's leg on the cotton sleeve lining, positioning the back of the knee over the popliteal opening and the back of the ankle over the ankle marking.

• Starting at the side opposite the clear plastic tubing, wrap the sleeve snugly around the patient's leg, beginning with the ankle and calf and then the thigh, and secure it with Velcro fasteners.
• Using the same procedure, apply the second sleeve.

Connect with a click

• Connect each sleeve to the tubing leading to the controller, making sure the tubing isn't kinked. Line up the blue arrows on the connectors and push the ends together firmly. Listen for a click, signalling a firm connection.
• Plug the compression controller into the wall outlet and turn on the power. The controller automatically sets the compression sleeve pressure at 45 mmHg, which is the midpoint of the normal range (35–55 mmHg).
• Check the audible alarm key. The green light should be lit, indicating that the alarm is working.
• When discontinuing the therapy, dispose of the sleeves, but store the tubing and compression controller according to local policy.

Practice pointers

• Be sure that there are no contraindications to therapy. If there are, discuss the situation with the doctor. (See *Contraindications to sequential compression therapy*.)

Two-finger test

• The sleeve should fit snugly, but you should still be able to insert two fingers between the sleeve and the patient's leg at the knee opening. Loosen or tighten the sleeve by readjusting the Velcro fastener.
• If you're applying only one sleeve—for example, if the patient has a cast—leave the unused sleeve folded in the plastic bag. Cut a small hole in the bag's sealed bottom edge, and pull the sleeve connector (the part that holds the connecting tubing) through the hole. Then you can join both sleeves to the compression controller.
• The compression sleeves should function continuously until the patient is fully ambulatory. Be sure to check the sleeves at least once each shift to ensure proper fit and inflation. (See *Documenting sequential compression therapy*.)

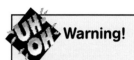 **Warning!**

Contraindications to sequential compression therapy

Consult with the doctor before use if the patient has:

• acute deep vein thrombosis (DVT)
• DVT diagnosed within the past 6 months
• severe arteriosclerosis or other ischaemic vascular disease
• massive oedema of the legs
• dermatitis
• vein ligation
• gangrene
• skin grafting.
   A patient with a pronounced leg deformity also would be unlikely to benefit from compression sleeves.

Elastic bandage application

Elastic bandages exert gentle, even pressure on a body part. By supporting blood vessels, these rolled bandages promote venous return and prevent pooling of blood that can lead to thrombophlebitis and pulmonary embolism.

Elastic bandages are used post-operatively, on bedridden patients, to minimize joint swelling after trauma, to secure a splint, or to immobilize a fracture. They also can provide haemostatic pressure and anchor dressings after surgical procedures such as vein stripping.

What you need

Elastic bandage of appropriate width ✻ tape or pins ✻ gauze pads or absorbent cotton.

Bandages usually come in 1 cm to 20 cm widths and 1.2–1.8 m lengths. The 10 cm width is adaptable to most applications. An elastic bandage with self-closures is also available.

Getting ready

Select a bandage that wraps the affected body part completely but isn't excessively long. In most cases, use a narrower bandage for wrapping the foot, lower leg, hand, or arm and a wider bandage for the thigh or torso. The bandage should be clean and rolled before application.

How you do it

• Check the medical notes and nursing care plan, examine the area to be wrapped for lesions or skin breakdown. If these conditions are present, consult the doctor or tissue viability nurse before applying the elastic bandage.
• Explain the procedure to the patient, provide privacy, and wash your hands thoroughly. Explain the procedure to the patient and family if the bandage is to be used at home. Position him comfortably, with the body part to be bandaged in normal functioning position to promote circulation and prevent deformity and discomfort. If the extremity has been dependent,

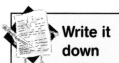

Write it down

Documenting sequential compression therapy

In your notes, record:

• date and time
• procedure
• patient's response to, and understanding of, the procedure
• status of the alarm and cooling settings
• signature.

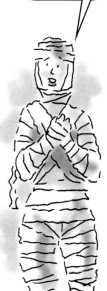

I think this bandage is too long!

elevate it for 15–30 minutes before application to facilitate venous return.
• Place gauze or absorbent cotton as needed between skin surfaces, such as toes or fingers, or under breasts and arms, to prevent skin irritation.
• Hold the bandage close to the part being bandaged with the roll facing upward in one hand and the free end of the bandage in the other hand.

That special twist

• Unroll the bandage as you wrap the body part using a spiral or spiral-reverse method and overlap each layer of bandage by one-half to two-thirds the width of the strip. (For an explanation of these and other techniques, see *Bandaging techniques*.)
• Wrap firmly, applying even pressure.
• When wrapping an extremity, anchor the bandage initially by circling the body part twice. To prevent the bandage from slipping out of place on the foot, or to go around a joint, wrap it in a figure eight around the foot and ankle before continuing. Remember to leave the toes (or fingers) exposed to detect impaired circulation.

Better than metal

• When you've finished wrapping, secure the end of the bandage with tape, pins or self-closures. Avoid using metal clips because they typically come loose and can injure the patient.
• Check distal circulation after the bandage is on and be sure to elevate a wrapped extremity for 15–30 minutes to facilitate venous return. (See *Complications of elastic bandages*.)
• Remove the bandage every 8 hours, or as per care plan, to inspect the skin for irritation or breakdown. It also should be changed at least once daily, and the area bathed and dried thoroughly.

Practice pointers

• If the bandage becomes loose and wrinkled, unwrap it and roll it up as you unwrap for reuse. Observe the area and provide skin care before rewrapping the bandage.
• Wrap an elastic bandage from the distal area to the proximal area to promote venous return. Avoid leaving gaps in bandage layers or exposed skin surfaces because this may result in uneven pressure on the body part. (See *Documenting elastic bandage application*.)

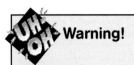 **Warning!**

Compli-cations of elastic bandages

Check distal circulation once or twice every 8 hours and assess the skin underneath.

Too tight

If the elastic bandage is too constricting, arterial obstruction can occur. This can cause a decreased or an absent distal pulse, blanching or bluish discoloration of the skin, dusky nail beds, numbness and tingling or pain and cramping, and cold skin. Oedema is caused by obstruction of venous return. Less serious complications include allergic reaction and skin irritation.

Bandaging techniques

Here are several techniques for applying elastic bandages.

Circular

Each turn encircles the previous one, covering it completely. Use this technique to anchor a bandage.

Spiral

Each turn partially overlaps the previous one. Use this technique to wrap a long, straight body part or one of increasing circumference.

Spiral-reverse

Anchor the bandage and then reverse direction halfway through each spiral turn. Use this technique to accommodate the increasing circumference of a body part.

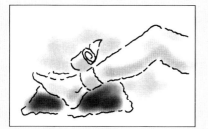

Figure eight

Anchor below the joint, and then use alternating, ascending and descending turns to form a figure eight. Use this technique around joints.

Recurrent

This technique includes a combination of recurrent and circular turns. Hold the bandage as you make each recurrent turn and then use the circular turns as a final anchor. Use this technique for a stump, a hand or the scalp.

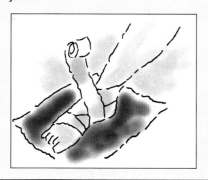
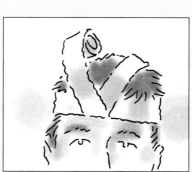
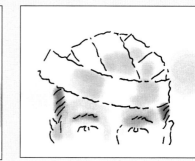

Pressure dressing application

Pressure dressing application is a temporary measure used for control of capillary or small-vein bleeding. In this procedure, a bulky dressing is held in place with a glove-protected hand and then bound into place with a pressure bandage or held under pressure by an inflated air splint.

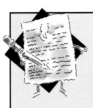

Write it down

Documenting elastic bandage application

In your notes, record:

- date and time of bandage application and removal
- application site and bandage size
- skin condition before application
- skin care provided after removal
- complications
- patient's tolerance of the treatment
- patient teaching provided.

Check, please!

A pressure dressing requires frequent checks for wound drainage to determine its effectiveness in controlling bleeding.

What you need

Two or more sterile gauze pads ✳ roller gauze ✳ adhesive tape ✳ clean disposable gloves ✳ metric ruler.

Getting ready

Obtain the pressure dressing quickly to avoid excessive blood loss, or have another staff member obtain the equipment while you apply manual pressure and monitor the patient. Use a clean cloth for the dressing if sterile gauze pads aren't available.

How you do it

- Quickly explain the procedure to the patient to help decrease his anxiety and gain permission, then put on gloves.
- Elevate the injured body part to help reduce bleeding.
- Place enough gauze pads over the wound to cover it. Don't clean the wound until the bleeding stops. For an extremity or a trunk wound, hold the dressing firmly over the wound and wrap the roller gauze tightly across it and around the body part to provide pressure on the wound. Secure the bandage with adhesive tape.
- Check pulse, temperature and skin condition distal to the wound site because excessive pressure can obstruct normal circulation.

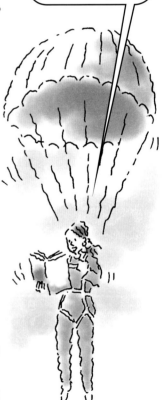

When applying the dressing, elevate the injured area to reduce bleeding.

- Check the dressing frequently to monitor wound drainage.
- Obtain expert care as soon as possible.

Practice pointers

- To apply a dressing to the neck, shoulder or another location that can't be tightly wrapped, apply tape directly over the dressing to provide the necessary pressure at the wound site.
- If the dressing becomes saturated, don't remove it because this will interfere with the pressure. Instead, reinforce the original dressing by applying an additional dressing over the saturated one and continue to monitor and record drainage. (See *Documenting pressure dressing application*.)

Pressure ulcer care

What is a pressure ulcer? The National Institute of Clinical Excellence in their document and guideline entitled *Pressure ulcer risk assessment and prevention* (2001) (derived from the Department of Health guideline, 1999) describes pressure ulcers as 'areas of damage to the skin and underlying tissue'. This guideline is generally accepted in the UK as the most up-to-date and evidence-based set of recommendations to follow when planning and implementing both training in, and the practice of assessing and preventing, pressure ulcers. Therefore the following section of this book is based upon their advice.

Use the key

Ideally, prevention is the key to avoiding extensive therapy. Preventive measures include risk-assessing each individual coming into the care setting within a 6-hour period. The following intrinsic and extrinsic factors are known to increase the patient's risk and should therefore be assessed: reduced mobility or immobility, sensory impairment, acute illness, level of consciousness, extremes of age, vascular disease, severe chronic or terminal illness, previous history of pressure damage, malnutrition and dehydration, pressure, shearing and friction—the latter three being extrinsic factors.

Inspect

As discussed in the Total care section in Chapter 1 (see *Waterlow score*), skin assessment should always be carried out, paying particular attention to the high-risk areas of the body: heels, sacrum, ischial tuberosities, parts of the body affected by anti-embolism stockings, femoral trochanters and all areas of the body affected by shearing, pressure or friction, either during normal daily activities, or due to clothing or mechanical devices and equipment.

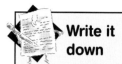

Write it down

Document-ing pressure dressing application

When the bleeding is controlled, record:

- date and time of dressing application
- whether reinforcement was necessary
- presence or absence of distal pulses
- integrity of distal skin
- amount of wound drainage
- complications
- your name and signature.

Look out and feel . . .

There are many factors to look out and feel for when performing skin inspection. Look for areas of purplish or bluish patches on dark-skinned people, red patches on light-skinned people, swelling, blisters, shiny areas, dry patches, cracks, calluses or wrinkles. The factors to feel for are hard areas, warm areas, cold areas and swollen skin, particularly over bony prominences. All of these signs may be indicative of pressure ulcer development and can be classified into different grades of ulcer using the European Pressure Ulcer Advisory Panel (EPUAP) Classification tool (2003). Your findings should therefore be acted upon as well as documented. (See *Documenting pressure ulcer assessment*.)

Preventing pressure ulcers

Once the initial assessment has been undertaken, it is essential to continue to monitor the patient's skin using the same technique as described above in order to prevent ulcers forming. Further methods of preventing the formation of ulcers are: using aids, positioning, seating and education.

No doughnut here

Provide the patient with appropriate pressure-relieving devices according to the risk assessment, Waterlow score and EPUAP classification. However, avoid seating the patient on a rubber or plastic doughnut, water-filled gloves or sheepskins, as they will increase localized pressure at vulnerable points, leading to an increased risk of pressure ulcer formation.

Positioning

The aim of repositioning is to ensure that prolonged pressure on bony prominences is minimized and that shearing and friction are minimized, with the effective use of moving and handling devices. Patients who have been determined to be at risk should be taught how and when to reposition if they are able, and those who are unable should be repositioned by clinical staff. This should be done according to a schedule or timing determined from the skin assessment and not from ritualistic methods, as these may not be sufficient to reduce the risk of ulcer formation. The repositioning should also take into consideration the patient's present condition, the plan of care and must prevent the patient sitting in a chair for more than 2 hours at a time.

Seating

Specialists with specific knowledge and who are competent and confident, such as occupational therapists, physiotherapists and

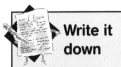

Write it down

Document-ing pressure ulcer assessment

Immediately after performing skin assessment it is essential to document the following in order that all members of the multidisciplinary team are aware of the patient's condition and risk status:

- date and time of assessment
- a detailed review and map of the body, indicating colour, heat and all other indicative factors—present or not—remember you are responsible for both your acts and omissions, write in detail or complete any risk assessment tools in place in your local area
- sign the entry in the notes.

Home care connection

Pressure ulcer prevention

Patients and relatives who are willing and able should be taught:

- the risk factors
- the sites of greatest risk
- how to inspect their skin or their relative's skin and recognize changes
- how to care for skin
- how to use pressure-relieving devices and aids
- methods for preventing pressure ulcers
- where further advice can be obtained
- to seek immediate assistance if changes have been recognized.

tissue viability nurses, should perform an assessment of the aids and equipment required by individual patients. They will take into account factors such as distribution of weight, length of time spent in a seated position (such as wheelchair users), postural alignment and foot support. As a student nurse, try to spend some time with these specialists, observing this type of assessment.

Education and training

Interprofessional training of all healthcare professionals is recommended, thus ensuring that a multidisciplinary approach is adopted for patient care. Employers, trusts and universities should offer this training locally. Once this training has been completed, healthcare professionals should pass on the knowledge and skills within their clinical area, ensuring that everyone is up to date and using evidence-based methods in care delivery. It is also important to involve patients and carers who are willing in the education and training process (see *Pressure ulcer prevention*).

Practice pointers

It is the responsibility of a registered healthcare professional to perform the initial and ongoing assessment; it is therefore mandatory that you attend a formal training programme in this procedure if you are a registered nurse. As a student, work with your mentor and the multidisciplinary team (MDT) to gain knowledge, skills practice and understanding of the grading system before you qualify; preparing you for your responsibility upon registration.

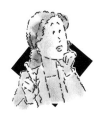

Quick quiz

1. When performing aseptic technique you should use:
   A. Disposable gloves
   B. Sterile gloves
   C. Polyurethane examination gloves

Answer: B. Sterile gloves should be used to prevent cross-infection and contamination.

2. Your patient with abdominal surgery states that he felt something 'pop' when he was getting back into bed. You examine his abdominal wound and find bowel protruding. You should:
   A. Tell him everything is normal.
   B. Get the patient back into a chair.
   C. Place the patient flat in bed and reassure him.

Answer: B. Place the patient flat in bed to reduce tension on the wound.

3. When removing sutures, you need to:
   A. Remove every other suture initially.
   B. Remove the middle sutures first.
   C. Remove the retention sutures last.

Answer: A. Remove every other suture initially to determine wound closure.

4. To irrigate a wound, direct the flow of irrigation fluid:
   A. Toward the wound.
   B. Away from the wound.
   C. Toward the centre of the wound.

Answer: B. Direct flow away from the wound to prevent contamination.

5. After applying anti-embolism stockings, it's important to:
   A. Check for circulation distally.
   B. Make sure the legs remain elevated for a short period.
   C. Remove the stockings periodically.

Answer: A. Circulation should be monitored to detect adequate perfusion.

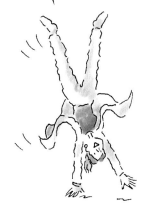

Time to flip from reviewing to testing. Try your hand at these quick quiz questions!

Scoring

☆☆☆ If you answered all five items correctly, yippee! You're the Anti Em of anti-embolism stocking application, you're De Bride of debridement, you're the . . . well, you get the picture—you're great!

☆☆ If you answered three or four items correctly, way to go! You're fit for wound care!

☆ If you answered fewer than three items correctly, don't worry. Just review the chapter and try again!

5 Medicines management

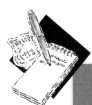

Just the facts

In this chapter, you'll learn:

♦ your responsibilities regarding drug administration

♦ how to safely administer drugs via various routes

♦ what patient care is associated with drug administration

♦ how to manage complications

♦ what patient teaching and documentation are associated with drug administration.

Essential skills clusters

Essential skills clusters associated with and specific to medicines management are:
• Medicines management—specific to all.
• Care, compassion and communication: associated with all numbers, 1–9.
• Organizational aspects of care: associated with numbers 10–21.
• Infection prevention and control: specific to numbers 22, 25 and 26.
• Nutrition and fluid management: specific to numbers 29 and 32**.

** Essential skills cluster No. 32, 'Safely administer fluids when fluids cannot be taken by mouth', is only applicable for entry to branch. All activities and practice in intravenous therapy administration by pre-registration nurses must be under direct supervision of a mentor.

Intravenous drug administration is covered in Chapter 8 of this book.

Terminology used in medicines management

Due to the use of abbreviations in healthcare and the publishing of the Standards for Medicines Management by the Nursing and Midwifery Council (NMC), you must understand what the following abbreviations and terms mean in order that you can interpret and follow the guidelines and legislation in place at this time.

• Patient-specific direction (PSD) is a written instruction by a prescriber determining a specific medication, its dose, time and course length for an individual patient.

• Patient medicines administration chart (PMAR) or medicines administration record (MAR), this has historically been referred to as a 'prescription chart' or 'drug chart'. However, it must be understood that this is not in fact a prescription, merely a direction (or delegation) from a registered and qualified prescriber to another appropriately trained and qualified practitioner to administer the medicines.

• Patient group direction (PGD) is the opposite to a PSD. It is a specific set of written instruction for the administration of a named medicine to specific groups of patients, e.g. vaccines.

Accountability and responsibility

There are many published guidelines, codes, policies and legislative acts that you must have a working knowledge of and adhere to when administering medications. These include:

Legislation

- Misuse of Drug Regulations 2001
- Misuse of Drugs (Safe Custody) Regulations 1973
- Misuse of Drugs (Supply to Addicts) Regulations 1997
- Prescription Only Medicines (Human Use) Order 1997
- Health Act 2006
- Controlled Drugs (Supervision of Management and Use) Regulations 2006.

Guidance and standards

- NMC Standards for medicine management 2008 (replacing the Guidelines for the administration of medicines 2004).

- NMC Essential skills clusters 2007, relating to the Standards for pre-registration nursing
- NMC Code of Conduct 2004.

Remember the following standard from the aforementioned Standards for medicine management:

> As a registrant you are accountable for your actions and omissions. In administering any medication, or assisting or overseeing any self-administration of medication, you must exercise your professional judgement and apply your knowledge and skill in the given situation. As a registrant, before you administer a medicinal product you must always check that the prescription or other direction to administer is . . .

then follows the list of safety checks you must make. This is covered in the MAR safety check section in this chapter. What this statement is saying is that you have been directed or delegated to administer these medicines. You are accountable and responsible for carrying out this task with the patients' best interests in mind and ensuring their safety at all times. Post-registration nurses should be given a period of training by their employer (often called medicines management training) and then assessed in this skill to ensure that they are both confident and competent in this task. The employer will hold a record of this training and the assessment outcome. Pre-registration nurses from 2008 must complete this training and assessment process prior to entry to the NMC register. This does not mean that they cannot be assessed again, the individual employer will follow their local medicines management policy.

Patient medicines administration record (MAR) safety checks

When checking the patient medicines administration record (MAR) (previously and commonly known as the prescription chart) it is imperative that you make sure that the direction is written safely and that it is safe to administer the drug.

Here is the process you should be following when checking the MAR:
- Check that the following are documented on the front of the record: patient's name, hospital number, date of birth, ward name, bed number, consultant's name and contact details.
- The patient's weight needs to be documented as drugs are often given according to weight.

- Allergies; ensure that all alergies the patient is aware of are noted, this means allergies to substances, foods or drugs. Remember, nurses are accountable for their acts and omissions, so also document, when applicable, that the patient has no known allergies—remember this doesn't mean he definitely doesn't have an allergy, it just means he doesn't know of any.
- Patients in hospital often have more than one MAR; this should be indicated on the front of the record; for example as 'no. 1 of 2 records'. Ensure you have both and administer from both!
- Check that the direction for each drug is legible, dated, and signed by a doctor; is the correct dose, has the route indicated and that the correct internationally recommended drug name is used.
- Stop and think, is it safe to administer the drug; do you know the patient's condition and the drug's indications, normal dose, cautions, interactions, side effects, etc.? If not, look it up using the patient's medical and nursing notes and the *British National Formulary* (BNF) (see *British National Formulary* section below).
- Now check that the drug has not already been given for the time you wish to administer it. Remember to check the PRN ('as required') section of the MAR as well as the regular section.
- Check the ID and allergy status of the patient against the wrist band of the patient, the patient's verbal response to being asked their name, etc. and the details on the MAR.

The *British National Formulary* (BNF)

Every clinical area where medications are dispensed or administered should have access to a copy of the BNF. This access may be through the internet or, of course, by having a copy of the actual reference book. The BNF is updated every 6 months, ensuring that any new findings about medicines already listed, or any new drugs, are included in the text.

The BNF should be your key reference when administering medications. As you have already read above, you are responsible and accountable for the medications you have given to the patient, so use the text to make an informed decision about administering the drug.

The BNF can provide you with information on the following:

- which drug group a medicine belongs to
- the indications for giving the drug
- the contraindications, when you wouldn't give the drug
- the cautions, when to take care, check the specific appendix, i.e. renal disease, hepatic disease, pregnancy or breastfeeding patients

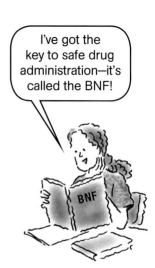

I've got the key to safe drug administration—it's called the BNF!

- the normal therapeutic dose for each medicine, the dose for all routes and adult and child doses are given
- the routes by which the drug can be given
- the interactions—how one drug reacts with another the patient is prescribed, is it safe to give?
- wound and elastic hosiery products, find out which dressing is best for which wound
- borderline substances: many people are surprised when they find this appendix as it gives lots of information on prescribed treatments such as build-up drinks and shakes, soups, etc.; they are prescribed so you are still responsible for administering them—find out here what they are
- intravenous drugs—how to reconstitute safely and administer
- advice and information to give to your patient when they commence a new drug or when they are taking medications home from hospital.

Tips on using the BNF

Many clinical staff do not use the BNF effectively, which means time is wasted and dangerous mistakes can be made, so here are a few tips and guidelines to help you.

Where is it?

When you find the medicine you are looking for in the main index at the back of the text you will notice there is often more than one page number listed for each drug; the page number printed in bold text is the main page for this drug, the other pages may only carry a fleeting reference to it—always go to the page printed in bold text first!

What is it?

To find out the drug group a medicine belongs to, look either at the top of the page or the title of the section you are reading; if you do not know anything about the drug group, read the paragraphs at the beginning of the section!

Watch out

When reading about the cautions for each drug you may find it useful to say to yourself 'be cautious of this drug in patients with...' before you read the paragraph listings, such as 'be cautious of this drug in patients with . . . renal disease', etc. Then if your patient has any of the cautions listed, go to the appropriate appendix, find the drug in the appendix (each appendix is listed alphabetically) and read to find out whether it is safe to give the drug to your patient, or what you may have to do to make it safe, for example you may have to obtain blood samples and check specific blood levels before safe administration.

What if . . .

If the patient is on more than one medicine, check the interactions appendix to find out if it is safe, or if the drugs will interact with one another, leading to enhanced or decreased effect or dangerous reactions.

Little known fact

Few people are aware that the advisory labels appendix (Appendix 9) exists. Practise using it. First, look up the drug name in the appendix index (be careful not to go too far in the text and end up in the main index—a common mistake). Against each drug you will find numbers again. These are not page numbers; these numbers refer to the numbered paragraphs (1–33) at the beginning of the chapter. For each number listed read the paragraph and pass this information on to the patient.

Basic drug calculations

There are three main drug calculation formulas you should know. These are used for calculating manual flow rates (drops per minute for intravenous infusions); calculating flow rates when infusion devices are used for intravenous infusions (millilitres per hour); and calculating stock dose calculations (how much volume to administer or how many tablets to give).

Drops per minute

This formula will assist you in working out how many drops per minute are required to administer an infusion over the directed time. To use the formula you will need to look at the patient's MAR and know:
- the type of fluid to be administered
- the type of infusion set required to administer it, and
- how many drops it takes for this infusion set to administer 1 ml, plus the volume of fluid to be administered and the time it is to be delivered in.

For example, the MAR directs you to administer 1 litre of 0.9% sodium chloride over 8 hours. Sodium chloride is a crystalloid fluid (low molecular weight) and thus a crystalloid-giving set should be used. Check the packaging of the crystalloid-giving set you use locally and you will find that the manufacturer's instruction will inform you of how many drops it takes to administer 1 ml of fluid (usually 20 drops per ml).

The formula should be run in order as indicated, starting at point 1 (the volume) and working through to point 8 (equals) to get the answer. Remember the line indicates that you need to divide the top figure by the bottom figure. For example:

(1) Volume to be infused (1,000 ml or 1 litre)

(5) 20 drops per ml

(2) _____ × (4)   (6) _____ = (8) 41.6 dpm (42 dpm)

(3) Time infusion to be administered (8 hours)

(7) 60 minutes

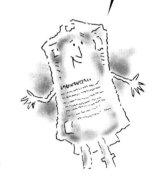

In other words, 1,000 divided by 8, multiplied by 20, divided by 60, equals 41.6 drops per minute, which would be rounded up to 42 drops per minute to administer.

The last part of the calculation directs you to divide your answer by 60 minutes; this is because up until this point you have worked out how many drops to administer over 1 hour. It would not be reasonable to stand and count drops for 1 hour to set the rate accurately, therefore by dividing the figure by 60 minutes you have concluded how many drops are required over a 1 minute time frame—much more reasonable! Remember you cannot deliver half a drop, therefore round up or down as appropriate any answer with a decimal point in it.

Likewise, if you are asked to administer 500 ml of plasma in 6 hours, plasma is a colloid (higher molecular weight fluid, it is thicker) thus when you check the packaging for a colloid administration set you will notice that it takes fewer drops to administer 1 ml of fluid (usually 15 drops). Use these figures to work out the number of drops you need to administer per minute. Remember, the formula should be run in order as indicated, starting at point 1 (the volume) and working through to point 8 (equals) to get the answer. Remember the line indicates that you need to divide the top figure by the bottom figure. For example:

(1) Volume to be infused (500 ml)

(5) 15 drops per ml

(2) _____ × (4)   (6) _____ = (8) 20.8 dpm (21 dpm)

(3) Time infusion to be administered (6 hours)

(7) 60 minutes

In other words, 500 divided by 6, multiplied by 15 and divided by 60, equals, a rate of 20.8 drops per minute, which would be rounded up to 21 drops per minute to administer.

Millilitres per hour

The formula used to calculate the number of millilitres (ml) per hour to administer a fluid using an infusion device is basically the first half of the previous calculation. The infusion device will only push through that amount of fluid in 1 hour. For example, following the same direction as in the previous section; to administer 1 litre of 0.9% sodium chloride in 8 hours, would be calculated as follows:

(1) Volume to be infused (1,000 ml)

(2) _____ = (4) 125 ml per hour.

(3) Time infusion to be administered
    (8 hours)

In other words, 1,000 divided by 8, equals a rate of 125 ml per hour to be set.

Stock dose formula

The stock dose formula is very useful as it can be used for calculating either how much fluid or liquid to draw up from a vial or bottle or how many tablets to administer. So lets have a look; lets say the direction on the patient's MAR requested that you 'Administer 12.5 mg of prochlorperazine via the intramuscular route'. You check out a vial of prochlorperazine from the stock cupboard. You notice that it actually comes in a 5 ml vial and in that vial there is 50 mg. How much do you draw up to administer? Don't panic—its easy, use the following; remember the formula should be run in order as indicated, starting at point 1 and working through to point 6 to get the answer. Note that the line indicates that you need to divide the top figure by the bottom figure:

(1) How much you want to give
    (12.5 mg)

(2) _____ × (4) (5) The volume in the vial (5 ml) = (6) 1.25 ml

(3) How much is in the vial (50 mg)

In other words, 12.5 mg, divided by 50 mg, multiplied by 5 ml, equals a dose of 1.25 ml to administer.

Remember, this is a specific dose you must administer, NEVER round it up or down—that could administer below or above the therapeutic dose and may lead to overdose of the patient! (See *Documenting flow rate control*.)

Per oral (PO) medications

Oral administration is usually the safest, most convenient, and least expensive method. For that reason, most drugs are administered by this route for patients who are conscious and able to swallow.

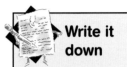

Write it down

Document-ing flow rate control

Record the original flow rate when setting up a peripheral line. If you adjust the rate, record the change, date and time.

Drugs for oral administration are available in many forms: tablets, enteric-coated tablets, capsules, syrups, elixirs, oils, liquids, suspensions, powders and granules. Some require special preparation before administration, such as mixing with water to make them more palatable; oils, powders and granules most often require such preparation.

What you need

The patient medicines administration record (MAR) ✳ prescribed medication ✳ medication pots ✳ medication trolley or individual pods by the bedside ✳ on the drug trolley: BNF, alcohol-based hand gel, gloves, jug of water, disposable cups, teaspoons, tablet cutter, 5 ml and 10 ml syringes, selection of build-up shakes and drinks brought from the fridge for the individual medication round, pharmacy order form, note paper, waste bag and sharps bin.

Dispensing the drug

• For each drug you are directed to administer check the direction is safe (see Patient medicines administration record safety check section at the beginning of this chapter). Wash your hands.
• If you do not know the indications, therapeutic dose, common side effects, cautions or effects for any of the medications, check this information in the BNF before you administer the drug; remember, you are accountable for administering it!
• If you are unaware of the patient's medical plan, nursing plan, past medical history or reason for admission, do not administer the medication—find out first!
• For each drug being administered, check you have the correct medication bottle or box and that the drug is safe to administer, by checking the labelling on both the outer and inner packaging for dose, route and expiry date information, to prevent administering the wrong drug or dose.
• Perform a stock dose calculation as required for each drug (see Basic drug calculations).
• Using a non-touch technique, dispense the required number of tablets or amount of fluid (use a syringe to draw up fluid) into a clean medication pot.
• Medication that you inadvertently touch or that falls on a high-risk surface (i.e. floor, bedside table) should be disposed of in the sharps bin, to minimize the risk of persons obtaining direct access to dangerous drugs.

dispose of them and document on an incident form, notify the pharmacy as per local policy.

• Keep in mind that the dispensing, administration and disposal of any controlled drugs must be counter signed by two nurses; this may be one registered nurse and a student nurse, depending on local guidelines and competency of both nurses. Remember to take the controlled drug record book to the bedside to complete; this record should not be signed until the drug is administered.

• If the patient questions you about his medication or the dosage, check his MAR again. If the medication is correct, reassure him. Make sure you tell him about any changes in his medication or dosage, and ask him to report anything he thinks may be an adverse effect.

• If the patient can't swallow a whole tablet or capsule, ask the pharmacist if the drug is available in liquid form or if it can be administered by another route. If not, ask him if you can crush the tablet or open the capsule and mix it with food—with the patient's prior consent and knowledge. Never hide drugs, you must inform the patient what you are giving them. Remember to contact the doctor and request that the prescription is changed prior to administration. (See *Documenting administration of oral medications*.)

Buccal, sublingual and translingual medications

Certain drugs are given buccally, sublingually or translingually to prevent their destruction or transformation in the stomach or small intestine. These drugs act quickly because the oral mucosa's thin epithelium and abundant vasculature allow direct absorption into the bloodstream.

What you need

Patient's MAR ✳ prescribed medication ✳ medication pots ✳ medication trolley or individual pots by the bedside ✳ on the drug trolley: BNF, alcohol-based hand gel, gloves, jug of water, disposable cups, teaspoons, tablet cutter, 5 ml and 10 ml syringes, selection of build-up shakes and drinks brought from the fridge for the individual medication round, pharmacy order form, note paper, waste bag and sharps bin.

Write it down

Documenting administration of oral medications

On the patient's medicines administration record, document:

• drug administration (by signing)
• any drug refusal, reason and your actions
• date and time
• patient's reaction.
 If the patient refuses a drug, document the refusal and notify the charge nurse and the patient's doctor, as needed. Also note if a drug was omitted or withheld for other reasons, such as radiology or laboratory tests, or if, in your judgement, the drug was contraindicated at that point in time. Check local policy for drugs that may be given when the patient is being held nil-by-mouth for surgery.
 Sign out all controlled drugs in the controlled drug book.

Dispensing the drug

- For each drug prescribed, check that the written direction is safe (see MAR safety check section at the beginning of this chapter). Wash your hands.
- If you do not know the indications, therapeutic dose, common side effects, cautions or effects for any of the medications, check this information in the BNF before you administer the drug; remember, you are accountable for administering it!
- If you are unaware of the patient's medical plan, nursing plan, past medical history or reason for admission, do not administer the medication—find out first!
- For each drug being administered, check you have the correct medication bottle or box and that the drug is safe to administer, by checking the labelling on both the outer and inner packaging for dose, route and expiry date information, to prevent administering the wrong drug or dose.
- Perform a stock dose calculation as required for each drug (see Basic drug calculations).
- Using a non-touch technique, dispense the required number of tablets or amount of fluid (use a syringe to draw up fluid) into a clean medication pot.
- Medication that you inadvertently touch or that falls on a high-risk surface (i.e. floor, bedside table), should be disposed of in the sharps bin, to minimize the risk of persons obtaining direct access to dangerous drugs.

How you do it

- Follow standard infection control practices throughout the procedure.
- Introduce yourself to the patient as necessary and gain permission and compliance.
- Confirm the patient's identity by asking his name and date of birth, while checking the name, date of birth and hospital number on his wristband and the MAR.
- Ask the patient if he has any allergies, and check that allergy documentation on the MAR is completed. Do not administer drugs if this is not completed—follow local policy to determine your actions in this situation.
- Assess the patient's condition, including level of consciousness and vital signs, as needed and indicated by the particular medication, and act according to your findings.

Buccal and sublingual administration

• For buccal administration, place the tablet in the buccal pouch, between the cheek and gum. For sublingual administration, place the tablet under the patient's tongue. (See *Placing drugs in the oral mucosa*.)

• Instruct the patient to keep the medication in place until it dissolves and not to chew or touch it with his tongue, to prevent accidental swallowing.

Translingual administration

• To administer a translingual drug, tell the patient to hold the medication canister vertically, with the valve head at the top and the spray orifice close to his mouth.

Don't give liquids to a patient receiving drugs by the buccal route. Some drugs take up to an hour to be absorbed after buccal administration.

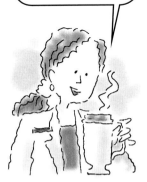

 Warning!

Placing drugs in the oral mucosa

Buccal and sublingual administration routes allow some drugs, such as nitroglycerin and methyltestosterone, to enter the bloodstream rapidly without being degraded in the GI tract.

What to do

To give a drug buccally, insert it between the patient's cheek and teeth (as shown below left). Ask him to close his mouth and hold the tablet against his cheek until the tablet is absorbed.

To give a drug sublingually, place it under the patient's tongue (as shown below right), and ask him to leave it there until it's dissolved.

Problem solving

Some buccal medications may irritate the mucosa. Alternate sides of the mouth for repeat doses to prevent continuous irritation of the same site. Sublingual medications—such as nitroglycerin—may cause a tingling sensation under the tongue. If the patient finds this annoying, try placing the drug in the buccal pouch instead.

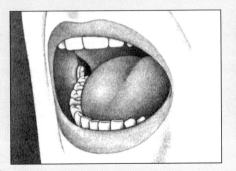

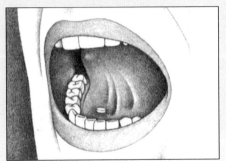

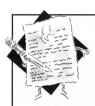

Write it down

Documenting administration of buccal, sublingual and translingual medications

On the patient's medicines administration record, document:

* drug administration (by signing)
* any drug refusal, reason and your actions
* date and time
* patient's reaction.

If the patient refuses a drug, document the refusal and notify the charge nurse and the patient's doctor, as needed. Also note if a drug was omitted or withheld for other reasons, such as radiology or laboratory tests, or if, in your judgement, the drug was contraindicated at that point in time.

Check local policy and indication to determine which drugs may be given when the patient is being held nil-by-mouth for surgery. For example, a patient with angina pain should take his GTN spray even when nil by mouth, as the indication and benefits outweigh the risk.

* Instruct him to spray the dose on to his tongue by pressing the button firmly and not to inhale. He should also wait 10 seconds or so before swallowing.

Practice pointers

* Inform the patient with angina to wet the nitroglycerin tablet with saliva and to keep it under his tongue until it has been fully absorbed. (See *Documenting administration of buccal, sublingual and translingual medications*.)

Topical (Top) medications: skin

* Topical drugs are applied 'into' or 'on top' of a surface or area.
* These surfaces include the skin, the eye and into the ear canal.

Topical drugs are applied directly to the skin surface and are absorbed through the epidermal layer into the dermis. They include lotions, pastes, ointments, creams, powders, shampoos, patches and aerosol sprays.

Most topical medications are used for local effects, although some are used for systemic effects. Typically, topical medications should be applied two or three times a day to achieve their therapeutic effect.

What you need

Patient's MAR ✳ prescribed medication ✳ gloves ✳ apron ✳ sterile gauze pads ✳ tongue depressor ✳ transparent semi-permeable dressing ✳ adhesive tape ✳ optional: goggles if using sprays.

Dispensing the drug

• For each drug you are directed to administer check the direction is safe (see MAR safety check section at the beginning of this chapter). Wash your hands.
• If you do not know the indications, therapeutic dose, common side effects, cautions or effects for any of the medications, check this information in the BNF before you administer the drug; remember, you are accountable for administering it!
• If you are unaware of the patient's medical plan, nursing plan, past medical history or reason for admission, do not administer the medication—find out first!
• For each drug being administered, check you have the correct medication bottle or box and that the drug is safe to administer, by checking the labelling on both the outer and inner packaging for dose, route and expiry date information, to prevent administering the wrong drug or dose.
• Perform a stock dose calculation as required for each drug (see Basic drug calculations).

How you do it

• Follow standard infection control practices throughout the procedure.
• Introduce yourself to the patient as necessary and gain permission and compliance.
• Confirm the patient's identity by asking his name and date of birth, while checking the name, date of birth and hospital number on his wristband and the MAR.
• Ask the patient if he has any allergies and check that allergy documentation on the MAR is completed. Do not administer drugs if this is not completed—follow local policy to determine your actions in this situation.
• Help the patient assume a comfortable position that allows access to the area to be treated. Perform skin assessment.
• If necessary, clean the skin of debris, including crusts, epidermal scales and old medication.
• Change gloves if soiled.

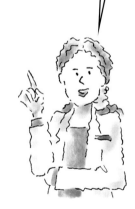

Help the patient into a comfortable position that allows access to the skin.

Applying paste, cream, or ointment
• Open the medication container and place the lid or cap upside down on a flat surface, remove a tongue blade or gauze from its sterile wrapper, and cover one end with medication from the tube or jar. Then transfer the medication from the tongue blade or gauze to your gloved hand, minimizing the risk of contaminating the tube or bottle.
• Apply the medication to the affected area with long, smooth strokes that follow the direction of hair growth; use a new tongue blade or gauze each time you remove medication from the container.

Applying other topical medications
• To apply shampoos, wet the patient's hair and wring out excess water, shake the bottle, and apply the proper amount as indicated by the label. Work the lather into the scalp, adding water as necessary. Leave the shampoo on the scalp as directed and then rinse thoroughly. A fine-tooth comb is used to remove nits, if necessary.
• To apply aerosol sprays, shake the container and hold it 15–30.5 cm from the skin, or according to the manufacturer's recommendation. Spray a thin film of the medication evenly over the treatment area.
• To apply prescribed powders, dry the skin surface, making sure to spread skin folds where moisture collects. Then apply a thin layer of powder over the treatment area.

Practice pointers
• Never apply medication without removing previous applications, to prevent skin irritation from medication accumulation.

Less is more

• Don't apply ointments to mucous membranes as liberally as you would to skin because mucous membranes are usually moist and absorb ointment more quickly than does skin.

The cover-up

• With certain medications (such as topical steroids), semi-permeable dressings may be contraindicated. Check the medication's information and cautions. If you're applying a topical medication to the patient's hands or feet, cover the site with white cotton gloves for the hands or terry cloth scuffs for the feet.
• Inspect the treated area frequently for adverse effects, such as signs of an allergic reaction. (See *Documenting administration of skin medications*.)

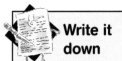

Write it down

Documenting administration of skin medications

On the patient's medicines administration record, document:

• drug administration (by signing)
• any drug refusal, reason and your actions
• date, time and site of application
• patient's reaction.
   If the patient refuses a drug, document the refusal and notify the charge nurse and the patient's doctor, as needed. Also note if a drug was omitted or withheld for other reasons, such as adverse condition of the skin, patient complaining of burning at the site of topical application, etc.

Topical medications: eye

Eye medications typically include drops and ointments. Eye drops can be used to anaesthetize the eye, dilate the pupil for examination, and stain the cornea to identify corneal abrasions, scars or abnormalities. Eye medications can also be used to lubricate, treat certain eye conditions and protect the vision of neonates.

What you need

Prescribed eye medication ✳ patient's MAR ✳ gloves ✳ warm water or normal saline solution ✳ sterile gauze pads ✳ facial tissues ✳ optional: ocular dressing.

Dispensing the drug

• For each drug you are directed to administer, check the direction is safe (see MAR safety check section at the beginning of this chapter). Wash your hands.
• If you do not know the indications, therapeutic dose, common side effects, cautions or effects for any of the medications, check this information in the BNF before you administer the drug; remember, you are accountable for administering it!
• If you are unaware of the patient's medical plan, nursing plan, past medical history or reason for admission, do not administer the medication—find out first!
• For each drug being administered, check you have the correct medication bottle or box and that the drug is safe to administer, by checking the labelling on both the outer and inner packaging for dose, route and expiry date information, to prevent administering the wrong drug or dose.
• Make sure the medication is labelled for ophthalmic use and check the expiration date. Remember to date the container the first time you use it and discard it in 2 weeks to avoid contamination.
• Inspect ocular solutions for cloudiness, discoloration and precipitation; don't use any solution that appears abnormal. If the tip of an eye ointment tube has crusted, turn the tip on a sterile gauze pad to remove the crust.

How you do it

• Follow standard infection control practices throughout the procedure.
• Introduce yourself to the patient as necessary and gain permission and compliance, provide privacy and maintain dignity by closing bed curtains or requesting the patient come to the treatment room.

Instilling eye medications

To instill eye drops, pull the lower lid down to expose the conjunctival sac. Have the patient look up and away, and then squeeze the prescribed number of drops into the sac. Release the patient's eyelid, and have him blink to distribute the medication.

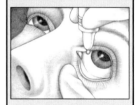

To apply an ointment, gently lay a thin strip of the medication along the conjunctival sac from the inner to the outer canthus. Avoid touching the tip of the tube to the patient's eye. Then release the eyelid, and have the patient roll his eye behind closed lids to distribute the medication.

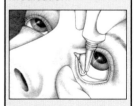

- Confirm the patient's identity by asking his name and date of birth, while checking the name, date of birth and hospital number on his wristband and the MAR.
- Ask the patient if he has any allergies and check that allergy documentation on the MAR is completed. Do not administer drugs if this is not completed—follow local policy to determine your actions in this situation.
- Make sure you know which eye to treat because different medications or doses may be ordered for each eye.
- If the patient is wearing an eye dressing, remove it by gently pulling it down and away from his forehead. Take care not to contaminate your hands.
- Remove any discharge by cleaning around the eye with sterile gauze pads moistened with warm water or normal saline solution, gently stroking from the inner to the outer canthus. Use a fresh sterile gauze pad for each stroke.
- Have the patient sit or lie in the supine position and tell him to tilt his head back and toward the side of the affected eye.

Instilling eye drops
- Remove the dropper cap from the medication container and draw the medication into it. Be careful to avoid contaminating the dropper tip or bottle top.
- Before instilling the eye drops, instruct the patient to look up and away to minimize the risk of touching the cornea with the dropper.

Steady as she goes
- You can steady the hand holding the dropper by resting it against the patient's forehead. Then, with your other hand, gently pull down the lower lid and instil the drops in the conjunctival sac. (See *Instilling eye medications.*)
- Instruct the patient to slowly close and open his eyelid to distribute the medicine, blinking may cause the drop to be expelled from the eye.

Practice pointers
- After instilling eye drops or ointment, tissue away the excess from the eye, using a fresh tissue for each eye; then, apply a new eye dressing if necessary. Return the medication to the storage area, making sure you store it according to the label's instructions, and then wash your hands.
- Document administration.

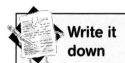

Write it down

Documenting administration of eye medication

On the patient's medicines administration record, document:

- drug administration (by signing)
- any drug refusal, reason and your actions
- date, time and which eye—right or left
- patient's reaction. If the patient refuses a drug, document the refusal and notify the charge nurse and the patient's doctor, as needed. Also note if a drug was omitted or withheld for other reasons, such as the consultant wishing to view the eye pre-medication administration, or if, in your judgement, the drug was contraindicated at that point in time.

None in the duct

- When administering an eye medication that may be absorbed systemically, gently press your thumb on the inner canthus for 1–2 minutes after instilling drops while the patient closes his eyes. This helps to prevent medication from flowing into the tear duct.
- To maintain the drug container's sterility, never touch the tip of the bottle or dropper to the patient's eyeball, lids or lashes.
- Teach the patient to instil eye medications and to review the procedure, asking for a return demonstration. (See *Documenting administration of eye medication*.)

Topical medications: eardrops

Eardrops treat infection or inflammation, soften cerumen (wax) for removal, produce local anaesthesia, or facilitate removal of an insect. Instillation of eardrops is usually contraindicated if the patient has a perforated eardrum, but it may be permitted with certain medications and adherence to aseptic technique. Some conditions may prohibit instillation of certain medications into the ear, such as hydrocortisone use in patients with viral or fungal infections.

What you need

Prescribed eardrops ✳ patient's MAR ✳ light source ✳ facial tissue or cotton-tipped applicator ✳ optional: gloves, cotton ball, bowl of warm water.

Dispensing the drug

- For each drug you are ordered to administer, check the direction is safe (see MAR safety check section at the beginning of this chapter). Wash your hands.
- If you do not know the indications, therapeutic dose, common side effects, cautions or effects for any of the medications, check this information in the BNF before you administer the drug; remember, you are accountable for administering it!
- If you are unaware of the patient's medical plan, nursing plan, past medical history or reason for admission, do not administer the medication—find out first!
- For each drug being administered, check you have the correct medication to administer, by checking the labelling on both the outer and inner packaging for dose, route and expiry date information, to prevent administering the wrong drug or dose.
- Make sure the medication is labelled for aural route use and check the expiration date.

How you do it

- Follow standard infection control practices throughout the procedure.
- Introduce yourself to the patient as necessary and gain permission and compliance, provide privacy and maintain dignity by closing bed curtains or requesting the patient come to the treatment room.
- Confirm the patient's identity by asking his name and date of birth, while checking the name, date of birth and hospital number on his wristband and the prescription chart.
- Ask the patient if he has any allergies and check that allergy documentation on the MAR is completed. Do not administer drugs if this is not completed—follow local policy to determine your actions in this situation.
- Make sure you know which ear to treat because different medications or doses may be ordered for each ear.
- Straighten the patient's ear canal. For an adult, pull the auricle of the ear up and back. (See *Positioning the patient for eardrop installation*.)
- Using a light source, examine the ear canal for drainage. If you find any, clean the canal with a tissue or cotton-tipped applicator, because drainage can reduce the medication's effectiveness.

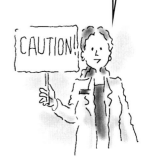

Yow! Test the medication's temperature by placing a drop on your wrist.

Ages and stages

Positioning the patient for eardrop instillation

Before instilling eardrops, have the patient lie on his side. Then straighten the patient's ear canal to help the medication reach the eardrum. For an adult, gently pull the auricle up and back. For a child under 3 years of age, gently pull the auricle down and back because the ear canal is straighter at this age.

Adult

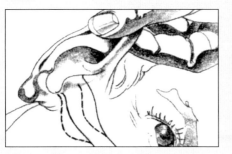

Child

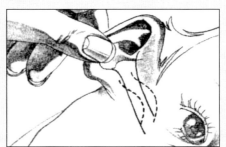

Aim for the canal

- To avoid damaging the ear canal with the dropper, gently support the hand holding the dropper against the patient's head.
- Straighten the patient's ear canal once again, and instil the prescribed number of drops. To avoid patient discomfort, aim the dropper so that the drops fall against the sides of the ear canal, not on the eardrum.
- Hold the ear canal in position until you see the medication disappear down the canal, then release the ear.

Need a magazine?

- Instruct the patient to remain on his side for 5–10 minutes to let the medication run down into the ear canal.
- If instructed by pharmacist/medication information leaflet or the BNF, tuck a cotton ball loosely into the opening of the ear canal to prevent the medication from leaking out. Be careful not to insert it too deeply into the canal because this would prevent drainage of secretions and increase pressure on the eardrum.
- Clean and dry the outer ear and, if ordered, repeat the procedure in the other ear after 5–10 minutes.
- Wash your hands.

Practice pointers

- To prevent injury to the eardrum, never insert a cotton-tipped applicator into the ear canal past the point where you can see the tip.

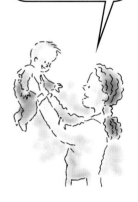

Be sure to pull the auricle down and back in a child under age 3.

Write it down

Documenting administration of eardrops

On the patient's medicines administration record, document:

- drug administration (by signing)
- any drug refusal, reason and your actions
- date, time and which ear—right or left
- signs or symptoms the patient experienced during the procedure, such as drainage, redness, vertigo, nausea and pain
- patient's reaction.

If the patient refuses a drug, document the refusal and notify the charge nurse and the patient's doctor, as needed. Also note if a drug was omitted or withheld for other reasons, the patient complaining of severe pain in the ear, or if, in your judgement, the drug was contraindicated.

After applying eardrops to soften the cerumen, irrigate the ear as ordered to facilitate cerumen removal.
• Teach the patient to instil the eardrops correctly so that he can continue treatment at home, if necessary. (See *Documenting administration of eardrops*.)

Transdermal medications

Through an adhesive patch or a measured dose of ointment applied to the skin, transdermal drugs deliver constant, controlled medication directly into the bloodstream for a prolonged systemic effect. Contraindications for transdermal drugs include skin allergies or skin reactions to the drug.

Transdermal drugs shouldn't be applied to broken or irritated skin because they increase irritation, or to scarred or callused skin, which might impair absorption.

What you need

Patient's MAR ✳ gloves ✳ prescribed medication (patch or ointment) ✳ application strip (if required) ✳ adhesive tape ✳ plastic wrap or semi-permeable dressing ✳ Biro pen.

Dispensing the drug

• For each drug you are directed to administer check the direction is safe (see MAR safety check section at the beginning of this chapter). Wash your hands.
• If you do not know the indications, therapeutic dose, common side effects, cautions or effects for any of the medications, check this information in the BNF before you administer the drug; remember, you are accountable for administering it!
• If you are unaware of the patient's medical plan, nursing plan, past medical history or reason for admission do not administer the medication—find out first!
• For each drug being administered, check you have the correct medication to administer, by checking the labelling on both the outer and inner packaging for dose, route and expiry date information, to prevent administering the wrong drug or dose.
• Make sure the medication is labelled for transdermal route use.

How you do it

• Follow standard infection control practices throughout the procedure.

- Introduce yourself to the patient as necessary and gain permission and compliance, provide privacy and maintain dignity by closing bed curtains or requesting the patient come to the treatment room.
- Confirm the patient's identity by asking his name and date of birth, while checking the name, date of birth and hospital number on his wristband and the MAR.
- Ask the patient if he has any allergies and check that allergy documentation on the MAR is completed, do not administer drugs if this is not completed—follow local policy to determine your actions in this situation.
- Remove previous patch.

Applying transdermal ointment

- Place the prescribed amount of ointment on the application strip, taking care not to get any on your skin.

Home care connection

Applying a transdermal medication patch

If the patient receives medication by transdermal patch, instruct him in its proper use.

A layered affair

- Explain that the patch consists of several layers. The layer closest to his skin contains a small amount of the drug and allows prompt drug introduction into the bloodstream. The next layer controls drug release from the main portion of the patch. The third layer contains the main dose. The outermost layer consists of an aluminized polyester barrier.
- Teach the patient to apply the patch to the upper arm or chest area or behind the ear. Warn him to avoid touching the gel or surrounding tape. Tell him to use a different site for each application to avoid skin irritation. If necessary, he can shave the site. Tell him to avoid any area that may cause uneven absorption, such as skin folds, scars, and calluses or any irritated or damaged skin areas. Also, tell him not to apply the patch below the elbow or knee.

More patch pointers

- Instruct the patient to wash his hands after application to remove any medication that may have rubbed off.
- Tell him to discard it if it leaks or falls off and then to clean the site and apply a new patch at a different site.
- Instruct the patient to apply the patch at the same time at the prescribed interval. Bedtime application is ideal because body movement is reduced during the night.

- Apply the prepared strip to any dry, hairless area of the body, but remember not to rub the ointment into the skin.
- If required, cover the application strip with the dressing.
- Write the date of application on the dressing.
- Instruct the patient to keep the area around the ointment as dry as possible.

Applying a transdermal patch

- Open the package and remove the patch.
- Without touching the adhesive surface, remove the clear plastic backing.
- Apply the patch to a dry, hairless area—following manufacturer's instructions or BNF instructions. (See *Applying a transdermal medication patch*.)
- Write the date, time and your initials on the dressing.

Practice pointers

- Re-apply daily transdermal medications at the same time every day to ensure a continuous effect, but alternate the application sites to avoid skin irritation. (See *Transdermal drug pointers*.)
- Review specific instructions with the patient regarding the type of medication, adverse effects and interactions.
- Instruct the patient to keep the area around the patch as dry as possible. (See *Documenting administration of transdermal medication*.)

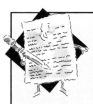

Write it down

Documenting administration of transdermal medication

On the patient's medicines administration record, document:

- drug administration (by signing)
- any drug refusal, reason and your actions
- date, time and site of application
- adverse reactions
- patient's response to the medication.

If the patient refuses a drug, document the refusal and notify the charge nurse and the patient's doctor, as needed. Also note if a drug was omitted or withheld for other reasons, or if, in your judgement, the drug was contraindicated at that point in time.

Sign out all controlled drugs in the controlled drug book.

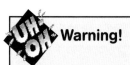

Warning!

Transdermal drug pointers

Topical medications may cause skin irritation, such as pruritus and a rash. Watch for these symptoms and for adverse reactions to the specific medication.

A few examples

Transdermal nitroglycerin medications may cause headaches and, in elderly patients, orthostatic hypotension.

Know what the drug is that you are administering and be alert to its effects, implications and adverse reactions.

Inhaled therapies: handheld

Handheld inhalers include the metered-dose inhaler (also known as a 'puffer' or 'aerosol inhaler'), the turbo-inhaler, the accuhaler and the nasal inhaler. These devices deliver topical medications to the respiratory tract, producing local and systemic effects. The mucosal lining of the respiratory tract absorbs the inhalant almost immediately.

Common inhalants are bronchodilators, used to improve airway patency and facilitate mucus drainage; mucolytics, which attain a high local concentration to liquefy tenacious bronchial secretions; and corticosteroids, used to decrease inflammation.

In order to monitor how the medication is working it is necessary to take a peak flow reading 5–10 minutes pre administration and 30 minutes post administration. These readings must be recorded on the appropriate document in the patient's nursing records.

What you need

Patient's MAR ✳ the inhaler ✳ prescribed medication ✳ normal saline solution (or another appropriate solution) for rinsing post inhalation (as necessary) ✳ optional: emesis basin. (See *Types of handheld inhalers*.)

Checking the direction

• For each inhaler pre check that the direction is safe (see MAR safety check section at the beginning of this chapter). Wash your hands.
• If you do not know the indications, therapeutic dose, common side effects, cautions or effects for any of the medications, check this information in the BNF before you administer the drug; remember, you are accountable for administering it!
• If you are unaware of the patient's medical plan, nursing plan, past medical history or reason for admission do not administer the medication—find out first!
• For each drug being administered, check you have the correct medication to administer, by checking the labelling on both the outer and inner packaging or on the inhaler canister for dose, route and expiry date information, to prevent administering the wrong drug or dose.
• Make sure the medication is labelled for inhalation route use.

Types of handheld inhalers

Handheld inhalers use air under pressure to produce a mist-containing medication. Drugs delivered in this form (such as mucolytics and bronchodilators) can travel deep into the lungs.

Inhalers with a spacer attachment provide greater therapeutic benefit for children and patients with poor coordination. A spacer attachment, an extension to the inhaler's mouthpiece, provides more dead-air space for mixing medication.

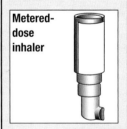

Metered-dose inhaler

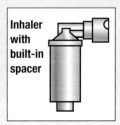

Inhaler with built-in spacer

How you do it

- Follow standard infection control practices throughout the procedure.
- Introduce yourself to the patient as necessary and gain permission and compliance, provide privacy and maintain dignity by closing bed curtains or requesting the patient come to the treatment room.
- Confirm the patient's identity by asking his name and date of birth, while checking the name, date of birth and hospital number on his wristband and the MAR.
- Ask the patient if he has any allergies and check that allergy documentation on the MAR is completed. Do not administer drugs if this is not completed—follow local policy to determine your actions in this situation.

Using a metered-dose inhaler

- Shake the inhaler bottle and remove the mouthpiece and cap.
- If the inhaler has not been used recently, spray it into the air first to check that it is working.
- Have the patient take a few deep breaths and then exhale gently; then immediately ask the patient to place the mouthpiece in his mouth and close his lips around it, creating a seal.

Fill 'er up

- Ask the patient to continue to breathe in slowly and deeply through the mouthpiece, then, as he breathes in, push the metal canister down into the inhaler shell to release the medication.
- Remove the mouthpiece from the patient's mouth, and tell him to hold his breath for 10 seconds (or as long as possible) and then ask him to exhale slowly through pursed lips.
- One press equals one puff of medication, so repeat according to the number of puffs prescribed.
- Rinse the mouthpiece with warm water to prevent accumulation of residue, dry and replace the cap.

Using a large volume spacer device

- Remove the cap from the inhaler and shake as above.
- Insert the inhaler into the back of the spacer device.
- Ask the patient to exhale gently and place the mouthpiece of the spacer in his mouth (as per metered-dose inhaler above).
- Press the inhaler canister into the inhaler holder as per above (this will release one 'puff' of medication into the device), at the same time as asking the patient to take one deep, slow breath in and then hold his breath for 10 seconds or for as long as possible.

- Ask the patient to remove the spacer device from his mouth and exhale.
- Repeat the process as necessary for the number of 'puffs' prescribed.

Using a turbo-inhaler
- Unscrew and remove the cover, while holding the inhaler upright twist the grip area forwards and backwards, as far as it will go, until you hear a 'click'.
- Ask the patient to breathe out gently and put the mouthpiece between his lips.
- Ask the patient to breathe in as deeply as possible, to pull in the drug.
- Have the patient remove the inhaler and breathe out slowly.
- Rinse the inhaler with warm water and replace the lid.
- Repeat the process as necessary for the number of puffs prescribed.
- See *Patient advice on discharge with a turbo-inhaler*.

Using an accuhaler
- Hold the outer casing of the circular accuhaler in one hand and push the grip away with the other hand, until you hear a 'click'.
- To make a dose available and move the dose counter forward, hold the accuhaler with the mouthpiece facing towards you and slide the lever away until again you hear a 'click'.
- Ask the patient to breathe out, gently.
- Holding the mouthpiece horizontally, ask the patient to put it between his lips and create a seal.
- Ask the patient to 'suck in' quickly and deeply.
- Remove the accuhaler and ask the patient to hold his breath for 10 seconds or for as long as possible.
- Close the mouthpiece by sliding the grip back towards you until you hear a 'click'.
- Repeat the process as necessary for the number of puffs prescribed.
- See *Patient advice on discharge with an accuhaler*.

Using a nasal inhaler
- Have the patient blow his nose to clear his nostrils.
- Shake the medication cartridge and then insert it in the adapter, removing the protective cap from the adapter tip.
- Hold the inhaler with your index finger on top of the cartridge and your thumb under the nasal adapter, pointing the adapter tip toward the patient.

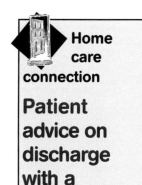

Home care connection

Patient advice on discharge with a turbo-inhaler

When a patient is taking a turbo-inhaler home upon discharge, inform him that it is essential that he does not run out of the drug. To aid him in this, most turbo-inhalers have a window at their top which will indicate either a red line when 20 doses remain or a dose counter informing the patient how many doses are left. Refer the patient to the asthma clinic in the primary care setting.

Home care connection

Patient advice on discharge with an accuhaler

- Remind and advise the patient that it is essential he does not run out of the drug.
- Show him the dose counter on top of the accuhaler—indicating that it informs him how many doses are left, NOT how many he has taken.

- When the dose meter gets to 5 or below the numbers are printed in red as a warning, the patient must contact his GP for a repeat prescription.

Cover one, then go

- Have the patient tilt his head back. Place the adapter tip into one nostril while occluding the other nostril with your finger.
- Instruct the patient to inhale gently as you press the adapter and the cartridge together firmly to release a measured dose of medication. Be sure to follow the manufacturer's instructions.
- Remove the inhaler and tell the patient to exhale through his mouth.
- Shake the inhaler, and repeat the procedure in the other nostril.
- Remove the medication cartridge from the nasal inhaler, and wash the nasal adapter in lukewarm water. Let the adapter dry thoroughly before reinserting the cartridge.

Practice pointers

- Teach the patient how to use the inhaler and explain that overdose can cause the medication to lose its effectiveness. Inform him of possible adverse reactions.
- If more than one inhalation is ordered, advise the patient to wait at least 30 seconds before repeating the procedure.
- Check the patient's inhaler technique and correct it as necessary every 6 months if he is attending your clinic. This is proven to maintain effective use of both the medication and the device.

Remind the patient that overdose causes the inhaler to lose its effectiveness.

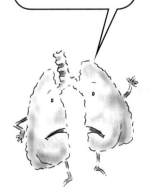

Steroid goes second

- If the patient is also using a steroid inhaler, instruct him to use the bronchodilator first and to then wait 5 minutes before using the steroid.

This allows the bronchodilator to open the air passages for maximum effectiveness. (See *Documenting administration of inhaler therapy*.)
• Also, when the patient is also using a steroid inhaler, instruct him to rinse his mouth after inhaler use. This prevents ulceration of the mouth caused by inhaled steroid therapy.

Inhaled therapies: nebulizers

A nebulizer is usually applied via a face mask with a chamber or bowl on the distal end. Liquid medications are placed in this chamber and then a driving gas (oxygen or medical air—check the MAR for directions) is forced through the liquid causing particulation of the drug (the majority of nebulizer therapy is administered using oxygen as the driving gas). The drug particles are then inhaled by the patient and, as with handheld inhalers, are delivered topically to the respiratory tract, producing local and systemic effects. Common inhalants are bronchodilators, used to improve airway patency and facilitate mucus drainage; mucolytics, which attain a high local concentration to liquefy tenacious bronchial secretions; and corticosteroids, used to decrease inflammation.

In order to monitor how the medication is working it is necessary to take a peak flow reading 5–10 minutes pre administration and 30 minutes post administration. These readings must be recorded on the appropriate document in the patient's nursing records.

What you need

Patient's MAR ✳ a nebulizer mask ✳ prescribed medication ✳ driving gas: oxygen or medical air as directed on the MAR.

Checking the direction

• For each medication pre check that the direction is safe (see MAR safety check section at the beginning of this chapter). Wash your hands.
• If you do not know the indications, therapeutic dose, common side effects, cautions or effects for any of the medications, check this information in the BNF before you administer the drug; remember, you are accountable for administering it!
• If you are unaware of the patient's medical plan, nursing plan, past medical history or reason for admission, do not administer the medication—find out first!
• For each drug being administered, check you have the correct medication to administer, by checking the labelling on both the

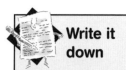

Write it down

Documenting administration of inhaler therapy

On the medicines administration record, document:

• pre-administration peak flow rate on the appropriate chart
• drug administration (by signing)
• any drug refusal, reason and your actions
• date and time
• patient's reaction and the post-administration peak flow rate.
  If the patient refuses a drug, document the refusal and notify the charge nurse and the patient's doctor, as needed. Also note if a drug was omitted or withheld for other reasons, or if, in your judgement, the drug was contraindicated at that point in time.

outer and inner packaging or on the vial for dose, route and expiry date information, to prevent administering the wrong drug or dose.
• Make sure the medication is labelled for inhalation or nebulizer route use.

How you do it

• Follow standard infection control practices throughout the procedure.
• Introduce yourself to the patient as necessary and gain permission and compliance.
• Confirm the patient's identity by asking his name and date of birth, while checking the name, date of birth and hospital number on his wristband and the MAR.
• Ask the patient if he has any allergies and check that allergy documentation on the MAR is completed. Do not administer drugs if this is not completed—follow local policy to determine your actions in this situation.
• Take and record a pre-administration peak flow reading.
• Open the bowl of the nebulizer mask.
• Squeeze the contents of the checked vial into the bottom bowl of the nebulizer mask.
• Re-attach the top half of the bowl, which will include the actual mask.
• If using air as a driving gas: switch on the air compressor unit and ensure the liquid medication is being particulated, you will notice a mist coming from the mask.
• If using oxygen as a driving gas: turn the oxygen flow meter to 2–4 litres until a mist is noted coming from the mask.
• Assist the patient to apply the mask and ensure a close fit by adjusting the elastic straps.

Don't document yet

• Repeat the process for each medication, each medication should take no longer than 10 minutes to administer; observe your patient regularly throughout this time.
• Only document administration when the nebulizer has been completed. (See *Documenting administration of nebulizer therapy*.)
• After 30 minutes take and record a post-administration peak flow to assist in monitoring effectiveness of the medication.

Practice pointers

• Depending on the patient's condition and oxygen requirements, it may be necessary to administer supplementary oxygen via a nasal cannula during nebulizer therapy, check the MAR and observe

Write it down

Documenting administration of nebulizer therapy

On the patient's medicines administration record, document:

• drug administration (by signing)
• any drug refusal, reason and your actions
• date and time of administration
• patient's reaction.

On the patient's vital signs record, document:

• The pre- and post-administration peak flow reading.

your patient for signs and symptoms of hypoxia (including oxygen saturation levels if indicated) during therapy, to prevent hypoxia and patient deterioration.

Inhaled therapies: oxygen

A patient needs oxygen therapy when the signs and symptoms of low oxygen levels in the blood (hypoxaemia) or low oxygen levels in the tissues (hypoxia) present as a result of a chronic or acute respiratory or cardiac episode.

Arterial blood gas (ABG) analysis (for paediatric patients, capillary blood gases), oximetry monitoring, and clinical examinations are used to determine if the patient is receiving enough oxygen.

Delivery systems

There are several ways to administer oxygen. The patient's disease, physical condition and age will help determine the most appropriate method; however, as oxygen must be prescribed by a doctor, nursing and allied health professionals must follow the direction in the patient's MAR—EXCEPT IN AN EMERGENCY when oxygen should be administered even without a prescription using a non-rebreath mask on 15 litres!

Oxygen administration devices can be categorized into two groups:

Variable

Variable oxygen delivery systems will deliver differing percentages of oxygen depending on how the patient is breathing (their respiratory pattern). Imagine, two patients in your care may be on the same prescription of oxygen using the same variable oxygen device such as a nasal cannula. However, one patient breathes only via his mouth and the other in through his nose and out through his mouth, can you see why they will receive different percentages of oxygen? It depends upon how much room air is pulled into the device and mixed with the 100% oxygen you started with. Because of this it is only possible to estimate what percentage of oxygen the patient is receiving, and the direction or prescription is therefore written in litres/minute (LPM) not in percentage.

Fixed

Fixed oxygen delivery systems, such as the Venturi system, have been designed and manufactured with a jet mixing port. This ensures that no matter what the patient's respiratory pattern, he will definitely receive the prescribed/directed amount of oxygen, as it limits the amount of room air pulled into the system and mixing with the oxygen you are delivering. Hence, when a variable delivery system is indicated on the MAR the direction will be written in percentage of oxygen to be administered.

What you need

The equipment needed depends on the direction in the MAR, which should indicate the type of delivery system to use (see *Oxygen delivery systems* and the Checking the direction section, below). Equipment includes selections from the following list: oxygen source (wall unit or cylinder) ✳ flow meter ✳ adapter, if using a wall unit, or a pressure-reduction gauge, if using a cylinder ✳ sterile humidity bottle and adapters ✳ sterile distilled water ✳ appropriate oxygen delivery system (a nasal cannula, partial rebreath mask, or non-rebreath mask for low-flow and variable oxygen concentrations; a Venturi mask, aerosol mask or tracheostomy collar for fixed oxygen concentrations) ✳ small-diameter and large-diameter connection tubing ✳ appropriate jet mixing port for Venturi mask ✳ pulse oximeter for continuous monitoring of patients receiving 40% oxygen or more.

Checking the direction

Check that the direction in the patient's MAR is complete and is safe; the direction in the patient's MAR should indicate:
- The date and time for administration and the doctor's signature.
- The percentage of oxygen to be administered (oxygen percentage can only be directed when a fixed oxygen delivery system is to be used), or the flow rate of oxygen to be delivered in LPM should be used when a variable oxygen delivery system is to be used.
- The oxygen delivery system to use, i.e. Venturi mask, nasal cannula.
- The aim of oxygen delivery. This may be written as an $SpaO_2$ to aim for (normally 96%; however, this aim must be achievable by the individual patient—if a patient's normal $SpaO_2$ is 90%, then it would be unlikely that they would ever achieve 96%, therefore the doctor should take this into consideration when writing the directive). Or it may be written, for example, as 'while on opiate analgesics' or 'while on PCA', etc.
- The need for humidification should be indicated; however, as best practice, oxygen should be humidified at the point of set-up if it is known that the patient will receive it for more than 6 hours. If the treatment period is unknown, then the maximum time oxygen should be given without humidification is 6 hours, reducing the risk of a dry mouth and infection.
- If you are unaware of the patient's medical plan, nursing plan, past medical history or reason for admission, do not administer the medication—find out first!

Oxygen delivery systems

Patients may receive oxygen through one of several administration systems, these systems belong to either the fixed oxygen delivery group or viariable oxygen delivery group.

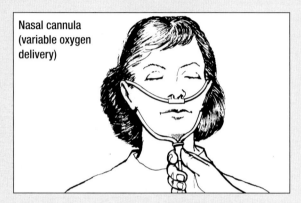

Nasal cannula
(variable oxygen
delivery)

Oxygen can be delivered at concentrations of less than 40% through a plastic cannula in the patient's nostrils; however, as it would be uncomfortable to deliver high-flow oxygen, a flow rate of no more than 4 litres per minute should be administered.

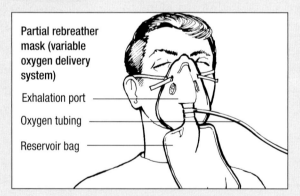

Partial rebreather mask (variable oxygen delivery system)

Exhalation port

Oxygen tubing

Reservoir bag

The patient inspires oxygen from a reservoir bag along with atmospheric air and oxygen from the mask. The first third of exhaled tidal volume enters the bag; the rest exits the mask. Because air entering the reservoir bag comes from the trachea and bronchi, where no gas exchange occurs, the patient rebreathes the oxygenated air he just exhaled. Forty to 60% oxygen could possibly be administered.

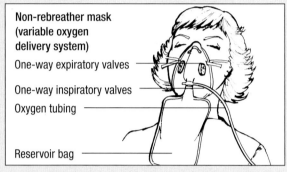

Non-rebreather mask
(variable oxygen
delivery system)

One-way expiratory valves

One-way inspiratory valves

Oxygen tubing

Reservoir bag

On inhalation, the one-way inspiratory valve opens, directing oxygen from a reservoir bag into the mask. On exhalation, gas exits the mask through the one-way expiratory valves and enters the atmosphere. The patient breathes air only from the bag. It is possible (remember it is a variable system) to deliver the highest possible oxygen concentration (60% to 90%) of any system short of intubation and mechanical ventilation, and should therefore be used in an emergency.

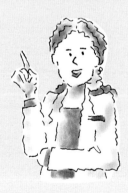

Oxygen delivery systems *(continued)*

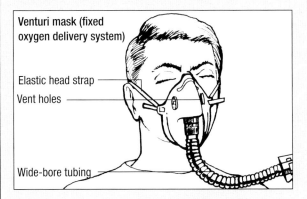

Venturi mask (fixed
oxygen delivery system)

Elastic head strap

Vent holes

Wide-bore tubing

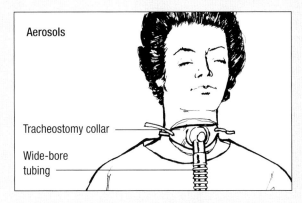

Aerosols

Tracheostomy collar

Wide-bore
tubing

The mask is connected to a Venturi device, which mixes a specific volume of air and oxygen. It delivers a highly accurate oxygen concentration despite the patient's respiratory pattern, hence it is a fixed oxygen delivery system.

A face mask, hood, tent or tracheostomy tube or collar is connected to wide-bore tubing that receives aerosolized oxygen from a jet nebulizer. It delivers high-humidity oxygen.

How you do it

- Follow standard infection control practices throughout the procedure.
- Introduce yourself to the patient as necessary, explain the procedure in order to gain permission and compliance, provide privacy and maintain dignity by closing bed curtains or requesting the patient come to the treatment room.
- Confirm the patient's identity by asking his name and date of birth, while checking the name, date of birth and hospital number on his wristband and the MAR.
- Ask the patient if he has any allergies and check that allergy documentation on the MAR is completed. Do not administer drugs if this is not completed—follow local policy to determine your actions in this situation.
- Assess the patient's condition (see A–G of assessment, Chapter 2). In an emergency situation, verify that he has an open airway before administering oxygen.

Safety first

- Check the patient's room to make sure it's safe for oxygen administration. Whenever possible, replace electrical devices with non-electric ones. (See *Caution: Oxygen in use*.)
- Help place the oxygen delivery device on the patient. Make sure it fits properly and is stable.

Measure your success

- Monitor the patient's response to oxygen therapy. Check his oxygen saturation levels continuously in an emergency and regularly as determined by the 'track and trigger system' in place in longer-term therapy. ABG values will be taken by an appropriately trained and competent person (doctor or advanced nurse practitioner) during initial adjustments of oxygen flow. Check the patient frequently for signs and symptoms of hypoxia, such as a decreased level of consciousness, increased heart rate, arrhythmias, restlessness, perspiration, dyspnoea, use of accessory muscles, yawning or flared nostrils, cyanosis and cool, clammy skin, and act upon your findings.
- Observe the patient's skin integrity to prevent skin breakdown on pressure points from the oxygen delivery device. Wipe moisture or perspiration from the patient's face and from the mask, as needed.

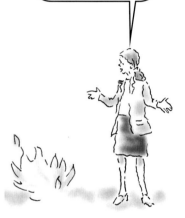

Hey! Oxygen is highly flammable. Use non-electric devices and make sure no one smokes.

Home care connection

Home oxygen therapy

If your patient will receive oxygen therapy after discharge, make sure he's familiar with the types of oxygen therapy and the services available. Together with the doctor and patient, help choose the device that's best suited to the patient. Remember to refer your patient to the oxygen at home service (if available) or the Primary Care Trust (they will ensure everything is set up), before the patient goes home.

If the patient will be receiving transtracheal oxygen therapy, teach him how to clean and care for the catheter. Advise him to keep the skin around the insertion site clean and dry to prevent infection.

Safety and supplies

No matter which device the patient uses, you'll need to evaluate his and his caregivers' ability and motivation to administer oxygen therapy at home. Make sure they understand the reason the patient is receiving oxygen and the safety issues involved. Teach them how to properly use and clean the equipment and supplies. Teach them about the safety issues too—no smoking around oxygen, no using aerosols either, what to do if they run out of oxygen, how to read the meter on the cylinder.

Ages and stages

Caution: Oxygen in use

If a child is receiving oxygen through an oxygen mist tent, remove all toys that may produce a spark, including those that are battery powered. Oxygen supports combustion, and the smallest spark can cause a fire.

Practice pointers

• Always administer oxygen (even without a prescription) in an emergency when the signs and symptoms of hypoxia are present, and use a non-rebreath mask.

• Never administer oxygen by nasal cannula at more than 4 LPM as it can be painful and uncomfortable for the patient.

• When monitoring a patient's response to a change in oxygen flow, check the pulse oximetry monitor values 20–30 minutes after adjusting the flow. In the interim, monitor the patient closely for an adverse response to the change in oxygen flow.

• Teaching and planning for home oxygen therapy should begin as soon as possible. (See *Home oxygen therapy* and *Documenting oxygen administration*.)

Per rectum (PR) medications

A rectal suppository is a small, solid, medicated mass that may be inserted to stimulate peristalsis or defecation; relieve pain, vomiting, or local irritation; reduce pyrexia; or induce relaxation. Rectal suppositories melt at body temperature and are absorbed slowly. They may be used when the medication interacts poorly with digestive enzymes, the patient is nil by mouth or because the medication has a taste too offensive for oral use.

An ointment is a semi-solid medication used to produce local effects. It may be applied externally to the anus or internally to the rectum. Rectal ointments commonly contain drugs that reduce inflammation or relieve pain and itching.

What you need

Rectal suppository or tube of ointment and applicator ✳ patient's MAR ✳ gloves ✳ water-soluble lubricant ✳ 10 cm × 10 cm gauze pads ✳ optional: bedpan, protective bed liner, stool chart.

Dispensing the drug

Store rectal suppositories in the refrigerator until needed to prevent softening and decreased effectiveness. A softened suppository is also difficult to handle and insert.

• For each suppository or ointment pre check that the direction is safe (see MAR safety check section at the beginning of this chapter). Wash your hands.

- If you do not know the indications, therapeutic dose, common side effects, cautions or effects for any of the medications, check this information in the BNF before you administer the drug; remember, you are accountable for administering it!
- If you are unaware of the patient's medical plan, nursing plan, past medical history or reason for admission, do not administer the medication—find out first!
- For each drug being administered, check you have the correct medication to administer, by checking the labelling on both the outer and inner packaging for dose, route and expiry date information, to prevent administering the wrong drug or dose.
- Make sure the medication is labelled for the PR route.

How you do it

- Follow standard infection control practices throughout the procedure.
- Introduce yourself to the patient as necessary and gain permission and compliance, provide privacy and maintain dignity by closing bed curtains or requesting the patient come to the treatment room.
- Confirm the patient's identity by asking his name and date of birth, while checking the name, date of birth and hospital number and bed number on his wristband and the MAR.
- Ask the patient if he has any allergies and check that allergy documentation on the MAR is completed. Do not administer drugs if this is not completed—follow local policy to determine your actions in this situation.
- Explain the procedure and the purpose of the medication to the patient and provide privacy and ensure as required that a commode or toilet is accessible.
- Wash your hands.

Position the patient and perform a DRE

- Place the patient on his left side with his knees drawn up towards his chest as far as possible. Drape him with the bedcovers to expose only the buttocks.
- If the indication of the medication is to empty the rectum, perform a digital rectal examination (DRE) with your gloved finger covered in lubricating jelly to ascertain whether the rectum is empty or full. If the rectum is empty, do not administer the medication as it is not required and will cause unnecessary distress, discomfort or pain.

Inserting a rectal suppository

- Put on gloves, remove the suppository from its wrapper, and lubricate it with water-soluble lubricant.
- Lift the patient's upper buttock with your non-dominant hand and have him take slow deep breaths.

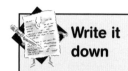

Write it down

Documenting use of rectal medications

On the patient's medicines administration record, document:

- drug administration (by signing)
- any drug refusal, reason and your actions
- date and time
- patient's reaction
- the result from laxative medications in the patient's nursing care plan or stool chart.

If the patient refuses a drug, document the refusal and notify the charge nurse and the patient's doctor, as needed. Also note if a drug was omitted or withheld for other reasons, for example empty rectum at point of DRE.

Here's the tough part

- Using your index finger, insert the suppository—blunt end first —about 7.6 cm, until you feel it pass the internal anal sphincter. Try to direct the blunt end toward the side of the rectum so that it contacts the membranes.
- Encourage the patient to retain the suppository for the appropriate length of time to be effective, retention is assisted by inserting the blunt end first.
- Give him the call bell and encourage him to call you should he require your assistance.
- Remove and discard your gloves and dispose of them as per local policy.
- Go back and check upon your patient regularly.
- Document administration. (See *Documenting use of rectal medications.*)

Applying rectal ointment

- Put on gloves and squeeze the directed amount of ointment slowly on to a gauze pad or your gloved hand and apply externally over the anal area.
- To apply internally, attach the applicator to the tube of ointment and coat the applicator with water-soluble lubricant.
- Lift the patient's upper buttock with your non-dominant hand to expose the anus and have him take several deep breaths through his mouth to relax the anal sphincters and reduce anxiety or discomfort during insertion.
- Gently insert the applicator, directing it toward the umbilicus, and slowly squeeze the tube to inject about 2.5 cm of the medication.
- Remove the applicator and place a folded 10 cm × 10 cm gauze pad between the patient's buttocks to absorb excess ointment.
- Detach the applicator from the tube and recap it. Then clean the applicator thoroughly with soap and warm water.

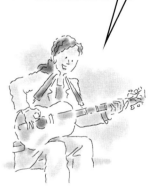

Do you know any good songs about rectal suppositories?

Practice pointers

- Because insertion of a rectal suppository may stimulate the vagus nerve, this procedure is contraindicated in patients with potential cardiac arrhythmias. It may have to be avoided in patients with recent rectal or prostate surgery because of the risk of local trauma or discomfort during insertion.

Mind the blinking light

- Make sure the patient's call button is handy, and watch for his signal because he may be unable to suppress the urge to defecate.
- Be sure to inform the patient that the suppository may discolour his next bowel movement. (See *Documenting use of rectal medications.*)

Enema administration

Enema administration involves instilling a solution into the rectum and colon. In a retention enema, the patient holds the solution within the rectum or colon for 30 minutes to 1 hour. In an irrigating enema, the patient expels the solution almost completely within 15 minutes. Both types of enema stimulate peristalsis by mechanically distending the colon and stimulating rectal wall nerves.

Enem-ies

Enemas are contraindicated, however, after recent colon or rectal surgery or myocardial infarction, and in a patient with an acute abdominal condition of unknown origin (such as suspected appendicitis). They should be administered cautiously to a patient with an arrhythmia.

What you need

The medicated solution ✳ enema administration bag with attached rectal tube and clamp ✳ I.V. pole ✳ gloves ✳ bed protector pads ✳ optional: bedpan with cover or bedside commode ✳ water-soluble lubricant ✳ toilet tissue ✳ clinical waste bag ✳ water ✳ washcloth ✳ soap and water.

Pre-packaged disposable enema sets are available, as are small-volume enema solutions in both irrigating and retention types.

Dispensing the drug

• Check the direction is safe (see MAR safety check section at the beginning of this chapter). Wash your hands.
• If you do not know the indications, therapeutic dose, common side effects, cautions or effects for any of the medications, check this information in the BNF before you administer the drug; remember, you are accountable for administering it!
• If you are unaware of the patient's medical plan, nursing plan, past medical history or reason for admission, do not administer the medication—find out first!
• For each drug being administered, check you have the correct medication to administer, by checking the labelling on both the outer and inner packaging for dose, route and expiry date information, to prevent administering the wrong drug or dose.
• Make sure the medication is labelled for the PR route.
• Prepare the prescribed type and amount of solution, as indicated. The standard volume of an irrigating enema for an adult is 750–1,000 ml. For an adult, warm the solution to 37.8°C to reduce patient discomfort.

Working toward the right solution

If preparing an irrigating enema, clamp the tubing and fill the solution bag with the prescribed solution. Unclamp the tubing, flush the solution through the tubing, and then reclamp it. Flushing detects leaks and removes air that could cause discomfort if introduced into the colon. Hang the solution container on the I.V. pole and take all supplies to the patient's room.

How you do it

- Follow standard infection control practices throughout the procedure.
- Introduce yourself to the patient as necessary, explain the procedure and the purpose of the medication, gain permission and compliance, provide privacy and maintain dignity by closing bed curtains or requesting the patient come to the treatment room.
- Confirm the patient's identity by asking his name and date of birth, while checking the name, date of birth and hospital number on his wristband and the MAR.
- Ask the patient if he has any allergies and check that allergy documentation on the MAR is completed. Do not administer drugs if this is not complete—follow local policy to determine your actions in this situation.
- Ensure that a commode or toilet is accessible, as required.
- Instruct the patient to breathe through his mouth to relax the anal sphincter, which will ease catheter insertion.
- Wash your hands and put on gloves. If there's a chance you could become soiled, put on a gown.
- Assist the patient into left-lateral position. This will facilitate the solution's flow by gravity into the descending colon. If contraindicated, or if the patient reports discomfort, reposition him on his right side.

Prep procedures

- Place bed protector pads under the patient's buttocks to prevent soiling the linen.
- Have a bedpan or commode nearby for the patient to use. If the patient can use the bathroom, make sure that it will be available when the patient needs it. Have toilet tissue within the patient's reach.
- If not pre-lubricated by the manufacturer, lubricate the distal tip of the rectal catheter with water-soluble lubricant to facilitate rectal insertion and reduce irritation.

Contraction reaction

- Separate the patient's buttocks and perform digital rectal examination (DRE) with a lubricated finger to ascertain the necessity of a laxative enema; if the rectum is empty, do not

Disconnect the tubing from the solution container, place the distal end in the bedpan, and reinsert the rectal end into the patient's anus. If gravity fails to drain the solution into the bedpan, instil 30–50 ml of warm water (40.6°C) for an adult. Then quickly direct the distal end of the tube into the bedpan. In both cases, measure the return to make sure all of the solution has drained.

• If the doctor orders enemas until returns are clear, give no more than three to avoid excessive irritation of the rectal mucosa. Notify the doctor if the returned fluid isn't clear after three administrations. (See *Documenting enema administration*.)

Per vagina (PV) medications

Vaginal medications include suppositories, creams, gels and ointments. These medications can be inserted as a topical treatment for infection or inflammation or as a contraceptive. Vaginal medications usually come with a disposable applicator and are most effective when the patient can lie down afterward to retain the medication.

What you need

Patient's MAR ✳ prescribed medication and applicator, if necessary ✳ water-soluble lubricant ✳ gloves ✳ small sanitary pad.

Dispensing the drug

• Check the direction is safe (see MAR safety check section at the beginning of this chapter). Wash your hands.

• If you do not know the indications, therapeutic dose, common side effects, cautions or effects for any of the medications, check this information in the BNF before you administer the drug; remember, you are accountable for administering it!

• If you are unaware of the patient's medical plan, nursing plan, past medical history or reason for admission, do not administer the medication—find out first!

• For each drug being administered, check you have the correct medication to administer, by checking the labelling on both the outer and inner packaging for dose, route and expiry date information, to prevent administering the wrong drug or dose.

• Make sure the medication is labelled for the PV route.

• If possible, plan to insert vaginal medications at bedtime, when the patient is recumbent.

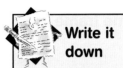

Write it down

Documenting enema administration

If you have administered an enema, be sure to record:

• date and time of administration
• type and amount of solution administered
• equipment used
• retention time
• approximate amount returned
• colour, consistency and amount of the return
• abnormalities within the return
• complications.

How you do it

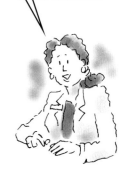

Give vaginal medications at bedtime, when the patient will be lying down.

- Follow standard infection control practices throughout the procedure.
- Introduce yourself to the patient as necessary, explain the procedure and the purpose of the medication, gain permission and compliance, provide privacy and maintain dignity by closing bed curtains or requesting the patient come to the treatment room.
- Confirm the patient's identity by asking her name and date of birth, while checking the name, date of birth and hospital number on her wristband and the MAR.
- Ask the patient if she has any allergies and check that allergy documentation on the MAR is completed. Do not administer drugs if this is not complete—follow local policy to determine your actions in this situation.
- Wash your hands.
- Ask the patient to void.
- Ask the patient if she would rather insert the medication herself. If so, provide appropriate instructions.
- Help her into the lithotomy position and expose only the perineum.

Inserting a suppository
- Remove the suppository from the wrapper, and lubricate it with water-soluble lubricant.
- Put on gloves and expose the vagina.
- With an applicator or the forefinger of your free hand, insert the suppository about 5 cm into the vagina.

Inserting ointments, creams or gels
- Insert the plunger into the applicator. Then attach the applicator to the tube of medication.
- Gently squeeze the tube to fill the applicator with the prescribed amount of medication, detach the applicator from the tube, and lubricate the applicator.
- Put on gloves and expose the vagina.
- Insert the applicator as you would a small suppository, and administer the medication by depressing the plunger on the applicator.

When you're done
- Remove and discard your gloves. Dispose of the applicator in the clinical waste and wash your hands.
- Document administration. (See *Documenting vaginal medication administration*.)
- Observe the patient for adverse effects.

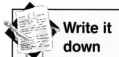

Write it down

Documenting vaginal medication administration

On the patient's medicines administration record, document:

- drug administration (by signing)
- any drug refusal, reason and your actions
- date and time
- patient's reaction.

Practice pointers

• Refrigerate vaginal suppositories that melt at room temperature.
• To prevent the medication from soiling the patient's clothing and bedding, provide a sanitary pad.
• Help the patient return to a comfortable position, and advise her to remain in bed as much as possible for the next several hours.

For the do-it-yourself type

• If possible, teach the patient how to insert the vaginal medication because she may have to administer it herself after discharge. Give her a patient-teaching sheet if one is available.
• Instruct the patient not to wear a tampon after inserting vaginal medication and also to avoid sexual intercourse during treatment.

Injection routes: subcutaneous (S.C.) injection

Subcutaneous (S.C.) injections are delivered into the adipose (fatty) tissues beneath the skin. The result is a slower and more sustained drug administration than I.M. injections. There's also less trauma to tissue and less risk of striking large blood vessels and nerves. Drugs and solutions are injected through short needles; common sites are the upper arms, anterior thigh, abdomen, upper hips, buttocks and upper back. (See *Subcutaneous injection sites.*)

What you need

Patient's MAR ✳ prescribed medication ✳ 25G (orange) needle ✳ gloves ✳ 1 ml or 3 ml syringe ✳ sharps container.

Dispensing the medication

• Check the direction is safe (see MAR safety check section at the beginning of this chapter). Wash your hands.
• If you do not know the indications, therapeutic dose, common side effects, cautions or effects for any of the medications, check this information in the BNF before you administer the drug; remember, you are accountable for administering it!
• If you are unaware of the patient's medical plan, nursing plan, past medical history or reason for admission, do not administer the medication—find out first!

Subcutaneous injection sites

Potential subcutaneous (S.C.) injection sites (indicated by the dotted areas) include the fat pads on the abdomen, upper hips, upper back, and lateral upper arms and thighs.

Preferred injection sites for insulin are the arms, abdomen, thighs and buttocks. For enoxiparin, the preferred injection site is the lower abdominal fat pad, just below the umbilicus.

If repeated, rotate

For S.C. injections administered repeatedly, such as insulin and enoxaparin, rotate sites. Choose one injection site in one area, move to a corresponding injection site in the next area, and so on. When returning to an area, choose a new site in that area.

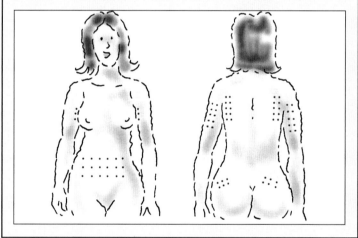

- For each drug being administered, check you have the correct medication to administer, by checking the labelling on both the outer and inner packaging for dose, route and expiry date information, to prevent administering the wrong drug or dose. Also check the medication for colour and clarity.
- Make sure the medication is labelled for the S.C. route.
- Chose equipment appropriate to the prescribed medication and injection site, and make sure it works properly.

If you use ampoules . . .

- Wrap an alcohol pad or piece of gauze around the ampoule's neck and snap off the top, directing the force away from your body.
- Attach a filter needle or 25G needle to the syringe and, using the non-touch technique, withdraw the medication.

- Tap the syringe to clear air from it.
- Before discarding the ampoule, again check the medication label against the patient's medication record, then discard the filter needle and the ampoule.
- Attach the appropriate sterile needle to the syringe.

But for vials . . .

- Reconstitute powdered drugs according to instructions, making sure all crystals have dissolved in the solution.
- Warm the vial by rolling it between your palms to help the drug dissolve faster.
- Wipe the stopper with a 70% alcohol pad and draw up the prescribed amount of medication.
- Read the medication label as you select the medication, as you draw it up, and after you've drawn it up, to verify the correct dosage.

How you do it

- Follow standard infection control procedures throughout administration and preparation.
- Introduce yourself to the patient as necessary, explain the procedure and the purpose of the medication, gain permission and compliance, provide privacy and maintain dignity by closing bed curtains or requesting the patient come to the treatment room.
- Confirm the patient's identity by asking his name and date of birth whilst checking the name, date of birth and hospital number on his wristband and the MAR.
- Ask the patient if they have any allergies and check allergy documentation on the MAR is completed, do not administer drugs if this is not complete—follow local policy to determine your actions in this situation
- Select an appropriate injection site and rotate sites for repeated injections, using different areas of the body unless contraindicated.
- Position and drape the patient.
- Clean the injection site if necessary with water, beginning at the centre of the site and moving outward in a circular motion. Allow the skin to dry.

Grasp and lift

- Loosen the protective needle sheath. With your non-dominant hand, grasp the skin around the injection site firmly to elevate the subcutaneous tissue.
- Holding the syringe in your dominant hand, insert the loosened needle sheath between the fourth and fifth fingers of your other hand while still pinching the skin around the injection site. Pull back the syringe with your dominant hand to uncover the needle.

Technique for subcutaneous injections

Before giving the injection, elevate subcutaneous tissue at the site by grasping it firmly. Insert the needle at a 90-degree angle to the skin surface, depending on needle length and the amount of subcutaneous tissue at the site. Most medications, such as enoxaparin and insulin, should always be injected at a 90-degree angle.

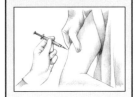

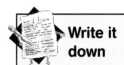

- Position the needle with its bevel up and tell the patient he'll feel a sharp scratch.
- Insert the needle quickly in one motion at a 90-degree angle. (See *Technique for subcutaneous injections*.)

Check and inject

- Inject drug.
- After injection, remove the needle gently but quickly at the same angle used for insertion, immediatly dispose of needle and syringe as one unit in the sharps bin.
- Check the site for bleeding and bruising, do not massage.

Practice pointers

- Never use medication that's cloudy or discoloured or contains a precipitate, unless the manufacturer's instructions allow it. If in doubt, check with the pharmacist.
- Prepared doses of subcutaneous medication will usually have an air bubble in the syringe—do not expel this air—it will rise to the top of the syringe when the syringe is inverted, thus ensuring the entire dose of medication is administered, the air pocket will remain in the needle.
- To avoid needle-stick injuries, don't re-sheath the needle and dispose of needle and syringe as one single unit immediately in the sharps bin.

Helpful hints

- The preferred site for heparin or anticoagulant injections is the lower abdominal fat pad, 5 cm beneath the umbilicus, between the right and left iliac crests.
- When injecting heparin or enoxaparin, leave the needle in place for 10 seconds, and then withdraw it; apply ice for 5 minutes if the patient bruises easily. Also, to prevent haemorrhages and bruising, don't rub or massage the site after the injection. (See *Documenting subcutaneous injection*.)

> **Write it down**
>
> ## Document-ing sub-cutaneous injection
>
> On the patient's medicines administration record, document:
>
> - drug administration (by signing)
> - any drug refusal, reason and your actions
> - date and time
> - patient's reaction. If the patient refuses a drug, document the refusal and notify the charge nurse and the patient's doctor, as needed. Also note if a drug was omitted or withheld for other reasons, or if, in your judgement, the drug was contraindicated at that point in time.

Injection routes: intramuscular (I.M.) injection

Intramuscular (I.M.) injections deposit medication deep into muscle tissue. This route of administration provides rapid systemic action and absorption of relatively large doses (up to 5 ml in appropriate sites).

I.M. injections are recommended for patients who can't take medication orally and for drugs that are altered by digestive juices. Because muscle tissue has few sensory nerves, I.M. injection allows less painful administration of irritating drugs.

What you need

Patient's MAR ✳ prescribed medication ✳ diluent (if required) ✳ 3 ml or 5 ml syringe ✳ 25G needle or filter needle for drawing up and 22–25G needle for administration ✳ gloves ✳ 70% alcohol pad ✳ gauze.

The prescribed medication must be sterile and the needle may be packaged separately or already attached to the syringe. Needles used for I.M. injections are longer than subcutaneous needles because they must reach deep into the muscle. Needle length also depends on the injection site, patient's size, and amount of subcutaneous fat covering the muscle. The needle gauge for I.M. injections should be larger to accommodate viscous solutions and suspensions.

I told you that injection might hurt a little bit.

Dispensing the drug

• Check the direction is safe (see MAR safety check section at the beginning of this chapter). Wash your hands.
• If you do not know the indications, therapeutic dose, common side effects, cautions or effects for any of the medications, check this information in the BNF before you administer the drug; remember, you are accountable for administering it!
• If you are unaware of the patient's medical plan, nursing plan, past medical history or reason for admission, do not administer the medication—find out first!
• For each drug being administered, check you have the correct medication to administer, by checking the labelling on both the outer and inner packaging for dose, route and expiry date information, to prevent administering the wrong drug or dose. Also check the medication for colour and clarity.
• Make sure the medication is labelled for the I.M. route.
• Chose equipment appropriate to the prescribed medication and injection site, and make sure it works properly.

For single-dose ampoules

- If using a glass ampoule, either use an ampoule opening device or wrap an alcohol pad around the ampoule's neck and snap off the top, directing the force away from your body.
- Attach a filter needle or 15G needle to the syringe and withdraw the medication.
- Tap the syringe to clear air from it.
- Before discarding the ampoule in the sharps bin, check the medication label against the patient's medication record, then discard the filter needle and the ampoule.
- Attach the appropriate needle for administration to the syringe using a non-touch technique.

For single-dose or multi-dose vials

- Reconstitute powdered drugs according to instructions, making sure all crystals have dissolved in the solution.
- Warm the vial by rolling it between your palms to help the drug dissolve faster.
- Wipe the stopper with a 70% alcohol pad, allow the alcohol to dry and then draw up the prescribed amount of medication (use Stock dose calculation).

How you do it

- Follow standard infection control practices throughout the procedure.
- Introduce yourself to the patient as necessary, explain the procedure and the purpose of the medication, gain permission and compliance, provide privacy and maintain dignity by closing bed curtains or requesting the patient come to the treatment room.
- Confirm the patient's identity by asking his name and date of birth, while checking the name, date of birth and hospital number on his wristband and the MAR.
- Ask the patient if he has any allergies and check that allergy documentation on the MAR is completed. Do not administer drugs if this is not complete—follow local policy to determine your actions in this situation.
- Put on gloves.
- Select an appropriate injection site. The gluteal muscles (gluteus medius and minimus and the upper outer corner of the gluteus maximus) are used most commonly used for healthy adults, although the deltoid muscle may be used for a small-volume injection (2 ml or less). Remember to rotate injection sites for patients who require repeated injections.

- Position and drape the patient appropriately, making sure the site is well exposed and that lighting is adequate.
- Loosen the protective needle sheath, but don't remove it.

Knock before entering

- After selecting the injection site, clean the skin at the site with a 70% alcohol pad in a circular motion to a circumference of about 5 cm from the injection site, and allow the skin to dry.
- With the thumb and index finger of your non-dominant hand, gently stretch the skin of the injection site taut (see Z track technique, below).
- While you hold the syringe in your dominant hand, remove the needle sheath by slipping it between the free fingers of your non-dominant hand and then drawing back the syringe.

> No need for speed. A slow, steady injection rate is best for I.M. administration.

Go deep

- Position the syringe at a 70- to 90-degree angle to the skin surface, with the needle a few inches from the skin. Tell the patient that he'll feel a 'sharp scratch' as you insert the needle. Then quickly and firmly exercise control and insert the needle through the skin and subcutaneous tissue, deep into the muscle.
- Support the syringe with your non-dominant hand, if desired. Pull back slightly on the plunger with your dominant hand to aspirate for blood. (See *I.M. injection complications.*) If no blood appears, slowly inject the medication into the muscle. A slow, steady injection rate allows the muscle to distend gradually and accept the medication under minimal pressure. You should feel little or no resistance against the force of the injection.
- After the injection, wait for several seconds to facilitate absorbtion of the drug then gently but quickly remove the needle at the same angle that you inserted and release the skin from your other hand. Apply pressure with gauze for 30 seconds, to stop bleeding and prevent haematoma formation.
- Dispose of the needle and syringe as one unit in the sharps bin.

Post-action rubdown

- Using a gloved hand, cover the injection site immediately with the gauze, apply gentle pressure.
- Remove the gauze and inspect the injection site for signs of active bleeding or bruising. If bleeding continues, apply pressure to the site.
- Watch for adverse reactions at the site for 10–30 minutes after the injection.

- Discard all equipment according to standard infection control precautions and your local policy. Don't re-sheath needles; dispose of them in an appropriate sharps container to avoid needle-stick injuries.

Practice pointers

- Never use medication that's cloudy or discoloured or contains a precipitate, unless the manufacturer's instructions allow it. If in doubt, check with the pharmacist.
- I.M. injections shouldn't be administered at inflamed, oedematous, sensitive or irritated sites, or at sites that contain moles, birthmarks, scar tissue or other lesions, and areas that twitch.
- The use of alcohol to prepare the skin before injection is argued within research and literature. It is advisable to check and follow local policy.

Stop the music

- I.M. injections may be contraindicated in patients with impaired coagulation mechanisms, occlusive peripheral vascular disease or oedema.

Heavy rotation

- Keep a rotation record that lists all available injection sites, divided into various body areas. Rotate from a site in the first area to a site in each of the other areas. Then return to a site in the first area that's at least 2.5 cm away from the previous injection site in that area.
- If you must inject more than 5 ml of solution, divide the solution and inject it at two separate sites.
- Dosage adjustments are usually necessary when changing from the I.M. route to the oral route. (See *Documenting I.M. injection*.)

Write it down

Documenting I.M. injection

On the patient's medicines administration record, document:

- drug administration (by signing)
- any drug refusal, reason and your actions
- date and time
- injection site
- patient's tolerance of the injection
- drug effects, including adverse reactions.

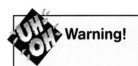 **Warning!**

I.M. injection complications

If blood appears in the syringe on aspiration, the needle is in a blood vessel. Stop the injection, withdraw the needle, prepare another injection with new equipment, and inject another site. Don't inject the bloody solution.

If you miss

Accidentally injecting concentrated or irritating medications into subcutaneous tissue, or other areas where they can't be fully absorbed, can cause sterile abscesses. Failing to rotate sites in patients who require repeated injections may lead to deposits of unabsorbed medications. Such deposits can reduce the desired pharmacological effect and cause abscess formation or tissue fibrosis.

Z-track technique

The Z-track method of intramuscular (I.M.) injection prevents leakage of irritating and discolouring medications into the subcutaneous tissue. It should always be used. Lateral displacement of the skin during the injection helps to seal the drug in the muscle. (See *Displacing the skin for Z-track injection*.)

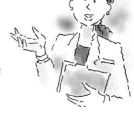

It's a low-tech solution, but ice works well for numbing sore injection sites.

Nasogastric (NG) tube route

A nasogastric (NG) tube or gastrostomy tube allows direct instillation of medication into the GI system of patients who can't ingest the drug orally. Before instilling the drug, you must check the patency and positioning of the tube. Oily medications and enteric-coated or sustained-release tablets or capsules are contraindicated for instillation through an NG tube.

What you need

Patient's MAR and fluid chart ✳ prescribed medication ✳ paper towel or gauze pads ✳ 2 × 50 or 60 ml catheter-tip syringe ✳ feeding tubing ✳ gloves ✳ diluent ✳ cup for mixing medication and fluid ✳ spoon ✳ 60 ml of water.

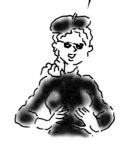

Dig this: The Z-track method is a cool way to prevent leakage into S.C. tissue.

Dispensing the drug

• Check the direction is safe (see MAR safety check section at the beginning of this chapter). Wash your hands.
• If you do not know the indications, therapeutic dose, common side effects, cautions or effects for any of the medications, check this information in the BNF before you administer the drug; remember, you are accountable for administering it!
• If you are unaware of the patient's medical plan, nursing plan, past medical history or reason for admission, do not administer the medication—find out first!
• For each drug being administered, check you have the correct medication to administer, by checking the labelling on both the outer and inner packaging for dose, route and expiry date information, to prevent administering the wrong drug or dose. Also check liquid medication for colour and clarity.

Displacing the skin for Z-track injection

Discomfort and tissue irritation may result from drug leakage into subcutaneous tissue. Displacing the skin helps prevent these problems.

Why do it

By blocking the needle pathway after an injection, the Z-track technique allows I.M. injection while minimizing the risk of subcutaneous irritation and staining from drugs such as iron dextran. The illustrations below show how to perform a Z-track injection.

How to do it

To begin, place your finger on the skin surface, and pull the skin and subcutaneous layers out of alignment with the underlying muscle. You should move the skin about 1 cm.

Insert the needle at a 90-degree angle at the site where you initially placed your finger. Inject the drug and withdraw the needle.

Finally, remove your finger from the skin surface, letting the layers return to normal. The needle track (shown by the dotted line) is now broken at the junction of each tissue layer, trapping the drug in the muscle.

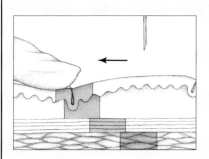
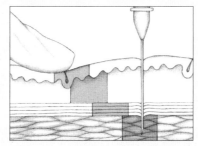
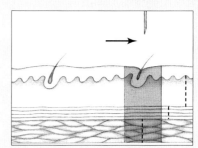

How you do it

- Gather all necessary equipment at the bedside. Liquids should be at room temperature so abdominal cramping doesn't occur.
- Follow standard infection control practices throughout the procedure.
- Introduce yourself to the patient as necessary, explain the procedure and the purpose of the medication, gain permission and compliance, provide privacy and maintain dignity by closing bed curtains or door of the individual patient room.
- Confirm the patient's identity by asking his name and date of birth, while checking the name, date of birth and hospital number on his wristband and the MAR.

- Ask the patient if he has any allergies and check that allergy documentation on the MAR is completed. Do not administer drugs if this is not complete—follow local policy to determine your actions in this situation.

Liquid don't crush

- Request liquid forms of medications, if available. However, if the prescribed medication is in effervescent tablet form, dilute them with liquid and bring the medication and equipment to the patient's bedside.
- Unpin the tube from the patient's gown and drape his chest with a paper towel or napkin.
- Elevate the head of the bed to a 30- to 45-degree angle, as tolerated.
- Clamp the tube, detach the feeding tube, and lay the end of the tube on the gauze pad, to keep it clean—this is not a sterile procedure—it is a clean procedure.

Flush, give, flush

- Draw up 30 ml of clean water in one of the 50 ml syringes, attach the syringe to the end of the tube and open the clamp.
- Deliver the water slowly and steadily to ensure patency of the tube and prevent overdose.
- Clamp the tube and draw up the medications in the other 50 ml syringe.
- Attach the syringe containing the medication to the tube, unclamp the tube and administer slowly and steadily, then re-clamp.
- If the patient does not have a nasogastric feed in progress, draw up a further 30 ml of clean water and repeat the first step again, ensuring that all medication has been administered and is not left in the tube. If you stopped a feed to administer the medication, attach it again and recommence the feed as directed in the patient's MAR.

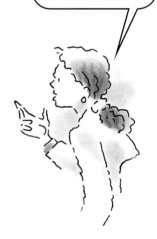

Slow and steady—that's the rule when delivering drugs through an NG tube.

How goes the flow?

- If the medication flows smoothly, slowly add more until the entire dose has been given. If the medication doesn't flow properly, don't force it. If you suspect that tube placement is inhibiting the flow, stop the procedure and re-evaluate tube placement.
- Watch the patient's reaction throughout the instillation. If he shows any sign of discomfort, stop the procedure immediately.
- Fasten the NG tube to the patient's gown, remove the towel or napkin, and replace linen as necessary.

• Document administration. (See *Documenting administration of NG route medications*.)

No time to lie down

• Leave the patient at a 30- to 45-degree angle, or have him lie on his right side with the head of the bed partially elevated for at least 30 minutes to facilitate flow and prevent oesophageal reflux.

Practice pointers

• The procedure is contraindicated if the tube is obstructed or improperly positioned, if the patient is vomiting around the tube, or if his bowel sounds are absent.

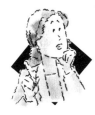

Quick quiz

1. Before instilling eye drops, you should instruct the patient to look:
    A.   Up and away.
    B.   Down and away.
    C.   Straight ahead.
Answer: A. Before instilling eye drops, instruct the patient to look up and away to minimize the risk of touching the cornea with the dropper.

2. You must straighten the patient's ear canal before instilling eardrops. How do you accomplish this in an adult patient?
    A.   Pull the auricle of the ear up and back.
    B.   Pull the auricle of the ear down and back.
    C.   Pull the auricle of the ear up and forward.
Answer: A. To straighten the ear canal of an adult, pull the auricle up and back; for an infant or young child, gently pull down and back.

3. After giving the patient his medication through a nasogastric (NG) tube, you should leave the head of his bed elevated for:
    A.   15 minutes.
    B.   30 minutes.
    C.   60 minutes.
Answer: B. After administering medication through an NG tube, leave the head of his bed elevated for at least 30 minutes.

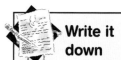

Write it down

Documenting administration of NG route medications

On the patient's medicines administration record, document:

• drug administration (by signing)
• any drug refusal, reason and your actions
• date and time.
  On the intake and output sheet, note:

• the volume of fluid instilled; remember to document the flush
• the type of fluid instilled.
  On the NG tube plan of care, document:

• date and time of procedure
• patient's tolerance of the procedure.
• patency state of the NG tube.

Guide to vitamins

Vitamin	Major functions	Food sources
B$_1$ thiamine	Appetite stimulation, blood building, carbohydrate metabolism, circulation, digestion, growth, learning ability, muscle tone and maintenance	Meat, fish, poultry, pork, brewer's yeast, brown rice, wheat germ, nuts, whole and enriched grains
B$_2$ (riboflavin)	Antibody and red blood cell formation, energy metabolism, cell respiration, epithelial, ocular and mucosal tissue maintenance	Meat, fish, poultry, milk, brewers yeast, eggs, fruit, green leafy veg, nuts, whole grains
B$_3$ (niacin)	Circulation, cholesterol level reduction, growth, hydrochloric acid production, metabolism (carbohydrates, protein and fat), sex hormone production	Eggs, lean meat, milk products, organ meat, peanuts, poultry, seafood, whole grains
B$_6$	Antibody formation, digestion, fat and protein utilization, amino acid metabolism, haemoglobin production	Meat, poultry, bananas, brewer's yeast, liver, fish, green leafy veg, peanuts, raisins, walnuts, wheat germ, whole grains
B$_{12}$	Blood cell formation, cellular and nutrient metabolism, iron absorption, tissue growth, nerve cell maintenance	Beef, eggs, fish, milk products, organ meat, pork
C (ascorbic acid)	Collagen production, digestion, fine bone and tooth formation, iodine conservation, healing, red blood cell formation, infection resistance	Fresh fruits and veg, especially citrus fruits and green leafy vegetables
Folic acid	Cell growth and reproduction, hydrochloric acid production, liver function, nucleic acid formation, protein metabolism, red blood cell formation	Citrus fruits, eggs, green leafy veg, milk products, organ meat, seafood, whole grains
Biotin	Cell growth, fatty acid production, metabolism, vitamin B utilization, skin, hair, nerve and bone marrow maintenance	Egg yolks, organ meats, whole grains, yeast, milk and seafood
A (retinol)	Body tissue repair, infection resistance, bone growth, nervous system development, cell membrane metabolism and structure	Fish, green and yellow fruits and veg, milk products
D	Calcium and phosphorus metabolism, myocardial function, nervous system maintenance, normal blood clotting	Bonemeal, egg yolks, organ meat, butter, liver oil, fatty fish
E	Ageing retardation, anticoagulation, dieresis, fertility, lung protection, muscle and nerve cell membrane maintenance, myocardial perfusion, serum cholesterol reduction	Butter, dark green veg, eggs, fruit, nuts, organ meats, vegetable oils, wheat germ
K	Liver synthesis of prothrombin and other blood clotting factors	Green leafy veg, yogurt, liver, sunflower oil

Source: *Nutrition made incredibly easy*, 2nd edn. Lippincott William & Wilkins, 2007.

Dietetic Service using the 'Malnutrition universal screening tool' (MUST) (Stratton, 2004). It should cover the following areas of questioning and physical assessment:
- Has the patient noticed any change to appetite or eating patterns recently?
- Has he avoided any foods and, if so, why? Is it due to experiencing difficulty in eating or swallowing?
- Has he suffered with any recent episodes of diarrhoea or vomiting?
- Has he lost any weight recently?

As many patients may not have actually weighed themselves recently, ask if they have noticed dentures or clothes becoming loose. Measure height and weight and calculate the body mass index (BMI). Consider the patient's past and present medical history and how these can impact upon the risk of malnutrition. From the answers received in response to these questions and physical assessments, a score can be formulated using the tool to identify patient's level of risk (relating to altered nutritional status). A care plan should then be established and implemented, specific to the individual need of the patient and may include referral to the Nutrition and Dietetic Service.

Further indicators

Malnutrition can be caused by many factors, any of which should cause you to consider the possibility of the patient requiring nutritional support and a referral to the Nutrition and Dietetic Service. These factors can be grouped into three areas:
- conditions incurring decreased nutrient intake: anorexia, dysphagia, nausea, vomiting, pain, difficulty in chewing, treatments, therapy, unconscious, neurological degeneration/disease
- conditions requiring increased nutrient intake: sepsis, trauma, burns, renal disease, wounds, liver disease, tremors
- conditions incurring increased loss of nutrients due to malabsorption: inflammatory bowel disorders, post-operative bowel surgery, fistulae, pancreatic disorders, liver disease and HIV-related illness.

From all of this information the form of additional nutritional support can be determined, as you have assessed the reason for the risk: is the patient already malnourished or is he likely to become malnourished? Plan and implement an appropriate nursing care plan if required, and remember to consider the need for a food observation chart (see *Documenting food intake*), a fluid balance chart (see *Completing a fluid balance chart* below) and possibly a referral to the nutrition team.

Write it down

Documenting food intake

When documenting and recording what the patient has eaten, it is important to be specific and include:

- the day, date and time
- the amount of each food, i.e. one teaspoon of mashed potato, half a portion of custard, four tablespoons of rice
- the effects on the patient, did he vomit?
- your name, designation and signature.

Types of diet

Diets for improving health

When caring for a patient's nutrition there are many differing types of diet you must be aware of, in order to: assist the patient to make the correct choices, assist in improving his health, and prevent deterioration of his condition. (See *Diets for health*.)

Diets for health

Diet name	Indication/aim	Description	Practice pointers
Fluid diet	Facial/oral injury or trauma	A fluid diet is thin enough to be drunk through a straw. Patients may be offered strained soup, strained custard, water, tea coffee, mild fruit juice, milky drinks as well as nutritional supplements	If the patient remains on a fluid diet for longer than 48 hours, refer to the dietician or clinical nurse specialist
Pureed/liquidized diet	Dysphagia, painful mouth and/or throat	Completely smooth food that has been pureed or liquidized so the food is still from the solid food groups. This food can be less appealing in presentation so encouragement is often required	These patients are at increased risk of nutritional deficiencies so encourage fruit juice, whole milk and at least 2 build-up drinks per day
Semi-solid or soft diet	Sore mouth or difficulty in chewing or swallowing lumps of food	Any food that can be chewed easily, e.g. mashed potato, banana, well-cooked vegetables, milk puddings, sponge and custard, ice cream	Avoid pastry, nuts, tough meats
Weight-reducing diet	Patient who is required to lose weight	Eating 3 meals per day with the correct proportions of food groups, no snacking, avoiding fried food, swapping whole milk for semi-skimmed or skimmed	Weight reduction may not be appropriate when the patient is in hospital, check with nutrition team or dieticians
Cholesterol-lowering diet	To reduce the risk of cardiac disease or prevent deterioration of cardiac disease. To improve general health	A diet low in saturated fats, reduced sugar and salt intake and an increase in fibre such as fruit, vegetables and wholegrain foods.	
Gluten-free diet	Coeliac disease or dermatitis herpetiformis	A diet that excludes wheat, rye, barley and oats	If the patient is unknown to the dietician locally, always refer on admission
Low-residue diet	Some digestive disorders	A diet low in fibre	

Adapted from the 'Ward Manual', with kind permission of the Nutrition and Dietetics Service, Waltham Forest PCT, London.

Vegetarian diets

There are three main types of vegetarians; vegan, lacto-vegetarian and lacto-ovo-vegetarian. See *Vegetarian diets* below for the different foods avoided and included in these diets.

Cultural/religious/traditional diets

Within the population of the UK today, there is enormous diversity of culture, traditions and religious beliefs. These can all influence eating habits and are therefore important for you to learn, as it is important that all patients receive food that is suitable and acceptable to them. Check with your local catering department as to how to obtain Kosher and Halal foods. See *Cultural, religious and traditional diets* below for further assistance.

> Different ethnic groups eat different diets; I must update my knowledge and not cause offence.

Vegetarian diets

	Foods included	Foods excluded
Vegan	• Soya milk and soya-based products • Quorn • Pulses • Nuts, nut butters and seeds • Cereals and grains • Fruit and vegetables	All animal flesh and animal products, including dairy and eggs
Lacto-vegetarian	• Milk and milk-based products • Vegetarian cheese • Quorn • Pulses and soya products • Nuts, nut butters and seeds • Cereals and grains • Fruit and vegetables	• Meat and poultry • Fish and shellfish • Eggs • Cheese made with animal rennet • Gelatine • Food colourings from animal sources (cochineal)
Lacto-ovo-vegetarian	As above, but includes eggs	

Adapted from the 'Ward Manual', with kind permission of the Nutrition and Dietetics Service, Waltham Forest PCT, London.

Cultural, religious and traditional diets

	Hindus	Muslims	Sikhs	Jewish	Seventh-day adventists
Meat and fish	No beef, lamb, chicken or white fish. Check with patient how strict they are as some may eat lamb, fish and chicken	No pork or products containing pork. Halal meat only. Little or no fish with fins and scales. No shellfish	No beef, little pork, some are lacto-vegetarians, but may eat chicken, lamb and fish	No pork or products containing pork. Kosher beef, lamb and poultry only. No shellfish	Often vegetarians. No pork. Only fish with fins and scales are eaten
Eggs	Not eaten by strict vegetarians	Usually eaten	Not a major part of the diet	Eaten	Eaten
Dairy	Important foods in the diet; milk, yogurt and curd cheese	Fairly important foods in the diet; milk and yogurt	Very important foods in the diet; yogurt and curd cheese (paneer)	Meat and dairy products must not be prepared, cooked or eaten together at the same meal, minimum of 3 hours before milk can be taken after eating meat. Only milk and mild products derived from Kosher species of animals (cows, lamb, etc.)	Fairly important foods in the diet; milk and yogurt
Other	No animal fats. Staples: pulses, cereals and chapattis made from flour or rice	No products containing gelatine, animal fats or emulsifiers derived from animal sources	No animal fats. Staples: pulses, cereals and chapattis made from flour or rice	All fruit and vegetables are Kosher, however some people may avoid specifics, e.g. broccoli and raspberries	Foods considered to be stimulants, e.g. tea, coffee, etc., are consumed

Adapted from the 'Ward Manual', with kind permission of the Nutrition and Dietetics Service, Waltham Forest PCT, London.

Preparing the environment and patient

Aiming for Michelin stars

Imagine you are eating out in a restaurant, café or bar; what do you expect? A clean, clutter-free and relaxing environment? Polite, efficient and friendly staff who are well presented and have knowledge of what they are serving? Hand-washing facilities? A table set with crockery, glasses, cutlery, condiments, napkins and fresh water? A choice of food on the menu, which, after ordering, arrives with you within a reasonable time frame and as it was described on the menu, i.e. hot or cold, sweet or savoury?

Patients in the hospital environment expect and should be provided with exactly these factors—after all, you could say they are 'eating out'! Therefore we should be striving to meet all of these targets.

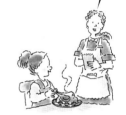

Is everything to your satisfaction madam?

Preparing the environment

The environment should be clean and clutter free. Ensure that there are no used commodes, urine bottles or specimens left in the ward or bed area; you wouldn't want to eat in a toilet environment, so why should your patients? Each patient should have a table to eat from; this could be a dining table in the ward area where patients who are fit and able can all sit together, or a single bed table by the patient's bed or chair. Whichever systems you use, ensure that the tables are cleaned down and set prior to the meal. A table should be set just as you would at home or if you were in a restaurant, with the following in easy reach of the patient: cutlery (appropriate for the patient), water, an appropriate drinking vessel, condiments (salt, if allowed, and pepper), eating aids (plate guard, etc.) and a napkin—never a plastic apron, towel or bib for an adult without their permission; would you wear any of these in a restaurant? And remember, patients look forward to meal times, when they see the environment being prepared the expectation is that it is happening soon, so don't set up too early. Think back again to the restaurant environment; you wouldn't expect to wait more than 15 minutes from ordering before receiving your starter, so 15 minutes prior to serving is a good guide to setting up. Ensure that all the equipment required to serve food is available.

Preparing yourself

Assuming that you are wearing your uniform or are dressed appropriately (cuffs above the elbow, hair off the collar, clean uniform, short well-kept nails, only a plain wedding band and stud earrings for jewellery) the following is all that is necessary. Make yourself aware of what type of diets your patients require (see Types of diet above). Know which patients require assistance with eating, are not eating or who require specific aids such as plate guards, large-handled cutlery, etc. Find out what is to be served; if you are unsure what ingredients are in a specific menu choice, find out; ask a colleague or telephone the catering department. Always ensure that you have performed hand hygiene prior to serving meals. Cover your uniform or clothes with an apron. Most hospital and care environments will advise you to wear a different colour of apron to that which you would wear to deliver clinical care, i.e. white aprons for clinical care and blue aprons for serving food. Anyone wearing a white uniform during food service could then be challenged: if they have not changed their apron between delivering clinical care and serving food, they could be putting the patient at risk.

Prepare the patient

Depending how menus are offered in your hospital, either assist the patient to complete their menu choice card the day before or inform them of what is available when the meals arrive. Advise them of what choices would be appropriate for their dietary needs in order to benefit their health, or to fit their cultural, religious or traditional beliefs. Prior to serving meals ensure that your patient has had the opportunity to meet his elimination needs and wash his hands; check the patient has his dentures in (if appropriate). Assist your patient into a suitable position to eat; to the dining table; out on to his chair by the bedside, upright in bed or on his side if he is being nursed horizontally. If your patient is not eating, offer a choice of closing bed curtains to either side, but not closing them in completely as this would be isolating.

Serving food

Hospitals in the UK use many differing systems to serve and deliver food; read and follow your local nutritional and mealtime policy and procedure document, this will have been devised in line with the Essence of Care and Benchmarking standards. However, the basic principles never change.

Basic principles of food service

Every member of nursing staff should be involved in the meal service and assistance with eating. Having 'protected patient mealtimes' mean that no staff breaks, doctors' rounds, investigations or multidisciplinary team (MDT) appointments should take place during meal times.

Rotate where you start service from, i.e. top end of the ward at breakfast, middle of the ward at lunch, far end of the ward at supper, middle of the ward for breakfast next morning, because it's not nice always being last!

If you are required to plate the food in the clinical area from a hot/cold locker, one member of staff should be in charge of the locker. She should:

• Empty the hot choices first from the hot lock on to the top of the locker, where they can be kept warm, and then the cold choices on to a cold surface (never place hot food on a cold surface or vice versa).

• Plate the meals according to the instructions taken from her colleagues who are taking orders and assisting patients.

• Know how many patients are vegetarian, require Halal or Kosher meals; ensure that these patients receive these meals and that they are not given to other patients first.

• Know what constitutes one portion and serve appropriately, so that there is enough food to go around.

• Always use a dedicated serving spoon/implement for each constituent.

• Ensure that food is not served to a patient requiring assistance until a member of staff is available, thus avoiding patients being left looking anxiously at food left for them, refusing to eat food because it is cold or actually eating foods that have gone cold.

Assisting the patient

Assisting your patient to eat, gain his nutritional requirement and enjoy his meal is a time of 1 : 1 care between you and your patient; it is not an opportunity for nursing staff to chat between themselves over the top of their patients. Concentrate and use the time to build up a rapport with your patient—you'll be amazed what you can find out! Before collecting the patient's meal from the locker, ensure that you know what foods he likes, doesn't like and has an allergy to, as well as how he normally eats, drinks, etc. Once you return with the meal make sure you are in a good position, you should be at eye level with your patient: if the patient is sitting, sit opposite him to maintain eye contact and prevent injury to your back through twisting. If the patient is sitting up in bed, elevate the bed height until the patient is at the same eye level as you, take down any bed side acting as a barrier between the patient and yourself—never lean over the top of a bedside (always raise the bed side when leaving the patient). (See *Questions to ask before, during and after feeding*.)

Questions to ask before, during and after feeding

	People eat in different ways
Do you like to eat meat and vegetables, etc. together on the fork/spoon, or do you only like one thing at a time?	Some people eat a little of different food groups in the same mouthful, some eat one thing at a time, some save their favourite until last!
How much would you like?	Before going to attain the meal from the locker, ascertain portion size. Patients can be put off by large portion sizes, give them small amounts in the first instance, you can always get them more!
Where would you like your gravy, on the meat and veg; only on the meat or at the side? Likewise with custard, condiments and sauces	Everyone likes sauces, juices and condiments on different foods, some like it on everything!
Would you like your soup in a mug or in a bowl? Would you like bread with your soup?	Many people like to enjoy a mug of soup as they find it warming; many patients can often manage a mug, whereas they cannot manage a bowl and spoon. Bread should always be offered with soup as an additional carbohydrate to aid nutrition
Do you eat with a spoon or a knife and fork?	Patients may have begun to adjust their eating habits prior to being admitted to hospital. If a patient prefers a spoon to eat, that is their choice—even if it is for meat and vegetables!
Do you usually drink before your meal, during your meal or after your meal?	Think about yourself and ask your colleagues, I'm sure you will find a mixture of all three
Between mouthfuls ask the patient, what would you like next? Offer a choice from the plate, i.e. peas, meat, potato or a mixture, or offer a drink if he told you that he drinks during his meal	Remember it is the patient who needs to enjoy his meal, not you. Never rush him and always offer him a choice
When the patient has eaten all of his plated meal, or he has informed you that he has eaten a sufficient amount, ask him: Would you like anything else? (If the answer is yes, and if it is appropriate, always ensure you fulfil this request.) Did you enjoy your meal? Was there anything you did not enjoy?	You can learn about your patient's likes and dislikes from this and also about the size of portions and meal choices he may require for future meals. Document the answers on the food chart

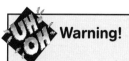

Warning!

Caution, choking

The main complication associated with feeding a patient is choking. Should your patient begin to show signs of choking (coughing, cyanosis, gasping for air, panic), then follow the United Kingdom Resuscitation Council algorithm for choking (2005):

Coughing patient
↓
Encourage cough
↓
When cough is ineffective, administer:
↓
5 back blows followed by 5 abdominal thrusts until airway is cleared, or
↓
should the patient become unconscious, commence Basic Life Support

Fluid recording: input and output

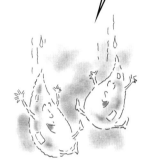

A few ml of fluid can make all the difference in fluid monitoring.

Recording your patient's fluid input and output is an essential tool to evaluate fluid balance or 'homeostasis'. Having identified that your patient is at risk of possible hypervolaemia (fluid overload) or hypovolaemia (low fluid) it is the nurse's responsibility to ensure that continuous, specific monitoring is carried out, evaluated and deficits reported as soon as possible (see *Cautions and specifics of fluid recording*). In order to do this most hospital and care settings use a fluid balance chart along with a care plan.

The care plan will be written specifically for an individual patient, having taken into account the reason why he is at risk (nil by mouth, restricted fluid intake due to cardiac aetiology, etc.), his present fluid status and the actions and care that need to be implemented by the nursing staff, i.e. daily weight, assessment of circulation (blood pressure, pulse, temperature, CVP), as well as a visual assessment (jugular vein pressure; sunken, dry eyes; skin assessment; mouth assessment). The fluid balance chart clearly identifies how much fluid the patient has taken in and has

---

Warning!

Cautions and specifics of fluid recording

When recording fluid intake and output, it is essential that you are accurate:

- Measure fluids that you give your patient to drink, never guess how much a cup holds.
- Always label I.V. lines and drains if the patient has more than one, use figures instead of 'left' and 'right', to prevent confusion.
- Always include small volumes that are administered, i.e. intravenous flush of 5 ml, PEG (percutaneous endoscopic gastrostomy) flush of 30 ml, these can accumulate rapidly and make a difference which will not be noted if you do not record them.
- You should document the minimum volume of urine to expect over the 1 hour period. Unless otherwise directed by the doctor, use the formula: 0.5 ml/kg/hour. For example, your patient weighs 100 kg therefore your sum would be 0.5 ml × 100 kg = 50 ml/hour minimum. You would report/escalate anything under this volume.

Only document fluid that has been administered. Or has been excreted. Be specific, do not guestimate; remember your patient is at risk of deterioration and you have a duty of care to your patient!

Fluid balance chart

Patient name: Complete with your patient's details   **Hospital Number:** important to complete 2nd identifier

Important Instructions: In this section add the obvious information you require, e.g. Fluid restriction 500 ml in 24 hours. Nil By Mouth, Urinary catheter on 1 hourly measurements

Date care plan started: insert the original date when the patient was identified as being at risk.

Fluid Chart from mid-day on _____ **to mid-day on** _____. Insert the date the fluid chart is being commenced and, as it is a 24 hour period beginning at mid-day, insert the next day's date too.

	Oral	IV 1	IV 2	NG/PEG	Cum Tot In	Cum Total Out	Urine	Faeces	Drain 1	Drain 2
	100	50		30	180	180	130			50
	100	50		30	360	360	130			50

Times: It is a period of 24 hours commencing from midday, therefore the first time noted on the chart is 1300 hours, all intake and output between 1200 hours and 1300 hours should be recorded along this horizontal column. Then continue for each hour. The last time noted is 1100 hours, however this shouldn't be completed until 1200 hours and will incorporate all fluid taken and fluid excreted between 1100 hours and 1200 hours.

Cumulative Totals; These columns should not be completed with hourly totals, but should be a continuous running total of how much intake and output the patient has had since the chart commenced. Look at the horizontal line for 1300 hours, you will note that the patient has taken in 100 ml of oral fluid, 50 ml of I.V. fluid and 30 ml of fluid via the parenteral route. The total of these (180) is documented in the 'cum total in' column, likewise with the output for that hour. Now look at 1400 hours, the same documentation has occurred, however the 'cum total in 'is the sum of the input for that hour + the previous' cum total' from the previous hour. This way, as the input and output totals are side by side it is easy to assess whether the patient is retaining fluid or excreting too much. (What goes in should be equal to what comes out.) This can then be acted upon hour by hour rather than waiting to the end of the 24 hour period, when reporting any deficits may be too late!

The totals section at the bottom of the chart should only be completed at 12 mid-day, it is then easier to refer back to each chart from previous days to assess the patient improvement or deterioration.

This diagram demonstrates the principles of completing a fluid balance chart. The fluid balance chart used in your local area may differ slightly, but the principles should remain unchanged.

excreted on an hour by hour basis, ensuring that any deficits can be noted quickly and appropriate actions taken. Each chart will include labelled vertical and time-specific horizontal columns to be completed and then totalled to check for the deficits. (See Completing a fluid balance chart.)

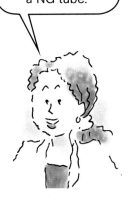

Post-surgery plans commonly include inserting a NG tube.

Nasogastric (NG) aspiration/ drainage tube insertion and removal

Inserted to decompress the stomach, an aspiration nasogastric (NG) tube prevents vomiting after major surgery. A NG tube typically is in place for 48–72 hours after surgery, by which time peristalsis usually resumes.

And that isn't all

The NG tube can also be used to assess and treat upper GI bleeding, collect gastric contents for analysis, perform gastric lavage, aspirate gastric secretions, and administer medications and nutrients (see NG feeding tube insertion and removal, below).

What you need

For NG tube insertion

Tube (usually size 12, 14, 16, or 18 French for a normal adult)
✷ towel or protective pad ✷ pen torch ✷ hypoallergenic
tape ✷ gloves and apron ✷ cup or glass of water with straw
(if appropriate) ✷ catheter-tip syringe ✷ pH indicator strips
✷ optional: ordered suction equipment, NG bung.

For NG tube removal

Gloves and apron ✷ catheter-tip syringe ✷ towel or protective pad
✷ adhesive remover ✷ optional: clamp or bung.

Getting ready

To ease insertion, increase a tube's flexibility by coiling it around
your gloved fingers for a few seconds. Check manufacturer's
instructions regarding lubrication instructions (for example, Ryles
tubes will require a lubricating jelly and others may only require that
you dip the tube into warm water to lubricate and aid insertion). It is
a clean technique, not an aseptic technique.

How you do it

• Provide privacy, wash your hands, put on gloves and apron.

Inserting an NG tube

• Check that the direction for this medical intervention is
documented in the medical notes.
• If the patient is conscious, explain the procedure to the patient to
gain permission. Tell him that he may experience some discomfort
and that swallowing will ease the tube's advancement.
• Establish and agree upon a non-verbal signal, such as the patient
raising his hand, to indicate that he wishes you to stop for a short
period.
• Gain co-operation and consent.
• Help the patient into an upright position unless contraindicated.
• Stand at the patient's side.
• Drape the towel or protective pad over the patient's chest.

Measure for measure

• To determine how long the NG tube must be to reach the
stomach, hold the end of the tube at the tip of the patient's nose.

Extend the tube to the patient's earlobe and then down to the xiphoid process.
• Mark this distance on the tubing with the tape or note the marking on the NG aspiration tube.
• To determine which nostril will allow easier access, use a penlight and inspect for a deviated septum or other abnormalities, if no abnormalities are found ask the patient if he has a preference.
• Lubricate the first 5–7 cm of the tube using manufacturer's instructions.
• Sit the patient in an upright position in bed.

Down the hatch

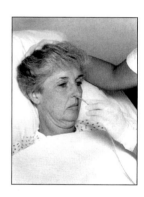

• Grasp the tube with the end pointing downward, curve it if necessary, and carefully insert it into the more patent nostril (as shown at right).
• Aim the tube downward and toward the ear closest to the chosen nostril. Advance it slowly to avoid pressure on the turbinates and resultant pain and bleeding.
• When the tube reaches the nasopharynx, you'll feel resistance. Instruct the patient to lower his head slightly to close the trachea and open the oesophagus. Then rotate the tube 180 degrees toward the opposite nostril to redirect it so that the tube won't enter the patient's mouth.

Take a sip

• Unless contraindicated, offer the patient a cup of water with a straw. Direct him to sip and swallow as you slowly advance the tube. This helps the tube pass to the oesophagus. (If you aren't using water, ask the patient to swallow.)

Ensuring proper tube placement

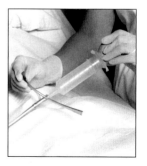

• Use a pen torch to examine the patient's mouth and throat for signs of a coiled section of tubing.
• As you carefully advance the tube and the patient swallows, watch for respiratory distress signs, which may mean the tube is in the bronchus and must be removed immediately. (See Practice pointers section, below, for further advice on confirming tube placement.)
• Stop advancing the tube when the mark reaches the patient's nostril.
• Attach a catheter-tip syringe to the tube and try to aspirate stomach contents (as shown at right). If you don't obtain stomach contents, position the patient on his left side to move the contents into the stomach's greater curvature, and aspirate again. (See *Confirming NG tube placement*.)

- If you still can't aspirate stomach contents, inject 10–20 ml of air and try to aspirate again. If still unable and the patient may drink, let him drink, wait a few minutes and try to aspirate again. If you are then still unable to aspirate, remove the tube and seek advice from a senior colleague or doctor.
- Once you have some aspirate, place some of it on the pH indicator strip. A pH of below 5.5 (or 5 if your paper has single gradings) indicates acid, confirming correct placement. Attach the drainage bag or suction device to the end of the tube.

Nobody move

- Secure the NG tube to the patient's cheek with hypoallergenic tape. If the patient's skin is oily, wipe the cheek with an alcohol pad and allow to dry.
- Do not adhere the tube to the nose.
- Remove your gloves and apron, wash your hands.
- To reduce discomfort from the weight of the tube and bag, fasten the bag to the patient's gown or clothing with a safety pin or clip designed for this purpose.

I'll be back

- Provide frequent nose and mouth care while the tube is in place.
- An NG tube may be inserted or removed at home. (See *Using an NG tube at home*.)

Removing an NG tube
- Explain the procedure to the patient and that it may cause some discomfort.
- Assess bowel function by auscultating for peristalsis or flatus.
- Help the patient into an upright position. Then drape a towel or protective pad across his chest to protect him from spills.
- Put on gloves and apron. Using a catheter-tip syringe, flush the tube with 10 ml of normal saline solution to ensure that the tube doesn't contain stomach contents that could irritate tissues during tube removal.
- Untape the tube from the patient's cheek, and then unpin it from his gown.
- Clamp the tube by folding it in your hand or using a clamp.

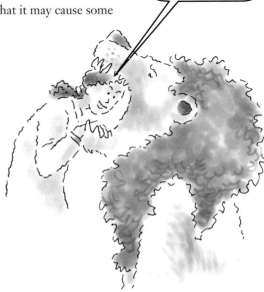

While the NG tube is in place, give frequent mouth care.

Warning!

Confirming NG tube placement

The following methods must NEVER be used:

- Auscultation of air insufflated through the feeding tube, commonly known as the 'whoosh test'.
- Testing acidity of aspirate using litmus paper.
- Interpreting absence of respiratory distress as an indicator of correct positioning.
- Monitoring bubbling at the end of the tube, *both the stomach and the lungs contain air*.
- Observing the appearance of feeding tube aspirate, *gastric contents can look very similar to respiratory secretions*.

Instead remember:

The most reliable way to check the position of the tube is to measure the pH (acidity/alkilinity) of the patient's stomach contents using pH indicator strips or paper. These have a colour code chart indicating the colour change of each pH reading; from pH 1 (acid), through pH 7 (neutral) to pH 14 (alkaline). These strips must be stored in a sealed container to keep them clean and dry.

1. Wash your hands before and after checking the tube position, remove the cap or plug from the tube.
2. Attach an appropriate syringe to the feeding tube, containing 10–20 ml of air for an adult patient.
3. Flush the air down the feeding tube in order to remove any water or feed.
4. Draw back the syringe slowly to obtain contents from the stomach (aspiration).
5. Place a few drops of the aspirate on to the pH strip/paper.
6. Match the colour change of the strip/paper with the colour code on the container to identify the pH of the aspirate.
7. A pH of below 5.5 (or below 5 if your paper has single gradings) indicates an acid reaction, meaning that the tube is correctly positioned in the stomach.
8. Radiological check if deemed necessary by local policy or procedure guidelines.

Pull slowly, then quickly

- Ask the patient to hold his breath to close the epiglottis. Then withdraw the tube gently and steadily. (When the distal end of the tube reaches the nasopharynx, you can pull it quickly.)
- Assist the patient with thorough mouth care, and clean the tape residue from his cheek with adhesive remover.
- Monitor the patient for signs of GI dysfunction.

Home care connection

Using an NG tube at home

If your patient will have a nasogastric (NG) tube in place at home, find out who will insert the tube. If he will have a home care nurse, ensure referral with full patient handover details has been made pre discharge. If the patient and home care nurse do not meet pre discharge, inform the patient who the home care nurse is (name and contact telephone number, minimum) and tell him when to expect her.

Make a list; check it twice

If the patient or a family member will perform the procedure, you'll need to provide additional instruction and supervision. Use this checklist to prepare teaching topics:

- ☑ how and where to obtain equipment needed for home intubation
- ☑ how to insert the tube
- ☑ how to verify tube placement by aspirating stomach contents
- ☑ how to correct tube misplacement
- ☑ how to prepare formula for tube feeding
- ☑ how to store formula, if appropriate
- ☑ how to administer formula through the tube
- ☑ how to remove and dispose of an NG tube
- ☑ how to clean and store a re-usable NG tube
- ☑ how to use the NG tube for gastric decompression, if appropriate
- ☑ how to set up and operate suctioning equipment
- ☑ how to troubleshoot suctioning equipment
- ☑ how to perform mouth care and other hygienic procedures.

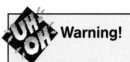

Warning!

Complications of NG intubation

Although nasogastric (NG) intubation is a common procedure, it does carry risks.

Long-term concerns

Potential complications of prolonged intubation include:

- oesophagitis
- oesophago-tracheal fistula
- gastric ulceration
- pulmonary and oral infection
- sinusitis
- pressure ulcer at the nostril/cheek.

Suction reactions

Additional complications of suction include electrolyte imbalances and dehydration. Vigorous suction may damage the gastric mucosa and cause significant bleeding, possibly interfering with endoscopic assessment and diagnosis.

Practice pointers

Down the wrong pipe

- Remember that absence of respiratory distress does not confirm correct placement, small-bore tubes may not cause distress. However, while advancing the tube, observe for signs that it has entered the trachea, such as choking or breathing difficulties in a conscious patient and cyanosis in an unconscious patient, or a patient without a cough reflex. If these signs occur, remove the tube immediately. Allow the patient time to rest; then try to reinsert the tube.

- After tube placement, vomiting suggests tubal obstruction or incorrect position. Assess immediately to determine the cause. (See *Complications of NG intubation* and *Documenting NG tube insertion and removal*.)

    For further information and updated advice on NG tube care and placement view the National Patient Safety Agency website: www.npsa.nhs.uk.

Nasogastric tube care

Providing effective NG tube care requires meticulous monitoring of both the patient and the equipment.

Monitoring the patient involves checking drainage from the NG tube and assessing GI function. Monitoring the equipment involves verifying correct tube placement and irrigating the tube to ensure patency and to prevent mucosal damage.

What you need

Irrigation fluid ✳ irrigant container ✳ 60 ml catheter-tip syringe ✳ suction equipment ✳ toothbrush and toothpaste ✳ hypoallergenic tape ✳ gloves and apron ✳ stethoscope ✳ protective pad or towel ✳ pH Indicator strips ✳ optional: kidney bowl.

Getting ready

Make sure the suction equipment works properly. When using a tube with suction, connect the larger, primary lumen (for drainage and suction) to the suction equipment and select the appropriate setting, as per medical instruction (usually low constant suction). If the doctor doesn't specify the setting, follow the manufacturer's directions.

How you do it

- Explain the procedure to the patient and gain consent, provide privacy and maintain the patient's dignity.
- Wash your hands and put on non-sterile gloves and an apron.

Irrigating an NG tube

- Aspirate stomach contents to check correct positioning.
- Measure the amount of irrigant in the syringe (usually 30 ml) to maintain an accurate intake and output record.

Write it down

Document- ing NG tube insertion and removal

In your notes, record:

- type and size of the nasogastric (NG) tube
- insertion date and time
- type and amount of suction, if used
- drainage characteristics, including amount, colour, character, consistency and odour
- patient's tolerance of the procedure
- your name, designation and signature.

Do it again

When you remove the tube, record:

- removal date and time
- colour, consistency and amount of gastric drainage
- patient's tolerance of the procedure
- your name, designation and signature.

- When using suction, unclamp and disconnect the tube from the suction equipment.
- Slowly instil the irrigant into the NG tube.
- Gently aspirate the solution with the syringe or connect the tube to the suction equipment. Report any bleeding.
- Reconnect the tube to suction after completing irrigation.

Instilling a solution through an NG tube
- If the doctor orders instillation, inject the solution—don't aspirate it—and record the amount as 'intake' on the fluid balance chart.
- Re-attach the tube to suction as ordered.

Monitoring patient comfort and condition
- Provide mouth care once per shift or as needed.
- Change the tape securing the tube daily or as needed. Clean the skin and apply fresh tape.
- Assess bowel sounds regularly (every 4–8 hours) to verify GI function.
- Measure the drainage amount and update the fluid balance chart as you administer and drain. Be alert for electrolyte imbalances with excessive gastric output.
- As well as assessing the pH of the aspirate pre-irrigation, also inspect gastric drainage and note its colour, consistency, odour and amount. Normal gastric secretions have no colour or appear yellow–green from bile and have a mucoid consistency. Immediately report any drainage with a coffee-bean colour; this may indicate bleeding. If you suspect that the drainage contains blood, use a screening test for occult blood according to local policy.

Practice pointers

- Irrigate the NG tube with 30 ml of irrigant in a 60 ml catheter-tip syringe before and after instilling medication. Wait about 30 minutes, or as ordered, after instillation before reconnecting the suction equipment to allow sufficient time for the medication to be absorbed.

Suction function

- If no drainage appears, check the suction equipment for proper function. Then, holding the NG tube over a protective pad, towel or a kidney bowl, separate the tube and the suction source. Check the suction equipment by placing the suction tubing in an irrigant container. If the apparatus draws the water, check the NG tube for

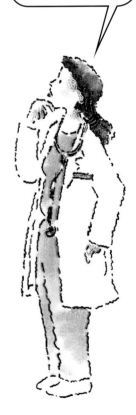

Do you feel resistance? The tube may be blocked—time to flush.

proper function. Be sure to note the amount of water drawn into the suction container on the fluid balance chart.
• If the patient ambulates, disconnect the NG tube from the suction equipment. Clamp the tube to prevent stomach contents from draining out of the tube. (See *Documenting NG tube care*.)

NG feeding tube insertion and removal

Inserting a feeding tube into the stomach or duodenum allows a patient who can't or won't eat to receive nourishment. The feeding tube also permits administration of supplemental feedings to a patient who has high nutritional requirements, such as an unconscious patient or one with extensive burns. The preferred feeding tube route is nasal, but the oral route may be used for patients with such conditions as a deviated septum or a head or nose injury.

Can't stomach this

The doctor may order duodenal feeding when the patient can't tolerate gastric feeding or when he expects gastric feeding to produce aspiration. Absence of bowel sounds or possible intestinal obstruction contraindicates using a feeding tube.

Flexibility rules!

Feeding tubes are made of silicone, rubber or polyurethane and have small diameters and great flexibility. To ease passage, some feeding tubes are weighted with tungsten, and some need a guide wire to keep them from curling in the back of the throat. These small-bore tubes usually have radio-opaque markings and a water-activated coating, which provides a lubricated surface.

What you need

For insertion
Feeding tube (6–18 French, with or without guide wire)
✳ protective pad or towel ✳ non-sterile gloves and apron
✳ hypoallergenic tape ✳ water ✳ facial tissues ✳ pen torch ✳ small cup of water with straw ✳ kidney bowel ✳ 60 ml Luer Lok syringe
✳ pH indicator strips ✳ sharps container.

Write it down

Document-ing NG tube care

- Record regularly confirmation of nasogastric (NG) tube placement (usually every 4–8 hours)
- Keep a precise record of fluid intake and output, including the instilled irrigant, in fluid input
- Track the irrigation schedule and note the actual time of each irrigation
- Describe drainage colour, consistency, odour and amount
- Note tape change times and the condition of the skin
- Document your name, designation, signature and accurate time.

During use
Mouthwash , toothpaste ✳ toothbrush.

For removal
Gloves and apron ✳ protective pad ✳ tube clamp/bung ✳ 60 ml
Luer Lok syringe ✳ clinical waste bag.

Getting ready

Have the appropriate-size tube available. Usually, the
doctor or nutrition nurse specialist orders the smallest-
bore tube that will allow free passage of the liquid
feeding formula. Read the instructions on the tubing
package carefully because tube characteristics vary
according to the manufacturer.

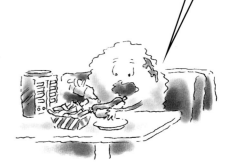

Feeding
tubes can help
patients with
high nutritional
requirements.
Waitress!

Check for cracks

Examine the tube to make sure it's free from defects,
such as cracks or rough or sharp edges.

How you do it

• Check that a direction to insert a feeding tube is documented in
the medical notes.
• Explain the procedure to the patient. Tell him he may
experience some discomfort and that swallowing will ease the tube's
advancement. Establish and agree upon a non-verbal signal, such as
the patient raising his hand, to indicate that he wishes you to stop
for a short period. Gain co-operation and consent.
• Provide privacy. Wash your hands, put on gloves and an apron.
• Assist the patient into an upright position if possible.
• Place a protective pad or towel over the patient's chest to protect
him from spills.

Inner tube

• To determine the tube length needed to reach the stomach, first
extend the distal end of the tube from the tip of the patient's nose to
his earlobe. Coil this portion of the tube around your fingers so the
end will remain curved until you insert it. Then extend the uncoiled
portion from the earlobe to the xiphoid process. Note the marking
on the tube.

Inserting the tube nasally
• Using the pen torch, assess nasal patency. Occlude one nostril,
then the other, to determine which has the better airflow. Offer

the patient a choice of which nasal cavity to use if there are no contraindications.

• Lubricate the curved tip of the tube (and the feeding tube guide, if appropriate) with a small amount of water to ease insertion and prevent tissue injury.

• Ask the patient to take a sip of water if appropriate and hold in their mouth.

• To advance the tube, insert the curved, lubricated tip into the nostril and direct it along the nasal passage toward the ear on the same side. When it passes the nasopharyngeal junction, turn the tube 180 degrees to aim it downward into the oesophagus. Tell the patient to lower his chin to his chest to close the trachea. Then instruct him to swallow the water he is holding in his mouth. This step may be repeated as necessary. This will ease the tube's passage. Advance the tube as he swallows.

> When I say so, swallow the water in your mouth. That will close your trachea— and help the tube go into the oesophagus.

Positioning the tube

• Keep passing the tube until the tape marking the appropriate length reaches the patient's nostril.

Ensuring proper tube placement

Check local policy regarding special instructions for high-risk groups of patients such as intensive care patients and neonates. An X-ray may be required for these patients or where aspiration of stomach contents has not been achieved. In these cases the guide wire should be left in place until the X-ray has been taken and tube placement confirmed.

• Use a pen torch to examine the patient's mouth and throat for signs of a coiled section of tubing.

• As you carefully advance the tube and the patient swallows, watch for respiratory distress signs, which may mean the tube is in the bronchus and must be removed immediately.

• Stop advancing the tube when the mark reaches the patient's nostril.

• Attach the Luer Lok syringe to the tube and try to aspirate stomach contents.

• If you don't obtain stomach contents, position the patient on his left side to move the contents into the stomach's greater curvature, and aspirate again. (See *Confirming NG tube placement* above.)

• If you still can't aspirate stomach contents, inject 10–20 ml (adult patient) of air and try to aspirate again. If still unable and the patient

may drink, let him drink, wait a few minutes and try to aspirate again. If you are then still unable to aspirate, remove the tube and seek advice from a senior colleague or doctor.
• Once you have some aspirate, place some of it on the pH indicator strip. A pH of below 5.5 (or 5 if your paper has single gradings) indicates acid, confirming correct placement.
• Remove the guide wire (if no special instruction is in place for the individual patient).

Tale of the tape

• Apply a skin preparation to the patient's cheek before securing the tube with tape. This helps the tube adhere to the skin and also prevents irritation.
• Tape the tube securely to the patient's cheek to avoid excessive pressure on his nostrils.

Removing the tube
• Wash your hands, put on gloves and an apron.
• Protect the patient's chest with a protective pad.
• Clamp or pinch the tube to prevent fluid aspiration during withdrawal, and withdraw it gently but quickly.
• Promptly cover and discard the used tube in the clinical waste.

Practice pointers

• Flush the feeding tube every 8 hours with up to 60 ml of water to maintain patency. Re-tape the tube daily and as needed. Inspect the skin for redness and breakdown.
• Provide nasal hygiene daily to remove crusted secretions. Also help the patient brush his teeth, gums and tongue with mouthwash or a mild toothpaste solution at least twice daily.
• When aspirating gastric contents to check tube placement, pull gently on the syringe plunger to prevent trauma to the stomach lining or bowel. (See *Documenting feeding tube insertion and removal*.)

Nasogastric tube feeding

This procedure involves delivery of a liquid feeding formula directly to the stomach, duodenum or jejunum. Typically it is indicated for a patient who can't eat normally because of dysphagia or oral or oesophageal obstruction or injury. Gastric feedings may also be given to an unconscious or intubated patient or to a patient recovering from GI tract surgery who can't ingest food orally.

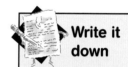

Write it down

Document-ing feeding tube insertion and removal

For tube insertion, record:

• insertion indications
• date and time
• tube type and size
• insertion site
• placement area
• confirmation of proper placement
• record any fluid aspirated or instilled on the fluid balance chart
• your name, designation and signature.

For tube removal, record:

• reason for removal
• removal date and time
• patient's tolerance of the procedure
• your name, designation and signature.

Transabdominal tube feeding

To access the stomach, duodenum or jejunum, the doctor may place a tube through the patient's abdominal wall. This procedure may be done surgically or percutaneously. The tube may be used for feeding during the immediate post-operative period or it may provide long-term enteral access. Typically, the doctor will suture the tube in place to prevent gastric contents from leaking.

PEG-ing the patient

In contrast, a percutaneous endoscopic gastrostomy (PEG) or jejunostomy (PEJ) tube can be inserted endoscopically without the need for laparotomy or general anaesthesia. A PEG or PEJ tube may be used for nutrition, drainage and decompression. (See *Caring for a PEG or PEJ site*, at the end of this section.)

What you need

For nasogastric feeding

Feeding formula ✳ I.V. pole ✳ 120 ml of water ✳ administration set ✳ towel or protective pad ✳ 60 ml catheter-tip syringe ✳ volumetric feeding device ✳ gloves and an apron.

For gastrostomy or jejunostomy feeding

Feeding formula ✳ administration set ✳ I.V. pole ✳ 60 ml catheter-tip syringe ✳ water ✳ optional: volumetric pump, Y-connector ✳ gloves and an apron.

Getting ready

Check the date on all formula containers. Discard expired commercial formula according to local policy. Always shake the container well to mix the solution thoroughly.

Warm, not hot …

- Let the formula warm to room temperature before administration. Cold formula can increase the chance of diarrhoea.
- Insert the administration set into the formula bottle and prime the line.

Letting the air out

- Open the flow clamp on the administration set to remove air from the lines, allow the fluid to run through the administration line until it reaches the distal point. This keeps air from entering the patient's stomach and causing distension and discomfort.

How you do it

- Provide privacy and wash your hands, put on gloves and an apron.
- Explain the procedure to the patient.
- Cover his chest with a towel or pad to protect him from spills.
- Assess the patient's abdomen for bowel sounds and distension.

Delivering a nasogastric feed

- Elevate the bed to prevent aspiration by gastro-oesophageal reflux and to promote digestion.

Tube check

- Check placement and patency of the feeding tube (as described in Positioning the tube, above) to be sure it hasn't slipped out since the last feeding. (See *Before you give that tube feed*.)
- Connect the administration tubing to the NG tube. Depending on the type of tube used, you may need to use an adapter to connect the two.
- Thread the administration line through the controller according to the manufacturer's directions.

No air allowed

- Open the flow clamp on the administration line, and adjust the flow rate appropriately, using the key pad on the pump. Set the alarms to identify occlusions and to alert you when the feed is almost complete, usually 50 ml, to prevent air from entering the tube and the patient's stomach. Never allow the feed to empty completely. NG feed regimes will be prescribed in the patient's notes. The initial rate of administration may be slow, but will gradually build to optimum feeding rate, depending on the patient's tolerance. Feeds are then usually maintained over 16–20 hours, allowing for a rest period. (See *Managing tube feeding problems*.)
- Never administer additional water unless it is part of the regime.

When dinner is done

- To discontinue nasogastric feeding, close the regulator clamp on the administration line and turn off the volumetric pump.
- Cover the end of the feeding tube with its plug or cap to prevent leakage and contamination of the tube.
- Leave the patient in a 30- to 90-degree upright position for at least 30 minutes.

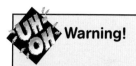

Warning!

Before you give that tube feed

Never give a tube feed until you're sure the tube is properly positioned in the patient's stomach. Administering a feed through a misplaced tube can cause formula to enter the patient's lungs.

Warning!

Managing tube feeding problems

Administering a tube feed isn't always problem-free. If your patient develops complications, you'll need to intervene quickly to avoid serious problems.

Complication	Interventions
Aspiration of gastric secretions	• Discontinue feeding immediately. • Perform tracheal suction of aspirated contents, if possible. • Notify the doctor and dietician. Prophylactic antibiotics and chest physiotherapy may be ordered. • Check tube placement before feeding, to prevent complications.
Tube obstruction	• Flush the tube with prescribed amount of water or carbonated fluid, i.e. soda water, pre and post feeding. If necessary, replace the tube. • Only ever administer liquid medications—do not crush tablets.
Oral, nasal or pharyngeal irritation or necrosis	• Provide frequent oral hygiene. • Change the tube's position. If necessary, replace the tube.

• Change equipment every 24 hours or according to local and national guidelines.

Delivering a gastrostomy feed
• Wait 12 hours after tube placement before commencing feed.
• Commence water or sterile feed at 30 ml/hour via an administration line and volumetric device for 12 hours.
• Commence prescribed feed at 30 ml/hour.

Delivering a jejunostomy feed
• Wait 24 hours post tube insertion.
• Feed as per gastrostomy, always use a volumetric pump and be aware that the rate prescribed is usually slower, as the feed is delivered continuously over 24 hours.
• Flush the jejunostomy tube every 4 hours with 10–20 ml of sterile water.

Practice pointers
• If the patient becomes nauseated or vomits, stop the feeding immediately.
• To reduce oropharyngeal discomfort from the tube, provide mouth care.

Something extra

- Always confirm correct tube placement before administering any drugs or fluid via an NG tube using the aspiration technique, as described in the above sections.

Advice from the experts

Caring for a PEG or PEJ site

The exit site of a percutaneous endoscopic gastrostomy (PEG) or percutaneous endoscopic jejunostomy (PEJ) tube requires routine observation and care. Follow these guidelines:

- Change the dressing daily while the tube is in place.
- After removing the dressing, carefully slide the tube's outer bumper away from the skin about 1.5 cm, as shown below left.
- Examine the skin around the tube. Look for redness and other signs of infection or erosion.
- Gently depress the skin around the tube and inspect for drainage, as shown below right. Expect minimal wound drainage initially after implantation. This should subside in about 1 week.

- Inspect the tube for wear and tear. A tube that wears out will need replacement.
- Clean the site with the prescribed cleaning solution—soap and water.
- Rotate the outer bumper 90 degrees (to avoid repeating the same tension on the same skin area), and slide the outer bumper back over the exit site.
- If leakage appears at the PEG site, or if the patient risks dislodging the tube, apply a sterile gauze dressing over the site. Don't put sterile gauze underneath the outer bumper. Loosening the anchor this way gives the feeding tube free play, which could lead to wound abscess.
- Record the date and time of the dressing change on the tape.

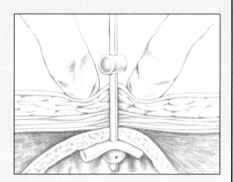

Outer bumper — Inner bumper

Abdominal wall — Stomach wall

• Liquid drugs only can be administered through the feeding tube. Never administer enteric-coated drugs or sustained-release medications, never crush tablets or open and dilute capsules in water before administering them.

• Be sure to flush the tubing after the administration of medication, to ensure full instillation of medication. Keep in mind that some drugs may change the osmolarity of the feeding formula and cause diarrhoea.

• For duodenal or jejunal feeding, most patients tolerate a continuous drip better than bolus feedings. Bolus feedings can cause complications such as hyperglycaemia and diarrhoea.

• For further advice on Nutritional Support see the National Collaborating Centre for Acute Care's Methods, evidence and guidance document on *Nutritional support for adults: oral nutrition support, enteral tube feeding and parenteral feeding*, which was commissioned by the National Institute for Clinical Excellence (2006). Available for download at www.nice.org.uk

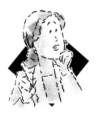

Quick quiz

1. What isn't a function of a nasogastric (NG) tube?
    A. Prevention of post-operative vomiting.
    B. Emptying of the stomach.
    C. Route for administration of tablets.

Answer: C. Only liquid medications can be administered via a feeding tube.

2. What shouldn't you do when confirming NG tube placement?
    A. Aspirate stomach contents.
    B. Use pH indicator paper
    C. Perform the woosh test.

Answer: C. When confirming tube placement, never using a woosh test, it is an outdated method.

3. A patient receiving a gastric feed should be placed in which position?
    A. Upright.
    B. Horizontal.
    C. Prone.

Answer: A patient receiving a gastric feed should be placed in an upright position to prevent aspiration.

4. Who should be involved in serving patient meals?
    A. Healthcare support workers.
    B. Only registered nurses.
    C. All nursing and support staff.

Answer: C. All staff on the ward should be involved in serving and assisting patients to receive their recommended diet.

5. What volume should you document on the fluid balance chart for a cup of water?
   A.   150 ml.
   B.   200 ml.
   C.   Depends on the cup. You need to be specific.

Answer: C. Depends on the cup. When monitoring patient's fluid balance it is essential to be specific, small mistakes can lead to harm being caused to the patient.

Scoring

☆☆☆ If you answered all five items correctly, marvellous! Your retention level is simply GI-ant!

☆☆ If you answered three or four items correctly, wonderful! You're as efficient as a well-placed NG tube.

☆ If you answered fewer than three items correctly, stay mellow. Remember, GI procedures may take some time to digest.

7 Continence, appliances and care

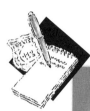

Just the facts

In this chapter, you'll learn:

♦ about renal and urology care procedures and how to perform them

♦ what patient care is associated with each procedure

♦ how to manage complications associated with each procedure

♦ about essential documentation for each procedure.

Essential skills clusters

Essential skills clusters associated and specific to continence are:
- Nutrition and fluid management: specific to numbers 29 and 32.
- Care, compassion and communication: associated with all.
- Organizational aspects of care: associated with all and specific to numbers 10–15 and 20.
- Infection prevention and control: associated with all.
- Medicines management: specific to numbers 36, 38–42.

Continence versus incontinence

In order to manage adult patients with incontinence it is first important to understand what continence is. Continence can be described as possessing the ability to store urine in the bladder or faeces in the bowel and have the ability excrete it voluntarily when appropriate. In other words, we as adults can store urine or faeces until we have the opportunity to release it.

So what is incontinence? There are many different classifications. The International Continence Society (Abrams *et al.*, 2002) describes the following classification:

- Urinary incontinence is the complaint of any involuntary leakage of urine.
- Stress urinary incontinence is the complaint of involuntary leakage on effort or exertion, or on sneezing or coughing.
- Urge urinary incontinence is the complaint of involuntary leakage accompanied by, or immediately preceded by, urgency.
- Mixed urinary continence is the complaint of involuntary leakage associated with urgency and also with exertion, effort, sneezing or coughing.
- Faecal incontinence is the involuntary loss of liquid or solid stool that is a social or hygienic problem.

Incontinence management

In adult patients, incontinence commonly follows loss of urinary or anal sphincter control or impairment of it. The incontinence can be transient or permanent, depending on the cause of the problem and the success of the treatment.

When treating a patient with urinary or faecal incontinence, a nurse specialist in continence will carefully assess the patient for underlying disorders. Treatment aims in the first instance are to control the incontinence through non-invasive therapy techniques, such as bladder or bowel retraining or other behaviour-management techniques, diet modification, drug therapy. Only once these have been tried without satisfactory outcomes for the patient, will invasive therapies and surgical intervention be considered.

Surgical options

Corrective surgery for urinary incontinence includes transurethral resection of the prostate in men, repair of the anterior vaginal wall or retropelvic suspension of the bladder in women, urethral sling, and bladder augmentation. (See *Artificial urinary sphincter implant* and *Correcting urinary incontinence with bladder retraining*.)

What you need

Bladder retraining record sheet ✳ gloves and apron ✳ stethoscope (to assess bowel sounds) ✳ moisture barrier cream ✳ incontinence

Artificial urinary sphincter implant

An artificial urinary sphincter implant helps restore continence to a patient with a neurogenic bladder.

Configuration and placement

An implant has a control pump, an occlusive cuff and a pressure-regulating balloon. The cuff is placed around the bladder neck, and the balloon is placed under the rectus muscle. Fluid in the balloon inflates the cuff. The surgeon places the control pump in the scrotum in men and in the labium in women.

Implant use

To void, the patient squeezes the bulb to deflate the cuff, which opens the urethra by returning fluid to the balloon. After voiding, the cuff re-inflates automatically, sealing the urethra until the patient needs to void again.

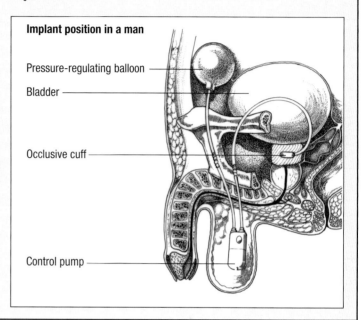

Implant position in a man

Pressure-regulating balloon

Bladder

Occlusive cuff

Control pump

---

pads ✻ bedpan ✻ specimen container ✻ label ✻ laboratory request form ✻ optional: stool collection kit, urinary catheter.

How you do it

• Whether the patient reports urinary or faecal incontinence or both, you'll need to perform initial and continuing assessments to plan effective interventions.

For urinary incontinence

• Ask the patient when he first noticed urine leakage and whether it began suddenly or gradually. Have him describe his typical urinary pattern: does he usually experience incontinence during the day or at night? Ask him to rate his urinary control: does he have moderate control, or is he completely incontinent? If he sometimes urinates with control, ask him to identify when and how much he usually urinates.

• Evaluate related problems, such as urinary hesitancy, frequency, and urgency; nocturia and decreased force or interrupted urine stream.

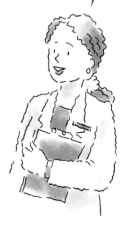

Note the onset, duration, severity and pattern of urinary incontinence.

Correcting urinary incontinence with bladder retraining

The incontinent patient typically feels frustrated, embarrassed and hopeless. Fortunately, he can correct the problem by retraining his bladder—a programme that aims to establish a regular voiding pattern. Follow these guidelines.

Assess elimination patterns

First, assess the patient's intake and voiding patterns and reason for each accidental voiding (such as a coughing spell). Use an incontinence monitoring record.

Establish a voiding schedule

Encourage the patient to void regularly, for example, every 2 hours. When he can stay dry for 2 hours, increase the interval by 30 minutes every day until he achieves a 3- to 4-hour voiding schedule. Teach the patient to practise relaxation techniques, such as deep breathing, which help decrease the sense of urgency.

Record results and remain positive

Keep a record of continence and incontinence on a bladder retraining sheet for about 5 days. This may reinforce the patient's efforts to remain continent. Remember, your own and your patient's positive attitudes are crucial to his successful bladder retraining.

Take steps for success

Here are some additional tips to boost the patient's success:

- Locate the patient's bed near a bathroom or portable toilet. Leave a light on at night. If he needs assistance getting out of bed or a chair, answer the call for help promptly.
- Teach him how to prevent urinary tract infections—for example by drinking plenty of fluids (at least 2 litres/day, unless contraindicated), drinking cranberry juice to acidify urine, wearing cotton underpants, and bathing with non-irritating soaps.
- Encourage him to empty his bladder completely before and after meals and at bedtime.
- Advise him to urinate whenever the urge arises and never to ignore it.
- Instruct him to take prescribed diuretics when he gets up in the morning.
- Advise him to limit the use of sleeping aids, sedatives and alcohol; they decrease the urge to urinate and can increase incontinence, especially at night.
- If he's overweight, encourage him to lose weight.
- Suggest exercises to strengthen pelvic muscles.
- Instruct him to increase dietary fibre to decrease constipation and incontinence.
- Monitor him for signs of anxiety and depression.
- Reassure him that periodic incontinent episodes don't mean that the programme has failed. Encourage persistence, tolerance and a positive attitude.

- Ask the patient to describe treatment he has used for incontinence, whether doctor prescribed or self-prescribed.

Know the environment

- Assess the patient's environment. Is a toilet, commode or bedpan readily available, and how long does the patient take to reach it?

After he's in the bathroom, assess his manual dexterity—for example, how easily does he manipulate his clothes?
- Evaluate the patient's mental status and cognitive function.
- Quantify the patient's normal daily fluid intake.
- Review the patient's medication and diet history for drugs and foods that affect digestion and elimination.
- Review or obtain the patient's medical history, noting especially the number and route of births and incidence of urinary tract infection (UTI), prostate disorders, spinal injury or tumour, cerebrovascular accident, and bladder, prostate or pelvic surgery. Also, check for signs and symptoms of delirium, dehydration, urine retention, restricted mobility, faecal impaction, infection, inflammation and polyuria.

Doing the inspection

- Put on gloves and an apron.
- Inspect the urethral meatus for obvious inflammation or anatomic defects. Have the female patient bear down while you note any urine leakage. Gently palpate the abdomen for bladder distention, which signals urine retention. If possible, have a urologist examine the patient.
- Label each specimen container prior to obtaining specimens (ensuring that cross-contamination is eliminated by preventing urine/faecal contact with your pen) for appropriate laboratory tests as ordered. Remove gloves and apron then wash your hands and send specimens to the laboratory with a request form.

Retraining the bladder

- Begin incontinence management by implementing an appropriate bladder retraining programme.
- Make sure the patient drinks plenty of fluids to ensure adequate hydration and to prevent UTIs. Restrict fluid intake after 6 p.m.
- Begin an exercise programme to strengthen the pelvic floor muscles and to help manage stress incontinence. (See *Strengthening pelvic floor muscles*.)
- To manage functional incontinence, frequently assess the patient's mental and functional status. Regularly remind him to void. Respond to his calls promptly, and help him get to the bathroom quickly. Provide positive reinforcement.

For faecal incontinence
- Ask the patient with faecal incontinence to identify its onset, duration, severity and pattern (for instance, determine whether it occurs at night or with diarrhoea). Focus the history on GI, neurological and psychological disorders.

Strengthening pelvic floor muscles

Stress incontinence usually results from weakening of the urethral sphincter. Teach pelvic floor exercises to help a patient prevent or minimize stress incontinence.

Teaching exercises

Explain how to locate pelvic floor muscles by tensing the muscles around the anus, as if to retain stool, and then tightening the muscles of the pelvic floor, as if to stop the flow of urine. When learned, these exercises can be done—10 seconds tensed and 10 seconds relaxed—anywhere, anytime. Remember that the quality of the exercises performed is more important than quantity.

Establishing a regimen

A typical regimen starts with 15 contractions in the morning and afternoon and 20 at night. An alternative would be 10 minutes three times per day, working up to 25 contractions as strength improves.

- Note the frequency, consistency and volume of stool passed in the past 24 hours. Obtain a stool specimen if ordered. Protect the patient's bed with an incontinence pad, appropriate to their needs and skin condition.
- Assess the patient for chronic constipation, GI and neurological disorders, and laxative abuse.
- Assess the patient's medication regimen. Check for drugs that affect bowel activity, such as aspirin, some anticholinergic anti-parkinsonian drugs, aluminium hydroxide, calcium carbonate antacids, diuretics, iron preparations, opiates, tranquillizers and tricyclic antidepressants.

Doing the inspection

- Check whether his abdomen is distended, and auscultate for bowel sounds. If not contraindicated, check for faecal impaction, which can contribute to overflow incontinence.

Retraining the bowel

- If the patient is neurologically capable, provide bowel retraining to control chronic incontinence.
- Advise the patient to eat plenty of fibre-rich foods, including lots of raw, leafy vegetables (such as carrots and lettuce), unpeeled fruits (such as apples), and whole grains (such as wheat or rye breads and cereals).
- Encourage adequate fluid intake.

- Teach the patient to gradually stop using laxatives. Point out that using laxatives to promote regular bowel movement may have the opposite effect, producing either constipation or incontinence over time. Suggest natural laxatives, such as prunes and prune juice, instead.
- Promote regular exercise by explaining how it helps to regulate bowel motility. Even a non-ambulatory patient can perform some exercises while sitting or lying in bed.

Practice pointers

- To rid the bladder of residual urine, teach the patient to perform Valsalva's (abdominal straining/bearing down) or Credé's (compression of the lower abdomen) manoeuvre or institute clean intermittent catheterization. Use an indwelling urinary catheter only as a last resort because of the risk of UTI.

Keeping it clean

- For faecal incontinence, provide and teach proper hygienic care to increase the patient's comfort and prevent skin breakdown and infection. Encourage the patient to clean the perineal area frequently (see Perineal Care, Chapter 1) and apply a moisture barrier cream. Control foul odours as well.

Boost his self-esteem

- Schedule extra time to provide encouragement and support for the patient, who may feel shame, embarrassment and powerlessness from loss of control. (See *Documenting incontinence management*.)

Colostomy and ileostomy care

A patient with a colostomy or an ileostomy must wear an external pouch to collect emerging faecal matter. Besides collecting waste matter, the pouch helps to control odour and protect the stoma and peristomal skin. Most disposable pouching systems can be used for between 1 and 7 days; some models last even longer. Your responsibilities include caring for the colostomy or ileostomy and teaching the patient self-care.

What you need

Pouching system ✳ stoma measuring guide ✳ stoma paste (if drainage is watery to pasty or stoma secretes excess mucus) ✳ plastic waste bag

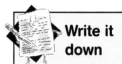

Write it down

Documenting incontinence management

In the patient's notes, record:

- all bladder and bowel retraining efforts, noting scheduled bathroom times, food and fluid intake, and elimination amounts, as appropriate
- duration of the patient's continent periods
- complications, including emotional problems and signs of skin breakdown and infection, as well as the treatments given for them
- referall to continence advisory service/ urologists
- your name, designation and signature.

✳ water ✳ washcloth and towel ✳ closure clamp ✳ toilet or bedpan ✳ water or pouch-cleaning solution ✳ gloves and apron ✳ facial tissues ✳ optional: ostomy belt, paper tape, mild non-moisturising soap, skin-shaving equipment, liquid skin sealant, pouch deodorant.

Catalogue of choices

Pouching systems may be drainable or closed-bottomed, disposable or reusable, adhesive-backed, and one-piece or two-piece. (See *Comparing ostomy pouching systems*.)

How you do it

• Provide privacy and emotional support.

Fitting the pouch and skin barrier
• For a pouch with an attached skin barrier, measure the stoma with the stoma-measuring guide. Select the opening size that matches the stoma.
• For an adhesive-backed pouch with a separate skin barrier, measure the stoma with the measuring guide and select the opening that matches the stoma. Trace the selected size opening on to the paper back of the skin barrier's adhesive side. Cut out the opening. (If the pouch has pre-cut openings, which can be handy for a round stoma, select an opening that's 0.3 cm larger than the stoma. If the pouch comes without an opening, cut the hole 0.8–1 cm wider than the measured tracing.) The cut-to-fit system works best for an irregularly shaped stoma.
• For a two-piece pouching system with flanges, see *Applying a skin barrier and pouch*.

Can't feel a thing

• Avoid fitting the pouch too tightly because the stoma has no pain receptors. A constrictive opening could injure the stoma or skin tissue without the patient feeling discomfort. Also avoid cutting the opening too big because this may expose the skin to faecal matter and moisture, leading to skin deterioration and excoriation.
• If the patient has a descending or sigmoid colostomy, has formed stools, and has an ostomy that doesn't secrete much mucus, he may choose to wear only a pouch. In this case, make sure the pouch opening closely matches the stoma size.
• Between 6 weeks and 1 year after surgery, the stoma will shrink to its permanent size. At that point, pattern-making preparations will be unnecessary unless the patient gains weight, has additional surgery, or injures the stoma.

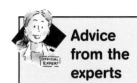

Advice from the experts

Applying a skin barrier and pouch

Fitting a skin barrier and ostomy pouch properly can be done in a few steps:

• Measure the stoma using a measuring guide
• Trace the appropriate circle carefully on the back of the skin barrier
• Cut the circular opening in the skin barrier. Bevel the edges to keep them from irritating the patient
• Remove the backing from the skin barrier, and moisten it or apply barrier paste as needed along the edge of the circular opening
• Centre the skin barrier over the stoma, adhesive side down, and gently press it to the skin
• Gently press the pouch opening on to the ring until it snaps into place.

Comparing ostomy pouching systems

Available in many shapes and sizes, ostomy pouches are fashioned for comfort, safety and easy application. A disposable closed-end pouch may meet the needs of a patient who irrigates, wants added security, or wants to discard the pouch after each bowel movement. Another patient may prefer a re-usable, drainable pouch. Some commonly available pouches are described here.

One-piece disposable pouch

The patient who must empty his pouch often (because the ostomy is overactive, produces very loose matter, or a for a new colostomy or ileostomy) may prefer a one-piece, drainable, disposable pouch with a closure clamp attached to a skin barrier (below left).

This odour-proof, plastic pouch comes with an attached adhesive seal. The bottom opening allows for easy draining. This pouch may be used permanently or temporarily, until stoma size stabilizes.

Also disposable and made of odour-proof plastic, a one-piece disposable closed-end pouch (below right) may come in a kit with adhesive seal, belt tabs, skin barrier or carbon filter for gas release. A patient with a regular bowel elimination pattern may choose this style.

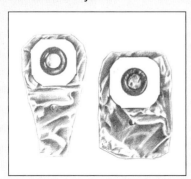

Two-piece disposable pouch

A two-piece disposable drainable pouch with separate skin barrier (below) permits frequent changes and minimizes skin breakdown. Also made of odour-proof plastic, this style comes with belt tabs and usually snaps to the skin barrier with a flange mechanism.

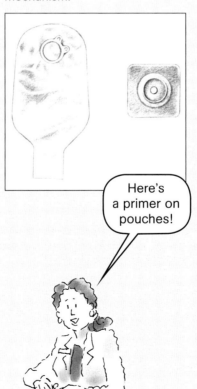

Here's a primer on pouches!

Reusable pouch

Typically made of sturdy, hypoallergenic plastic, the reusable pouch (below) comes with a separate custom-made faceplate and O-ring. Some reusable pouches have pressure valves for releasing gas. The device has a 1- to 2-month life span, depending on how frequently the patient empties the pouch.

Reusable equipment may benefit a patient who needs a firm faceplate. However, many reusable ostomy pouches aren't odour-proof and an additional odour spray will be required.

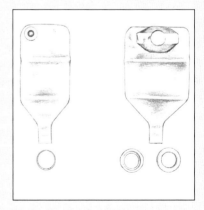

Applying or changing the pouch
- Collect all equipment.
- Wash your hands and provide privacy.
- Explain the procedure to the patient because the patient will eventually perform the procedure himself.
- Put on gloves and an apron.

Out with the old

- Remove and discard the old pouch in a plastic bag. Wipe the stoma and peristomal skin gently with a facial tissue.
- Carefully wash the peristomal skin with mild soap and water and dry it by patting gently. Allow the skin to dry thoroughly. Inspect the peristomal skin and stoma. If necessary, shave surrounding hair (in a direction away from the stoma) to promote a better seal and avoid skin irritation from hair pulling against the adhesive.
- If applying a separate skin barrier, peel off the paper backing of the prepared skin barrier, centre the barrier over the stoma, and press gently to ensure adhesion.
- You may want to outline the stoma on the back of the skin barrier (depending on the product) with a thin ring of stoma paste, to provide extra skin protection. (Skip this step if the patient has a sigmoid or descending colostomy, formed stools, and little mucus.)

Peel and press

- Remove the paper backing from the adhesive side of the pouching system and centre the pouch opening over the stoma. Press gently to secure.
- For a pouching system with flanges, align the lip of the pouch flange with the bottom edge of the skin barrier flange. Gently press around the circumference of the pouch flange, beginning at the bottom, until the pouch securely adheres to the barrier flange. (The pouch will click into its secured position.) Holding the barrier against the skin, gently pull on the pouch to confirm the seal between flanges.

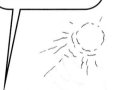

Body warmth improves adherence and softens a rigid skin barrier.

Warm to the task

- Encourage the patient to stay quietly in position for about 5 minutes to improve adherence. The patient's body warmth also helps to improve adherence and soften a rigid skin barrier.
- Attach an ostomy belt to further secure the pouch, if desired. (Some pouches have belt loops, and others have plastic adapters for belts, although these types of ostomy pouches are becoming less common with the improvement in adhesives.)

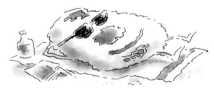

- Leave a bit of air in the pouch to allow drainage to fall to the bottom.
- Apply the closure clamp, if necessary.
- If desired, apply paper tape in a picture-frame fashion to the pouch edges for additional security.

Emptying the pouch
- Put on gloves and an apron. Tilt the bottom of the pouch upward and remove the closure clamp.
- Turn up a cuff on the lower end of the pouch and allow it to drain into the toilet or bedpan.
- Wipe the bottom of the pouch and re-apply the closure clamp.
- If desired, the bottom portion of the pouch can be rinsed with cool tap water. Don't aim water up near the top of the pouch because this may loosen the seal on the skin.
- A two-piece flanged system can also be emptied by unsnapping the pouch. Let the drainage flow into the toilet.

Gas release

- Release flatus through the gas release valve if the pouch has one. Otherwise, release flatus by tilting the pouch bottom upward, releasing the clamp, and expelling the flatus. To release flatus from a flanged system, loosen the seal between the flanges.

Practice pointers

- After performing and explaining the procedure to the patient, encourage the patient's increasing involvement in self-care.
- Use commercial pouch deodorants, if desired. However, most pouches are odour-free, and odour should only be evident when you empty the pouch or if it leaks. Before discharge, suggest that the patient avoid odour-causing foods. (See *Documenting colostomy and ileostomy care.*)

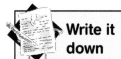

Write it down

Documenting colostomy and ileostomy care

In the patient's notes, record:

- date and time of the pouching system change
- character of drainage, including colour, amount, type and consistency
- appearance of the stoma and peristomal skin
- patient teaching
- patient's response to self-care, and evaluation of his learning progress
- your name, designation and signature.

Male urinary incontinence device

Many patients don't require an indwelling urinary catheter to manage their incontinence. For male patients, a male incontinence device reduces the risk of urinary tract infection from catheterization, promotes bladder retraining when possible, helps prevent skin breakdown and infection, and improves the patient's self-image.

The device consists of a condom catheter secured to the shaft of the penis and connected to a leg bag or drainage bag. It has no contraindications, but it can cause skin irritation and oedema.

> I would like to apply a simple device to help you manage your continence.

What you need

Condom catheter (sheath) ✳ drainage bag ✳ extension tubing ✳ incontinence sheath holder ✳ commercial adhesive strip ✳ gloves and apron ✳ basin ✳ soap ✳ washcloth ✳ towel ✳ optional: adhesive remover.

Getting ready

Fill the basin with lukewarm water. Then bring the basin and the remaining equipment to the patient's bedside.

How you do it

• Explain the procedure to the patient, wash your hands thoroughly, put on gloves and apron, ensure privacy and dignity are maintained.

Applying the device
• If the patient is circumcised, wash the penis with soap and water, rinse well, and pat dry with a towel. If the patient isn't circumcised, gently retract the foreskin, and clean beneath it. Rinse well but don't dry because moisture provides lubrication and prevents friction during foreskin replacement. Replace the foreskin to avoid penile constriction.
• If necessary, shave the base of the penis to prevent the adhesive strip from pulling pubic hair.

Making it stick

• If you're using a pre-cut commercial adhesive strip, insert the glans penis through its opening, and position the strip 2.5 cm from the scrotal area. If you're using uncut adhesive, cut a strip to fit around the shaft of the penis. Remove the protective covering from one side of the adhesive strip and press this side firmly to the penis to enhance adhesion. Remove the covering from the other side of the strip.

Positioning the catheter

• Position the rolled condom catheter at the tip of the penis, with its drainage opening at the urinary meatus. Allow 2.5–5 cm of space

at the tip of the penis to prevent erosion and to allow for expansion when the patient voids.
• Unroll the catheter upward, past the adhesive strip on the shaft of the penis. Then gently press the sheath against the strip until it adheres. (See *How to apply a condom catheter*.)
• After the condom catheter is in place, secure it with an incontinence sheath holder.
• Using extension tubing, connect the condom catheter to the leg bag or drainage bag. Remove and discard your gloves and apron and wash your hands.

Removing the device
• Put on gloves and an apron. Simultaneously roll the condom catheter and adhesive strip off the penis, and then discard them. Also remove and discard the incontinence sheath holder.
• Clean the penis with lukewarm water, rinse thoroughly, and dry. Check for swelling or signs of skin breakdown.
• Remove the leg bag by closing the drain clamp, unlatching the leg straps, and disconnecting the extension tubing at the top of the bag. Discard your gloves and apron and wash your hands.

Practice pointers

• Inspect the condom catheter for twists and the extension tubing for kinks to prevent obstruction of urine flow, which could cause the condom to balloon and eventually dislodge. (See *Documenting use of a male incontinence device*.)

Female indwelling catheter insertion

An indwelling urinary catheter provides the patient with continuous urine drainage. It's inserted into the bladder and a balloon is inflated at the catheter's distal end to prevent it from slipping out. Insert the catheter with extreme care to prevent injury and infection.

What you need

Sterile indwelling catheter (latex or silicone 10–14 French [larger French gauge if requested by clinician]) ✳ syringe filled with 10 ml of normal saline solution ✳ 10 ml syringe ✳ protective pad ✳ two pairs of sterile gloves ✳ sterile drape ✳ apron ✳ sterile gauze ✳ sterile urine receptacle (kidney bowl) ✳ Normasol solution ✳ sterile anaesthetic gel (such as Instillagel) ✳ sterile drainage collection bag

How to apply a condom catheter

Apply an adhesive strip to the shaft of the penis about 2.5 cm from the scrotal area.

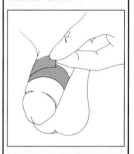

Then roll the condom catheter on to the penis past the adhesive strip, leaving about 1 cm clearance at the end. Press the sheath gently against the strip until it adheres.

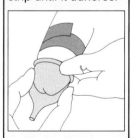

✳ clinical waste bag ✳ optional: urine-specimen container and laboratory request form, leg band with Velcro closure, gooseneck lamp pillows or rolled blankets or towels.

At your disposal

Pre-packaged sterile disposable catheterization packs that usually contain all the necessary equipment are available. Many urinary catheters now come with a syringe in the sterile packaging, pre-filled with 10 ml of normal saline solution, but remember if the patient is requiring a change of catheter you will require an empty 10 ml sterile syringe to remove the water from the catheter you wish to remove.

In case of contamination

In addition, gather an extra pair of sterile gloves and an extra catheter of an appropriate size to be readily available at the bedside in case of contamination during insertion.

Getting ready

Check the medical and nursing records to determine if a catheter size or type has been specified. Then wash your hands, select the appropriate equipment, and assemble it at the patient's bedside.

How you do it

• Explain the procedure to the patient and provide privacy. Check her vital signs and ask when she voided last. Percuss and palpate the bladder to establish baseline data. Ask if the patient feels the urge to void. Make sure she isn't allergic and that there are no contraindications to administering the local anaesthetic (lignocaine); if she is allergic, obtain another local anaesthetic agent, seek advice from the pharmacy if necessary.
• Place a gooseneck lamp next to the patient's bed so that you can see the urinary meatus clearly in poor lighting.

Assume the position

• Place the female patient in the supine position, on top of the protective pad, with her knees flexed and separated and her feet flat on the bed. If she finds this position uncomfortable, have her flex one knee and keep the other leg flat on the bed. (See *Positioning for catheter insertion*.)
• Ask the patient to hold the position to give you a clear view of the urinary meatus and to prevent contamination of the sterile field.

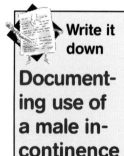

Write it down

Document-ing use of a male in-continence device

• Record the date and time that the incontinence device was applied and removed
• Also, note skin condition and the patient's response to the device, including voiding pattern, to assist with bladder retraining
• Record your name, designation and signature.

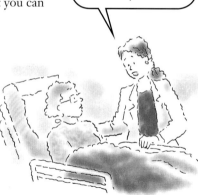

I would like you to lie flat, with your knees flexed and separated.

Sterile fieldwork

- Wash your hands, put on apron and open the sterile catheterization pack and place all sterile equipment on to this (as described in Aseptic technique, Chapter 4). Pour the Normasol solution over the low-linting cotton balls and into the galley pot provided in the catheterization pack.
- Open and apply first pair of sterile gloves.
- Separate the labia majora and labia minora as widely as possible with the thumb, middle and index fingers so you have a full view of the urinary meatus. Keep the labia well separated throughout the procedure, so they don't obscure the urinary meatus or contaminate the area when it's cleaned, you may find it useful to use sterile dry gauze to hold the labia open.
- With your other hand, pick up a sterile, low-linting cotton ball and wipe one side of the urinary meatus with a single downward motion. Wipe the other side with another sterile cotton ball in the same way. Then wipe directly over the meatus with still another sterile cotton ball. Take care not to contaminate your sterile glove— use a non-touch aseptic technique.
- Open the local anaesthetic solution, expel the air in the syringe and apply a drop of gel over the area of the urethral meatus and wait for 30 seconds. (Instillagel in particular has dilating properties and thus will assist in dilating the urethral meatus and making it easier to view.)
- Insert the rest of the local anaesthetic into the urethral meatus. While this is taking effect remove the first pair of gloves and wash or gel your hands.
- Apply the second pair of sterile gloves and place the sterile field in front of the patient's perineum. Place the sterile kidney bowl on this sterile field. Take care not to contaminate your gloves.

Female facts

- Again, separate the labia majora and labia minora as widely as possible with the thumb, middle and index fingers so you have a full view of the urinary meatus. Keep the labia well separated throughout the procedure, so they don't obscure the urinary meatus; you may find it useful to use sterile dry gauze to hold the labia open.

Advanced class

- Pick up the catheter in your gloved hand (sterile catheter in sterile glove, don't worry) and curl it around your hand so that you have approximately 5–6 cm protruding, direct this towards and insert into the urethral meatus.

Ages and stages

Positioning for catheter insertion

The older female patient may need pillows or rolled towels or blankets for positioning support. If necessary, ask her to lie on her side with one knee drawn up to her chest during catheterization (as shown below). This position also may be helpful for disabled patients or post-op orthopaedic patients.

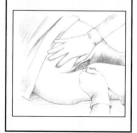

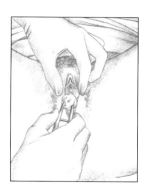

Indwelling catheter care and removal

Catheter care should be performed while administering patient hygiene care needs and immediately after perineal care. When the patient's condition warrants catheter removal, you will also be required to remove the indwelling catheter.

Difference of opinion

Because some studies suggest that catheter care increases the risk of infection and other complications rather than reduces it, many healthcare providers do not recommend daily catheter care. Thus, individual policy dictates whether a patient receives such care. Regardless of the catheter care policy, the equipment and the patient's genitalia require inspection twice daily and a closed system should always be maintained.

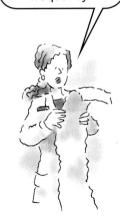

Check local policy regarding catheter care, the procedure and the frequency.

What you need

For catheter care

Non-sterile gloves and apron ✳ gauze pads ✳ basin and water ✳ leg bag ✳ collection bag ✳ adhesive tape ✳ optional: specimen container. Commercially prepared catheter care kits containing all necessary supplies are available.

For catheter removal

Apron ✳ gloves ✳ alcohol pad ✳ 10 ml syringe with a Luer Lok ✳ bedpan ✳ protective pad ✳ optional: clamp for bladder retraining.

Getting ready

Wash your hands and bring all equipment to the patient's bedside. Open the gauze pads, place several in the basin with warm water.

How you do it

- Explain the procedure to the patient, gain permission, provide privacy and maintain dignity.

Catheter care

- Wash your hands, put on gloves and apron.
- Make sure that the lighting is adequate so that you can see the perineum and catheter tubing clearly.

- Inspect the catheter for any problems, and check the urine drainage for mucus, blood clots, sediment and turbidity. Then pinch the catheter between two fingers to determine if the lumen contains any material. If you notice any of these conditions (or if your local policy requires it), obtain a urine specimen and notify the doctor.
- Inspect the outside of the catheter where it enters the urinary meatus for encrusted material and suppurative drainage. Also inspect the tissue around the meatus for irritation or swelling.

Wipe away

- Then use a saturated, sterile gauze pad to clean the outside of the catheter and the tissue around the meatus. To avoid contaminating the urinary tract, always clean by wiping away from—never toward—the urinary meatus. Use a dry gauze pad to remove encrusted material. Don't pull on the catheter while you're cleaning it. This can injure the urethra and the bladder wall. It can also expose a section of the catheter that was inside the urethra, so that when you release the catheter the newly contaminated section will re-enter the urethra, introducing potentially infectious organisms.
- Remove your gloves.
- Most drainage bags have a plastic clamp on the tubing to attach them to the sheet. If this isn't available, wrap a rubber band around the drainage tubing, insert a safety pin through a loop of the rubber band, and pin the tubing to the sheet below bladder level. Then attach the collection bag, below bladder level, to the bed frame.

Catheter removal

- Wash your hands. Assemble the equipment at the patient's bedside. Explain the procedure to the patient and tell her that she may feel slight discomfort. Tell her that you'll check her periodically during the first 6–24 hours after catheter removal to make sure she resumes voiding.
- Put on gloves and apron. Attach the syringe to the Luer Lok mechanism on the catheter. Place a protective pad under the patient's buttocks.

Deflating the balloon

- Pull back on the plunger of the syringe. This deflates the balloon by aspirating the injected fluid. The amount of fluid injected is usually indicated on the tip of the catheter's balloon lumen as well as in the patient's medical and nursing records.
- Before removing the catheter, offer the patient a bedpan. Then hold the catheter with the gauze and gently ease it from the urethra. Inspect the balloon to be sure that it's intact. If it isn't, report this to the doctor.
- Measure and record the amount of urine in the collection bag before discarding it.

Home care connection

Teaching about leg bags

A urine drainage bag attached to the leg gives a catheterized patient greater mobility. Because the bag is hidden under clothing, it also may help him feel more comfortable about catheterization. Leg bags usually are worn during the day and connected at night to a standard collection device.

If your patient will be discharged with an indwelling catheter, teach him how to attach and remove a leg bag. To demonstrate, gather a bag with a short drainage tube, two straps, an alcohol pad, adhesive tape (if necessary) and a clamp.

Attaching the leg bag

When teaching the patient how to attach the leg bag, follow these steps:

- Provide privacy and explain the procedure. Emphasize that a leg bag is smaller than a standard collection device and may have to be emptied more frequently.
- Remove the protective covering from the tip of the drainage tube. Then show the patient how to clean the tip with an alcohol pad, wiping away from the opening to avoid contaminating the tube. Show him how to attach the tube to the catheter.
- Place the drainage bag on the patient's calf or thigh. Have him fasten the straps securely (as shown), and show him how to tape the catheter to his leg.

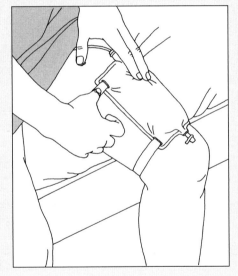

Let's not get complicated

To avoid complications, provide the following guidelines:

- To prevent a full leg bag from damaging the bladder wall and urethra, instruct the patient to empty the bag when it's only half full.
- To prevent infection, tell the patient to wash the leg bag with soap and water or antibacterial solution before each use.

Practice pointers

- Your local policy may require the use of specific cleaning agents for catheter care, so check the policy manual before beginning this procedure. A doctor's direction or prescription will also be needed to apply antibiotic ointments to the urinary meatus after cleaning.

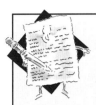

Write it down

Documenting indwelling catheter care and removal

When providing care for a patient with an indwelling catheter, document your name, designation and signature as well as:

- care you performed
- changes to the plan of care
- patient complaints
- condition of the perineum and urinary meatus
- characteristics of urine in the drainage bag
- whether a specimen was sent for laboratory analysis
- fluid intake and output. (Usually, an hourly record is required for critically ill patients and haemodynamically unstable patients with renal insufficiency.)

Catheter removal

Be sure to record:

- date and time of catheter removal
- patient's tolerance of the procedure
- when and how much the patient voided after removal (usually for first 24 hours)
- associated problems.

Bladder retraining

Document:

- date and time the catheter was clamped and released
- volume and appearance of urine.

Stay low

- Avoid raising the drainage bag above bladder level. This prevents reflux of urine, which may contain bacteria. Ensure the system is cared for when the patient is moved from bed to bed, bed to chair, bed to trolley.
- If the patient will be discharged with an indwelling catheter, teach her how to use a leg bag. (See *Teaching about leg bags*.)
- When changing catheters after long-term use (usually 6 weeks), you may need a larger size catheter because the meatus enlarges, causing urine to leak around the catheter. (See *Documenting indwelling catheter care and removal*.)

Catheter irrigation

To avoid introducing microorganisms into the bladder, you should irrigate an indwelling catheter only when necessary. The procedure is generally performed to remove an obstruction—such as a blood clot that develops after bladder, kidney or prostate surgery.

What you need

Prescribed irrigating solution ✳ sterile receptacle or basin ✳ 50 ml catheter-tip syringe ✳ two alcohol pads ✳ sterile gloves and apron ✳ protective pad ✳ intake–output (fluid balance) sheet ✳ optional: basin of warm water.

We pause for this commercial message

Commercially packaged kits containing sterile irrigating solution, a graduated receptacle, and a 50 ml catheter-tip syringe are available.

Getting ready

Check the expiration date on the irrigating solution. To prevent spasms during instillation of solution, warm it to room temperature. If necessary, place the container in a basin of warm water. Never heat the solution on a burner or in a microwave oven. Hot irrigating solution can injure the patient's bladder.

How you do it

• Wash your hands, put on apron and assemble the equipment at the bedside. Explain the procedure to the patient and provide privacy.
• Place the protective pad under the patient's buttocks to protect the bed linen.
• Create a sterile field at the patient's bedside by opening the sterile equipment tray or pre-packaged kit. Using an aseptic technique, open the irrigating fluid bottle.

Fill 'er up

• Place the tip of the syringe into the solution. Pull back the plunger and fill the syringe with the appropriate amount of solution (usually 30 ml).
• Open the package of alcohol pads; then put on sterile gloves. Clean the juncture of the catheter and drainage tube with an alcohol pad to remove as many bacterial contaminants as possible.

Don't let go

• Disconnect the catheter and drainage tube by twisting them in opposite directions and carefully pulling them apart without creating tension on the catheter. Don't let go of the catheter—hold it in your

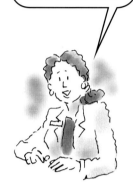

Perform catheter irrigation to remove an obstruction such as a blood clot.

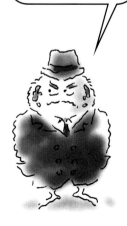

I'm always looking for new territory. Be careful when performing catheter irrigation or I'll take over.

hand. Then place the end of the drainage tube on the sterile field, making sure not to contaminate the tube.
- Twist the catheter-tip syringe on to the catheter's distal end.

Flash flood

- Slowly push the plunger of the syringe to instil the irrigating solution through the catheter. If necessary, refill the syringe and repeat this step until you've instilled the prescribed amount of irrigating solution.
- Remove the syringe and direct the return flow from the catheter into the basin or bowl. Don't let the catheter end touch the drainage in the receptacle or become contaminated in any other way.
- Wipe the end of the drainage tube and catheter with the remaining alcohol pad.
- Wait a few seconds until the alcohol evaporates; then re-attach the drainage tubing to the catheter.
- Dispose of all used supplies using local policy guidelines.

Practice pointers

- Catheter irrigation requires a strict aseptic technique to prevent bacteria from entering the bladder. The ends of the catheter and drainage tube and the tip of the syringe must be kept sterile throughout the procedure.

In-stall-ation

- If you encounter resistance during instillation of the irrigating solution, don't try to force the solution into the bladder. Instead, stop the procedure and notify the doctor. If an indwelling catheter becomes totally obstructed, obtain permission to remove it and replace it with a new one to prevent bladder distention, acute renal failure, urinary stasis and subsequent infection. (See *Documenting catheter irrigation*.)

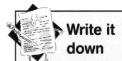

Write it down

Document-ing catheter irrigation

In your notes, record:

- time of irrigation
- amount, colour and consistency of return urine flow
- patient's tolerance of the procedure
- any resistance met during instillation of the solution
- your name, designation and signature.

If the return flow volume measures less than the amount of solution instilled, note this on the fluid intake and output balance sheets as well as in your notes, and notify the doctor.

Continuous bladder irrigation

Continuous bladder irrigation can help prevent urinary tract obstruction by flushing out small blood clots that form after prostate or bladder surgery. It may also be used to treat an irritated, inflamed or infected bladder lining.

Triple threat

This procedure requires placement of a triple-lumen catheter. One lumen controls balloon inflation, one allows irrigant inflow, and one

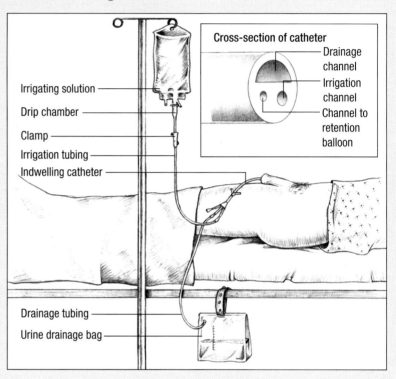

Set-up for continuous bladder irrigation

In continuous bladder irrigation, a triple-lumen catheter allows irrigating solution to flow into the bladder through one lumen and flow out through another, as shown in the inset. The third lumen is used to inflate the balloon that holds the catheter in place.

Irrigating solution

Drip chamber

Clamp

Irrigation tubing

Indwelling catheter

Drainage tubing

Urine drainage bag

Cross-section of catheter

Drainage channel

Irrigation channel

Channel to retention balloon

allows irrigant outflow. The continuous flow of irrigating solution through the bladder also creates a mild tamponade that may help prevent venous haemorrhage. (See *Set-up for continuous bladder irrigation*.)

What you need

One 4-litre container or two 2-litre containers of irrigating solution (usually normal saline solution) or the prescribed amount of medicated solution ✳ Y-type tubing made specifically for bladder irrigation ✳ alcohol pad ✳ I.V. pole ✳ gloves and apron ✳ continuous bladder irrigation documentation.

Getting ready

Before starting continuous bladder irrigation, double-check the irrigating solution against the doctor's directions. If the solution contains medication, check the patient's chart to make sure he isn't allergic to the drug.

How you do it

- Wash your hands. Assemble all equipment at the patient's bedside. Explain the procedure to the patient, gain permission, maintain dignity and provide privacy.
- Insert the spike of the Y-type tubing into the container of irrigating solution. (If you have a two-container system, insert one spike into each container.)
- Squeeze the drip chamber on the spike of the tubing.
- Open the flow clamp and flush the tubing to remove air, which could cause bladder distension. Then close the clamp.

Hanging out

- To begin, hang the bag of irrigating solution on the I.V. pole.
- Clean the opening to the inflow lumen of the catheter with the alcohol pad.
- Insert the distal end of the Y-type tubing securely into the inflow lumen (third port) of the catheter.
- Make sure the catheter's outflow lumen is securely attached to the drainage bag tubing.
- Open the flow clamp under the container of irrigating solution, and set the drip rate as ordered.
- To prevent air from entering the system, don't let the primary container empty completely before replacing it.

Close this, open that

- If you have a two-container system, simultaneously close the flow clamp under the nearly empty container and open the flow clamp under the reserve container. This prevents reflux of irrigating solution from the reserve container into the nearly empty one. Hang a new reserve container on the I.V. pole and insert the tubing, maintaining asepsis.
- Empty the drainage bag about every 4 hours, or as often as needed. Use a sterile technique to avoid the risk of contamination.

Practice pointers

- Check the inflow and outflow lines periodically for kinks, to make sure the solution is running freely. If the solution flows rapidly, check the lines frequently.

Go all out—measure and assess

• Measure the outflow volume accurately. It should equal or, allowing for urine production, slightly exceed the inflow volume. If inflow volume exceeds outflow volume post-operatively, suspect bladder rupture at the suture lines or renal damage, and notify the doctor immediately.

• Also assess outflow for changes in appearance and for blood clots, especially if irrigation is being performed post-operatively to control bleeding. If drainage is bright red, irrigating solution should usually be infused rapidly with the clamp wide open until drainage clears. Notify the doctor at once if you suspect haemorrhage. If drainage is clear, the solution is usually given at a rate of 40–60 drops/minute. The doctor typically specifies the rate for antibiotic solutions. (See *Documenting continuous bladder irrigation*.)

Nephrostomy and cystostomy tube care

A nephrostomy tube drains urine directly from a kidney when a disorder inhibits the normal flow of urine. The tube is usually placed percutaneously, although sometimes it's surgically inserted through the renal cortex and medulla into the renal pelvis from a lateral incision in the flank. Draining urine with a nephrostomy tube also allows kidney tissue damaged by obstructive disease to heal.

Creating a diversion

A cystostomy tube drains urine from the bladder, diverting it from the urethra. This type of tube is used after certain gynaecological procedures, bladder surgery, prostatectomy and for severe urethral strictures or traumatic injury. Inserted about 5 cm above the symphysis pubis, a cystostomy tube may be used alone or with an indwelling urethral catheter. Care involves changing the dressing daily (or more often if it becomes soiled) and irrigating the tube if necessary.

What you need

For dressing changes

Normasol solution ✳ gauze pads ✳ sterile basin ✳ waste bag ✳ protective pad ✳ clean gloves (for dressing removal) ✳ sterile gloves (for new dressing) ✳ apron ✳ forceps ✳ pre-cut drain dressings or

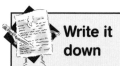

Write it down

Document-ing continuous bladder irrigation

Each time you finish a container of irrigating solution, record the date, time and amount of fluid given on the patient's intake and output record.

Each time you empty the drainage bag, record the time and amount of drainage, appearance of the drainage and any patient complaints.

transparent semi-permeable dressings ✳ adhesive tape (preferably hypoallergenic).

For nephrostomy-tube irrigation
3 ml syringe ✳ alcohol pad ✳ normal saline solution.
Commercially prepared sterile dressing kits may be available.

Getting ready

Wash your hands and assemble all equipment at the patient's bedside, put on the apron. Open several packages of gauze pads, place them in the sterile basin, and pour the Normasol solution over them. If you're using a commercially packaged dressing kit, open it using aseptic technique. Fill the basin with solution.

Cleanliness isn't next to the other equipment

Open the waste bag and place it away from the other equipment to avoid contaminating the sterile field.

How you do it

• Provide privacy and explain the procedure to the patient, gain permission.

Changing a dressing
• Help the patient to lie on his back (for a cystostomy tube) or on the side opposite the tube (for a nephrostomy tube) so that you can see the tube clearly and change the dressing more easily.
• Place the protective pad under the patient to absorb excess drainage and keep him dry.

Changing hands (just gloves really)

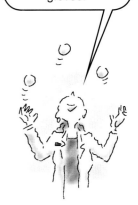

As a nurse, I sure could use four hands at times! For these tube changes, however, I need two sets of gloves.

• Put on the non-sterile gloves. Carefully remove the tape around the tube, and then remove the wet or soiled dressing. Discard the tape and dressing in the waste bag. Remove the gloves and discard them in the bag. Wash your hands.
• Put on the sterile gloves. Pick up a saturated pad or dip a dry one into the bowl of solution.
• To clean the wound, wipe only once with each pad, moving from the insertion site outward. Discard the used pad in the waste bag. Don't touch the bag, to avoid contaminating your gloves.

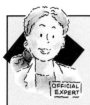

Advice from the experts

Taping a nephrostomy tube

To tape a nephrostomy tube directly to the patient's skin, follow these steps:

- Cut a wide piece of hypoallergenic adhesive tape twice lengthwise to its midpoint.

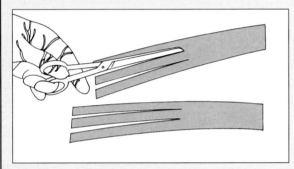

- Apply the uncut end of the tape to the skin so that the midpoint meets the tube.
- Wrap the middle strip around the tube in spiral fashion.

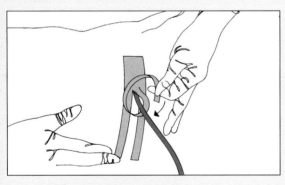

- Tape the other two strips to the patient's skin on both sides of the tube. For greater security, repeat this step with a second piece of tape, applying it in the reverse direction. You may also apply two more strips of tape perpendicular to and over the first two pieces.

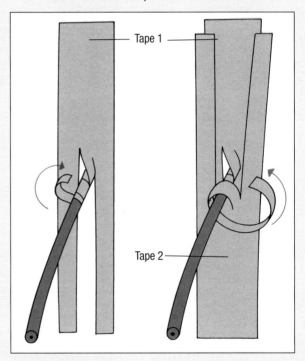

Tape 1

Tape 2

Dropping anchor

Always apply another strip of tape lower down on the tube in the direction of the drainage tube to further anchor the tube. Don't put tension on any sutures that prevent tube distension.

All dressed up

- Pick up a sterile drain dressing and place it around the tube. If necessary, overlap two drain dressings to provide maximum absorption. Or, depending on your local policy, apply a transparent semi-permeable dressing over the site and tubing to allow observation of the site without removing the dressing.
- Secure the dressing with hypoallergenic tape. Then tape the tube to the patient's lateral abdomen to prevent tension on the tube. (See *Taping a nephrostomy tube*.)
- Dispose of all equipment appropriately.

Irrigating a nephrostomy tube
- Fill the 3 ml syringe with the normal saline solution.
- Clean the junction of the nephrostomy tube and drainage tube with the alcohol pad and disconnect the tubes.

Small serving

- Insert the syringe into the nephrostomy tube opening, and instil 2–3 ml of saline solution into the tube. Never irrigate a nephrostomy tube with more than 5 ml of solution because the capacity of the renal pelvis is usually between 4 and 8 ml.
- Slowly aspirate the solution back into the syringe. To avoid damaging the renal pelvis tissue, never pull back forcefully on the plunger.
- If the solution doesn't return, remove the syringe from the tube and re-attach it to the drainage tubing to allow the solution to drain by gravity.
- Dispose of all equipment following local policy or guidelines.

Practice pointers

- Change dressings once a day or more often if needed.
- When necessary, irrigate a cystostomy tube as you would an indwelling urinary catheter. Be sure to perform the irrigation gently to avoid damaging any suture lines.
- Check a nephrostomy tube frequently for kinks or obstructions. Suspect an obstruction when the amount of urine in the drainage bag decreases or the amount of urine around the insertion site increases. Pressure created by urine backing up in the tube can damage nephrons. Gently curve a cystostomy tube to prevent kinks.
- Typically, a cystostomy tube for a post-operative urologic patient should be checked hourly for 24 hours to ensure adequate drainage and tube patency. (See *Documenting nephrostomy and cystostomy care*.)

Write it down

Document-ing neph-rostomy and cystostomy care

In your notes, record:

- colour and amount of drainage from the nephrostomy or cystostomy tube
- drainage colour changes (as they occur)
- drainage colour, amount and characteristics from each tube, if the patient has more than one tube
- amount and type of irrigant used (if irrigation is necessary)
- whether a complete return was obtained
- your name, designation and signature.

Urinary diversion stoma care

Urinary diversions provide an alternative route for urine flow when a disorder, such as an invasive bladder tumour, impedes normal drainage.

Temporary diversion

In conditions requiring temporary urinary drainage or diversion, a suprapubic or urethral catheter is usually inserted to divert the flow of urine temporarily. The catheter remains in place until the incision heals.

Permanent addition

A permanent urinary diversion is indicated in any condition that requires a total cystectomy (removal of the bladder). Ileal conduit (also known as ileal loop or ileal bladder) and continent urinary diversion are the two types of permanent urinary diversions with stomas. These procedures usually require the patient to wear a urine-collection appliance and to care for the stoma created during surgery. (See *Types of permanent urinary diversion.*)

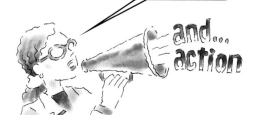

Let's take it from the beginning. Places! Nurse, I want you at the patient's bedside . . . and... action

What you need

Soap and warm water ✳ waste bag ✳ protective pad ✳ hypoallergenic paper tape ✳ alcohol pads ✳ urine collection container ✳ catheter (usually #14 or #16 French) ✳ ruler ✳ scissors ✳ urine-collection appliance (with or without anti-reflux valve) ✳ graduated container (jug) ✳ gauze ✳ washcloth ✳ skin barrier in liquid, paste, wafer or sheet form ✳ appliance belt ✳ two pairs of gloves ✳ optional: adhesive solvent, irrigating syringe, tampon.

Commercial break

Commercially packaged stoma care kits are available. In place of soap and water, you can use adhesive remover pads, if available, or cotton gauze saturated with adhesive solvent.

Getting ready

Assemble all the equipment on the patient's over-bed table. Tape the waste bag to the table for ready access. Provide privacy for the patient, and wash your hands, put on gloves and apron. Measure

Types of permanent urinary diversion

The two main types of permanent urinary diversions are the ileal conduit and the continent urinary diversion. The steps involved in creating each are described here.

Ileal conduit

A segment of the ileum is excised, and the two ends of the ileum that result from this excision are sutured closed. Then the ureters are dissected from the bladder and anastomosed to the ileal segment. One end of the ileal segment is closed with sutures; the opposite end is brought through the abdominal wall, forming a stoma.

Continent urinary diversion

A tube is formed from part of the ascending colon and ileum. One end of the tube is brought to the skin to form the stoma. At the internal end of this tube, a nipple valve is constructed so urine won't drain out unless a catheter is inserted through the stoma into the newly formed bladder pouch. The urethral neck is sutured closed.

Another recently developed type of continent urinary diversion is 'hooked' back to the urethra, obviating the need for a stoma.

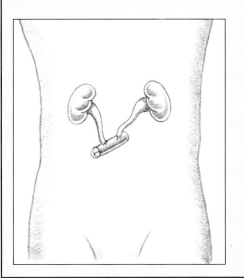

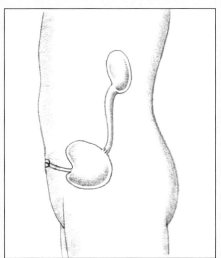

the diameter of the stoma with a ruler. Cut the opening of the appliance with the scissors—it shouldn't be more than 0.3–0.4 cm larger than the diameter of the stoma. Moisten the faceplate of the appliance with a small amount of solvent or water to prepare it for adhesion.

Performance art

Performing these preliminary steps at the bedside allows you to demonstrate the procedure and show the patient that it isn't difficult, which will help him relax.

How you do it

• Wash your hands again. Explain the procedure to the patient as you go along, and offer constant reinforcement and reassurance to counteract negative reactions that may be elicited by stoma care.
• Place the bed in a low position so the patient's abdomen is flat. This position eliminates skin folds that could cause the appliance to slip or irritate the skin and allows the patient to observe or participate.
• Put on the gloves and place the protective pad under the patient's side, near the stoma. Open the drain valve of the appliance being replaced to empty the urine into the graduated container. Then, to remove the appliance, apply soap and water or adhesive solvent as you gently push the skin back from the pouch. If the appliance is disposable, discard it into the waste bag. If it's reusable, clean it with soap and lukewarm water and let it air-dry.

Adhere to this: avoid adhesive

• To avoid irritating the patient's stoma, avoid touching it with adhesive solvent. If adhesive remains on the skin, gently rub it off with a dry gauze pad.
• To prevent a constant flow of urine on to the skin while you're changing the appliance, wick the urine with an absorbent, lint-free material. (See *Wicking urine from a stoma*.)

Wash and dry

• Use a washcloth and water to carefully wash off any crystal deposits that may have formed around the stoma. If urine has stagnated and has a strong odour, use soap to wash it off. Be sure to rinse thoroughly to remove any oily residue that could cause the appliance to slip.
• Follow your local skin care protocol to treat any minor skin problems.
• Dry the peristomal area thoroughly with a gauze pad because moisture will keep the appliance from sticking. Remove any hair from the area with scissors or an electric razor to prevent hair follicles from becoming irritated when the pouch is removed, which can cause folliculitis.

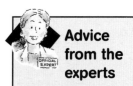

Advice from the experts

Wicking urine from a stoma

Use a piece of rolled, cottonless gauze or a tampon to wick urine from a stoma. Working by capillary action, wicking absorbs urine while you prepare the patient's skin to hold a urine-collection appliance.

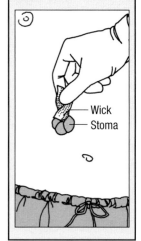

Wick
Stoma

• Inspect the stoma to see if it's healing properly and to detect complications. Inspect the peristomal skin for redness, irritation and intactness.

Skin sense

• Apply the skin barrier. If you apply a wafer or sheet, cut it to fit over the stoma. Remove any protective backing and set the barrier aside with the adhesive side up. If you apply a liquid barrier (such as Skin-Prep), saturate a gauze pad with it and coat the peristomal skin. Move in concentric circles outward from the stoma until you've covered an area 5 cm larger than the wafer. Let the skin dry for several minutes—it should feel tacky. Gently press the wafer around the stoma, sticky side down, smoothing from the stoma outward.
• If you're using a barrier paste, open the tube, squeeze out a small amount, and then discard it. Then squeeze a ribbon of paste directly on to the peristomal skin about 1.3 cm from the stoma, making a complete circle. Make several more concentric circles outward. Dip your fingers into lukewarm water, and smooth the paste until the skin is 0.6–1.3 cm thick. Then discard the gloves, wash your hands, and put on new gloves.
• Remove and discard the material used for wicking urine.
• Now place the appliance over the stoma, leaving only a small amount (1–2 cm) of skin exposed.
• Secure the faceplate of the appliance to the skin with paper tape, if recommended. To do this, place a piece of tape lengthwise on each edge of the faceplate so that the tape overlaps on to the skin.

Buckle up

• Apply the appliance belt, making sure that it's on a level with the stoma. If the belt is applied above or below the stoma, it could break the bag's seal, rub or injure the stoma. The belt should be loose enough for you to insert two fingers between the skin and the belt. If the belt is too tight, it could irritate the skin or cause internal damage. Some devices do not require a belt. Instead, the pouch has a ridge that fits over the rim of barrier adhesive and snaps securely into place.
• Dispose of the used materials following local policies and procedures.

Practice pointers

• Tell the patient to empty the appliance through the drain valve when it's one-third to one-half full to prevent the weight of the urine from loosening the seal around the stoma.

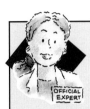

Advice from the experts

Caring for the patient with a continent urinary diversion

In a continent urinary diversion (an alternative to the traditional ileal conduit), a pouch created from the ascending colon and terminal ileum serves as a new bladder, which empties through a stoma. To drain urine continuously, several drains are inserted into this reconstructed bladder and left in place for 3–6 weeks until the new stoma heals. The patient will be discharged from the hospital with the drains in place. He'll return to have them removed and to learn how to catheterize his stoma.

First hospitalization

After the patient undergoes the procedure, follow these steps:

- Immediately after surgery, monitor intake and output from each drain. Stay alert for decreased output, which may indicate that urine flow is obstructed.
- Watch for common post-operative complications, such as infection and bleeding. Also watch for signs of urinary leakage, which include increased abdominal distention and urine appearing around the drains or midline incision.
- Using an irrigating syringe, irrigate the drains as ordered.
- Clean the area around the drains daily—with sterile water. Apply a dry, sterile dressing to the area. Use pre-cut drain dressings around the drain to absorb leakage.
- To increase the patient's mobility and comfort, connect the drains to a leg bag.

Second hospitalization or outpatient visit

When the patient requires care after the initial hospitalisation, follow these steps:

- After the patient's drains are removed, teach the patient how to catheterize the stoma. Gather the following equipment on a clean towel: catheter (14 or 16 French), water-soluble lubricant, washcloth, stoma covering (non-adherent gauze pad or panty liner), hypoallergenic adhesive tape and an irrigating solution (optional).
- Apply water-soluble lubricant to the catheter tip to ease insertion.
- Remove and discard the stoma cover. Using the washcloth, clean the stoma and the area around it, starting at the stoma and working outward in a circular motion.
- Hold the urine-collection container under the catheter; then slowly insert the catheter into the stoma. Urine should begin to flow into the container. If it doesn't, gently rotate the catheter or redirect its angle. If the catheter drains slowly, it may be plugged with mucus. Irrigate it with sterile saline solution or sterile water to clear it. When the flow stops, pinch the catheter closed and remove it.

Home care

When the patient goes home, provide these instructions:

- Teach the patient how to care for the drains and their insertion sites during the 3–6 weeks he'll be at home before their removal, and teach him how to attach them to a leg bag. Also teach him how to recognize signs and symptoms of infection and obstruction.
- After the drains are removed, teach the patient how to empty the pouch and how to establish a routine. Initially, he should catheterize the stoma and empty the pouch every 2–3 hours. Later, he should catheterize every 4 hours while awake and also irrigate the pouch each morning and evening, if ordered. Instruct him to empty the pouch whenever he feels a sensation of fullness.

Night collection

- Instruct the patient to connect his appliance to a urine-collection container before he goes to sleep. The continuous flow of urine into the container during the night prevents the urine from accumulating and stagnating in the appliance.
- If the patient has a continent urinary diversion, make sure you know how to meet his special needs. (See *Caring for the patient with a continent urinary diversion*.)
- Inform the patient about support services provided by ostomy clubs and nurses in the community. (See *Documenting urinary diversion stoma care*.)

Quick quiz

1. During catheter care, all of the following steps help avoid contaminating the urinary tract, except:
- A. Cleaning by wiping away from the urinary meatus.
- B. Exposing and cleaning a section of the catheter that was inside the urethra.
- C. Using a dry gauze pad to remove encrusted material.

Answer: B. Exposing a section of the catheter that was inside the urethra can cause this newly contaminated section to introduce potentially infectious organisms when it re-enters the urethra.

2. If drainage from continuous bladder irrigation is bright red, you should infuse the irrigating solution at:
- A. 40 to 60 drops/minute.
- B. 20 to 60 drops/minute.
- C. A rapid rate with the clamp wide open.

Answer: C. If drainage is bright red, run the irrigating solution rapidly until drainage clears. Continuous flow of irrigating solution through the bladder helps create a mild tamponade that may help prevent haemorrhage. Notify the doctor if you suspect haemorrhage.

3. What's the total volume of solution that can be safely used to irrigate a nephrostomy tube?
- A. 2 to 3 ml.
- B. 5 to 10 ml.
- C. 10 to 20 ml.

Answer: A. Never irrigate a nephrostomy tube with more than 5 ml of solution because renal pelvis capacity usually is between 4 and 8 ml.

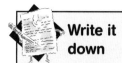

Write it down

Document-ing urinary diversion stoma care

- Record the appearance and colour of the stoma and whether it's inverted, flush with the skin or protruding
- If it protrudes, note by how much it protrudes above the skin (the normal range is 1.3–2 cm)
- Record the appearance and condition of the peristomal skin, noting any redness or irritation or complaints of itching or burning
- Record your name, designation and signature, plus the time of the care episode.

4. What's the best patient positioning during urinary diversion stoma care?

    A.   Low position.

    B.   High position.

    C.   Left lateral position.

Answer: A. Low position eliminates skin folds that could cause the appliance to slip or irritate the skin and lets the patient observe or participate in the care.

5. If inflow or outflow during continuous bladder irrigation is slow or absent, you should take all of the following steps, except:

    A.   Checking the tubing for kinks.

    B.   Repositioning the patient.

    C.   Lowering the solution.

Answer: C. Raising, not lowering, the solution may increase the flow rate of the solution by increasing the pressure of gravity.

Scoring

☆☆☆   If you answered all five items correctly, super! You're as smooth as a perfect catheter insertion.

☆☆   If you answered three or four items correctly, cool! You've got a ken for kidney procedures.

☆   If you answered fewer than three items correctly, that's okay. Just read the chapter again, and you'll begin to filter all the important facts.

⑧ Enhanced skills

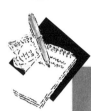

Just the facts

In this chapter, you'll learn:

♦ how enhanced skills such as venepuncture, I.V. cannulation and I.V. therapy administration are performed

♦ about patient care, complications and patient teaching that are associated with each procedure

♦ about essential documentation for each procedure.

'Enhanced skills' are undertaken by registered nurses or healthcare professionals who have undertaken further theoretical and practical training post-registration to gain further underpinning knowledge, competency and confidence in performing these procedures or skills. Post-registration nurses who undertake these skills must be able to provide documented evidence that they are confident and competent in these skills. This is usually in the form of a competency programme document, completed during and after the course of study, i.e. for a venepuncture course—attended the theoretical training, practised skill in simulation, practised skill in a clinical area under supervision until both the supervisor and candidate are happy that competence and confidence have been achieved. It could also be in the form of a reflective diary, a piece of writing documenting what has been learnt and how this has been achieved. It is worth noting that a 'Certificate of attendance' does not provide this evidence, it only gives evidence that you attended the teaching—not that you gained any knowledge.

Pre-registration nurses cannot perform these procedures and therefore essential skills cluster referencing is not included in this chapter, it is not applicable. However, there are guidelines and standards which are applicable. such as:

• *Standards for infusion therapy*, Royal College of Nursing (2005).
• *Standards for medicines management*, Nursing and Midwifery Council (2007).
• Local policies and procedures, individual to each employer.

For further information on intravenous therapy, please refer to the text *I.V. therapy made incredibly easy*, another in this series of 'Made Incredibly Easy' books.

Venepuncture

Venepuncture is an aseptic technique (performed using a non-touch technique) which involves piercing a vein with a needle and collecting a blood sample in an evacuated tube. You will use predominantly the three major veins located in the antecubital fossa (the triangular area that lies anterior to and below the elbow) of the arm (the basilic, median cubital and the cephalic veins). However, metacarpal and digital veins may also be pierced using a butterfly access device.

What you need

Single use or non-porous tourniquet (latex-free, if required) ✳ gloves (clean, not sterile) and apron ✳ evacuated tubes and needle holder ✳ 70% alcohol, pre-injection swab ✳ 20G or 21G needle for the forearm or 25G butterfly device for the wrist, metacarpal veins and digital veins ✳ sharps container ✳ colour-coded collection tubes containing appropriate additives ✳ laboratory request form ✳ gauze pads ✳ adhesive plaster. (See *Guide to colour-top collection tubes*.)

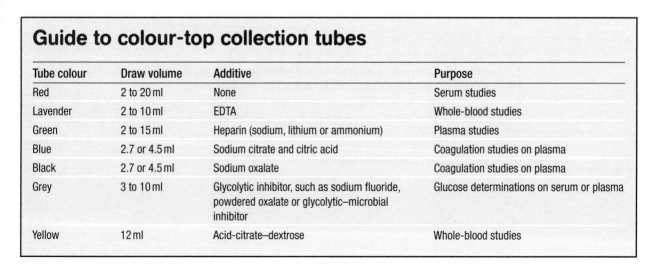

> Anterior to and below the elbow—that's the usual spot for venepuncture.

Guide to colour-top collection tubes

Tube colour	Draw volume	Additive	Purpose
Red	2 to 20 ml	None	Serum studies
Lavender	2 to 10 ml	EDTA	Whole-blood studies
Green	2 to 15 ml	Heparin (sodium, lithium or ammonium)	Plasma studies
Blue	2.7 or 4.5 ml	Sodium citrate and citric acid	Coagulation studies on plasma
Black	2.7 or 4.5 ml	Sodium oxalate	Coagulation studies on plasma
Grey	3 to 10 ml	Glycolytic inhibitor, such as sodium fluoride, powdered oxalate or glycolytic–microbial inhibitor	Glucose determinations on serum or plasma
Yellow	12 ml	Acid-citrate–dextrose	Whole-blood studies

Getting ready

Assemble all of the above equipment on a clean non-porous equipment tray to take to the patient. To assemble the needle and holder, hold the evacuated tube system needle in both hands and twist to open, only the covered needle will be exposed, direct this covered needle into the needle holder and screw together; DO NOT unsheath the needle at this point, in order to maintain asepsis. Select the appropriate tubes you require according to the laboratory request form.

How you do it

• Introduce yourself to the patient as necessary; confirm the patient's name, hospital number and date of birth verbally using the request form. Inform the patient that you would like to collect a blood sample, explain the procedure and gain his permission; this will also ease his anxiety and ensure his cooperation. Ask him if he's ever felt faint, sweaty or nauseated when having blood taken (see *Complications of venepuncture*) and take appropriate action.
• Wash your hands thoroughly, put on gloves and apron.
• If the patient is on bed rest, ask him to lie in a supine position with his head slightly elevated and his arms at his sides; if he's ambulatory, ask him to sit in a chair and support his arm on an armrest or a pillow.

The best site

• Apply a single-use or non-porous tourniquet approximately 5 cm proximal to the antecubital fossa or wrist. By impeding venous return to the heart while still allowing arterial flow, a tourniquet produces venous dilation. If the tourniquet fails to dilate the vein, have the patient open and close his fist repeatedly. Then ask him to relax before you insert the needle as insertion when the fist is clenched may increase the discomfort/pain felt.
• Assess the patient's veins to determine the best puncture site. (See *Common venepuncture sites*.) Palpate across the antecubital fossa for an appropriate vein (use the second and third fingers of your dominant hand), and visually inspect the area for a vein. An appropriate vein will feel soft, bouncy and full and, depending upon the vein's proximity to the skin surface, may be visible. You should not inject near to valves or junctions and try to avoid veins running over bony prominences.

Don't cancel

• Clean the venepuncture site with 70% alcohol swab for 30 seconds and allow the alcohol to dry; not allowing the alcohol to dry pre-insertion will cancel out any benefit of cleaning. Wipe

Warning!

Complications of venepuncture

Complication	Reduce the risk by:
Faint	• asking the patient if they have ever fainted previously when having blood taken; if yes, then ask the patient to lie down to have the blood taken • reassuring the patient • asking the patient to take deep breaths during the procedure (in through the nose and out through the mouth)
Pain and needle phobia	• using local anaesthetic cream and waiting the required time for it to take effect before taking a sample • inserting the needle quickly through the skin—slow insertion will causing tearing of the skin by the needle and increase the pain experienced by the patient • reassuring the patient throughout the procedure and warning him before you inject: 'sharp scratch coming' • avoiding bony prominences ensuring alcohol from pre-injection swab is dry before injection • asking the patient to relax his hand pre-injection
Mechanical phlebitis (inflammation of the vein)	• never injecting into a thrombosed, sclerosed or inflamed vein • never repositioning the needle under the skin if the first attempt was unsuccessful, take a new needle and holder and inject either above the previous attempt site or in a different area altogether
Hitting an artery	• ensuring that you perform visual inspection as well as physical palpation to choose an appropriate vein • removing the tourniquet and repalpating the site; an artery will continue to feel full and bouncy, a vein will constrict back to normal size
Haematoma (collection of blood in the tissues)	• using appropriate equipment, never use a needle and syringe • removing the tourniquet before you remove the needle • ensuring the limb is well supported • checking anticoagulant therapy and past medical history of the patient pre-procedure
Infection	• maintaining asepsis throughout procedure • cleaning the skin using 70% alcohol swab and ensuring alcohol on the skin is dry before injection

in a circular motion, spiralling outward from the site to avoid introducing potentially infectious skin flora into the vessel during the procedure.
• Immobilize the vein by pressing just below the venepuncture site with your thumb and drawing the skin taut; this is especially relevant when taking blood from an older person because, as tissue and muscle are lost, the veins become free-floating.

'aye-up' lad

• Position the needle with the needle bevel (the eye of the needle) facing upwards ('eye up' or 'eye to the sky') and the shaft parallel to the path of the vein and at a suitable angle to the arm (this may be

Common venepuncture sites

These illustrations show the most common sites for venepuncture. The best sites are the veins in the forearm, followed by those on the hand.

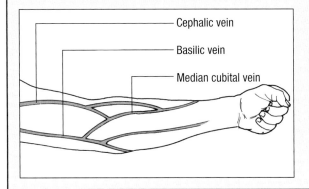

Cephalic vein

Basilic vein

Median cubital vein

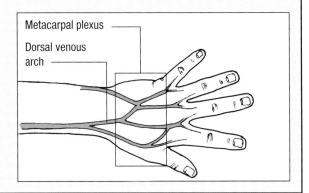

Metacarpal plexus

Dorsal venous arch

anything between 20 degrees and 45 degrees, depending again upon the vein's proximity to the skin surface.
• Warn the patient that he is about to feel the needle, 'sharp scratch' would be appropriate. Be aware that many patients are offended when inappropriate terminology, loaded with sexual innuendo, is used. Maintain your professionalism at all times.
• Insert the needle into the vein quickly. Some evacuated systems allow you to see a 'flash back of blood' just above the needle, informing you that you are in the vein, but unfortunately some do not. Whichever system you are using, once you are satisfied that you are in the vein grasp the holder securely to stabilize it in the vein, and push the collection tube down into the needle holder until the needle punctures the covered needle inside the holder.

Gentle rotation

• Continue to fill the required tubes, removing one and inserting another. Gently rotate each tube as you remove it to help mix the additive with the sample. Try not to push the needle further into the vein or pull it out of the vein when applying and removing the tubes. Blood will flow into the tube automatically.
• When you have filled the last required tube, remove it from the needle holder to release the vacuum.

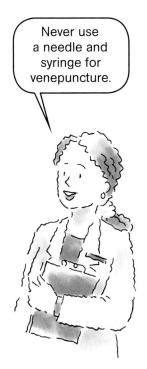

Never use a needle and syringe for venepuncture.

• Remove the tourniquet as soon as blood flows adequately, to prevent stasis and haemoconcentration, which can impair test results. If the flow is sluggish, leave the tourniquet in place longer, but always remove it before withdrawing the needle.
• After you have drawn the sample, place a gauze pad over the puncture site (without pressing on the needle), slowly and gently remove the needle from the vein, dispose of the needle and holder as a single unit immediately into the sharps container and then apply pressure using the gauze pad.

Gentle pressure

• Apply gentle pressure to the puncture site for 2–3 minutes or until bleeding stops, the patient may be able to apply this pressure himself, request that he keeps his arm straight. This prevents extravasation into the surrounding tissue, which can cause a haematoma.
• After bleeding stops, apply an adhesive plaster, if the patient has no allergies.
• Finally, check the venepuncture site for complications, and action your findings.
• Label the specimen while at the bedside to prevent mix-up of samples and patients, and send it to the laboratory with the appropriate request form.
• Remove gloves, clean the tourniquet if non-disposable (as per manufacture's instruction) and dispose of equipment appropriately.
• Document the procedure in the patient's notes. (See *Documenting venepuncture.*)

Practice pointers

• Never collect a venous sample from an arm that's already being used for I.V. therapy or blood administration, because this may affect test results.
• Never collect a venous sample from an infection site because this may introduce pathogens into the vascular system.
• Never collect blood from oedematous areas, arteriovenous shunts, arms affected by mastectomy and/or axillary clearance/ lymph node removal, and sites of previous haematomas or vascular injury (such as the side affected by a cerebrovascular accident).
• Always fill the purple-coloured tube last as it contains potassium as an additive and could alter the patient's potassium level result.
• Cotton- or fibre-covered tourniquets should only be used if washed at 90 degrees between uses to prevent infection.

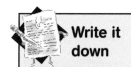

Write it down

Document-ing vene-puncture

In the patient's notes, record:

• date, time and site of the venepuncture
• number of tubes acquired and reason for acquisition
• time the sample was sent to the laboratory
• adverse reactions to the procedure and actions taken
• your name, signature and designation against the entry.

High visibility

- If the patient has large, distended, highly visible veins, perform venepuncture without a tourniquet to minimize the risk of haematoma formation. If the patient has a clotting disorder or is receiving anticoagulant therapy, maintain firm pressure on the venepuncture site for at least 5 minutes after withdrawing the needle, to prevent haematoma formation.
- Avoid using veins in the patient's legs for venepuncture, if possible, because this increases the risk of thrombophlebitis.

Blood culture

Blood cultures are performed to detect bacterial invasion (bacteraemia) and the systemic spread of such an infection (septicaemia) through the bloodstream. In this procedure, a technician, doctor or nurse who is competent and confident performs the above venepuncture procedure using a butterfly needle and holder at the patient's bedside. But, rather than using evacuated blood tubes, will use glass sample bottles: one contains an anaerobic (without oxygen) medium and the other an aerobic (with oxygen) medium. The bottles are incubated to encourage any organisms present in the sample to grow in the media. Blood cultures allow identification of about 67% of pathogens within 24 hours and up to 90% within 72 hours.

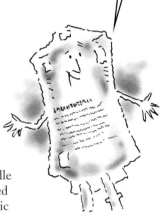

Don't collect a sample from a site that's already being used for I.V. therapy.

Timing may be everything

Although some authorities consider the timing of culture collections debatable and possibly irrelevant, others advocate drawing three blood samples at least 1 hour apart. Know your own establishment's policy and procedure. The first of these samples should be collected at the earliest sign of suspected bacteraemia or septicaemia. To check for suspected bacterial endocarditis, three or four samples may be collected at 30-minute intervals before starting antibiotic therapy.

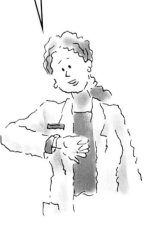

Many clinicians suggest drawing blood samples at least 1 hour apart.

What you need

Single-use or non-porous tourniquet (latex-free if required) ✳ gloves ✳ 70% alcohol swabs ✳ evacuated tube system butterfly and holder ✳ two blood culture bottles (50 ml bottles for adults or 20 ml bottles for infants and children), one aerobic bottle and one anaerobic bottle ✳ laboratory request form ✳ gauze pads ✳ small adhesive plaster (hypoallergenic if required) ✳ sharps container.

Getting ready

Assemble all of the above equipment on a non-porous equipment tray to take to the patient. To assemble the butterfly needle and holder, open the packaging of the butterfly needle and extension set—carefully, as the covered needle will be exposed—direct this covered needle into the needle holder and screw together; DO NOT unsheath the butterfly needle at this point, in order to maintain asepsis. Check the expiration dates on the culture bottles, and replace outdated bottles.

How you do it

• Introduce yourself to the patient as necessary; confirm the patient's name, hospital number and date of birth verbally, using the request form. Inform the patient that you would like to collect a series of blood samples to check for infection.
• Explain the procedure and gain his permission; this will also ease his anxiety and ensure his cooperation. Ask him if he's ever felt faint, sweaty or nauseated when having blood taken (see *Complications of venepuncture*) and take appropriate action.
• Wash your hands thoroughly, put on gloves and an apron.
• If the patient is on bed rest, ask him to lie in a supine position with his head slightly elevated and his arms at his sides; if he's ambulatory, ask him to sit in a chair and support his arm on an armrest or a pillow.
• Tie a tourniquet approximately 5 cm proximal to the area chosen. (See Venepuncture, above.)

Clean and dry

• Clean the venepuncture site with 70% alcohol swab for 30 seconds and allow the alcohol to dry; not allowing the alcohol to dry pre-insertion will cancel out any benefit of cleaning and cause unnecessary discomfort. Wipe in a circular motion, spiralling outward from the site to avoid introducing potentially infectious skin flora into the vessel during the procedure.
• Immobilize the vein by pressing just below the venepuncture site with your thumb and drawing the skin taut; this is especially relevant when taking blood from an older person because, as tissue and muscle are lost, the veins become free-floating.
• Perform a venepuncture as described in the Venepuncture section of this chapter above, remember that the butterfly system will allow you to identify correct placement of the needle in the vein by showing a 'flashback' of blood in the extension tubing.

> After cleaning the venepuncture site with 70% alcohol you must allow it to dry—not doing so would cancel the cleaning effect.

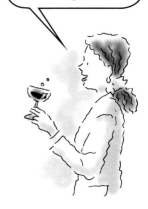

• Wipe the diaphragm tops of the culture bottles with a 70% alcohol pre-injection swab and insert the first bottle into the needle holder. Remove the bottle when the sample is acquired and insert the second bottle into the needle holder to acquire the second sample.

• When you have filled the second bottle remove it from the needle holder to release the vacuum.

• Remove the tourniquet as soon as blood flows adequately, to prevent stasis and haemoconcentration which can impair test results. If the flow is sluggish, leave the tourniquet in place longer; remove it before removing the second bottle.

• After you have drawn the sample, place a gauze pad over the puncture site (without pressing on the butterfly needle), slowly and gently remove the butterfly needle from the vein, push the sheath cover up over the needle and dispose of the butterfly needle, extension and holder as a single unit immediately into the sharps container and then apply pressure using the gauze pad.

Culture ID

• Apply gentle pressure to the puncture site for 2–3 minutes or until bleeding stops. The patient may be able to apply this pressure himself; request that he keeps his arm straight during this time. This prevents extravasation into the surrounding tissue, which can cause a haematoma.

• After bleeding stops, apply an adhesive plaster, if the patient has no allergies.

• Finally, check the venepuncture site for complications, and action your findings.

• Label the specimen bottles while at the bedside, to prevent mix-up of samples and patients. Refrigerate the samples and call for collection or transport immediately to the laboratory, with the appropriate request form. Never put glass blood culture bottles in an air chute system.

• Remove gloves and apron, clean the tourniquet if non-disposable (as per manufacturer's instructions), wash your hands and dispose of equipment appropriately.

• Document the procedure in the patient's notes. (See *Documenting blood culture collection.*)

Practice pointers

• If repeating the cultures at a later date and time, obtain them from a different site.

• Avoid using existing blood lines for cultures unless the sample is drawn when the line is inserted or catheter sepsis is suspected.

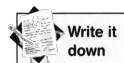
Write it down

Document-ing blood culture collection

In the patient's notes, record:

• the date and time of blood sample collection
• the anatomical site used
• name of the test
• number of bottles used
• patient's temperature
• adverse reactions to the procedure
• your name, designation and signature.

Arterial puncture for ABG analysis

Obtaining an arterial blood sample requires percutaneous puncture of the brachial, radial or femoral artery, or withdrawal of a sample from an arterial line. When collected, the sample can be analysed to determine arterial blood gas (ABG) values.

Breathing check

ABG analysis evaluates ventilation by measuring blood pH and the partial pressures of arterial oxygen (PaO_2) and partial pressure of arterial carbon dioxide ($PaCO_2$). Blood pH measurement reveals the blood's acid–base balance. PaO_2 indicates the amount of oxygen that the lungs deliver to the blood, and $PaCO_2$ indicates the lungs' capacity to eliminate carbon dioxide. ABG samples are also analysed for oxygen content and saturation, and for bicarbonate values.

Special training required

Most ABG samples can be collected by a respiratory technician or advanced nurse practitioner who has received theoretical and practical training to achieve competence. Collection from the femoral artery, however, is usually performed by a doctor. Before attempting a radial puncture, Allen's test should be performed. (See *Performing Allen's test*.)

What you need

Plastic Luer Lok pre-heparinized ABG syringe and needle with integral safety sheath/bung (usually 20–22G) ✳ gloves and apron ✳ linen protection (incontinence pad) ✳ sterile kidney bowl or wound dressing pack ✳ 70% alcohol pre-injection swab ✳ two 5 cm × 5 cm gauze pads ✳ biro pen ✳ laboratory request form ✳ adhesive bandage ✳ optional: for topical application pre-injection 1% lidocaine or 4% tetracaine gel.

Getting ready

Prepare everything you need before approaching the patient. Wash your hands thoroughly, this is an aseptic procedure; open the ABG equipment using a non-touch technique and drop into the sterile kidney bowl (or use a sterile wound dressing pack).

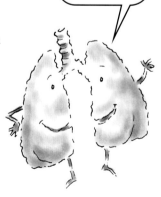

Arterial blood gas analysis is a common way to evaluate a patient's ventilation.

Performing Allen's test

Rest the patient's arm on the bed or bed table, and support his wrist with a rolled towel. Have him clench his fist. Then, using your index and middle fingers, press on the radial and ulnar arteries. Hold this position for a few seconds.

Without removing your fingers from the patient's arteries, ask him to unclench his fist and hold his hand in a relaxed position. The palm will be blanched because pressure from your fingers has impaired the normal blood flow.

Release pressure on the patient's ulnar artery. If the hand becomes flushed, which indicates blood filling the vessels, you can safely proceed with the radial artery puncture. If the hand doesn't flush, perform the test on the other arm.

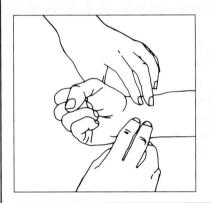 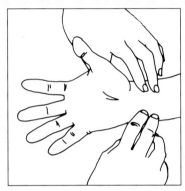 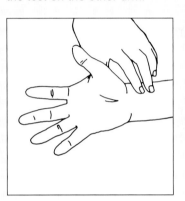

How you do it

- Tell the patient that you need to collect an arterial blood sample, and explain the procedure to help ease anxiety, gain permission and promote cooperation. Tell him that the needle stick will cause some discomfort but that he must try to remain still during the procedure.
- After washing your hands and putting on gloves, place a rolled towel or pillow (covered with the protective pad) under the patient's wrist for support. Locate the artery and palpate it for a strong pulse.

Site cleaning

- Clean the puncture site with the 70% alcohol pad. Don't re-palpate the injection site.
- Using a circular motion, clean the area, starting in the centre of the site and spiralling outward, apply it with friction for 30 seconds or until the final pad comes away clean. Allow the skin to dry.
- Palpate the artery above the intended injection site with the index and middle fingers of one hand while holding the syringe over the puncture site with the other hand.

pain, numbness or tingling in the affected arm. Watch for bleeding at the puncture site. If injury or complication has occurred, or is suspected, inform the doctor and complete and incident form.
• Document the procedure. (See *Documenting arterial puncture.*)

Practice pointers

• If the patient is receiving oxygen, make sure that his therapy has been under way for at least 15 minutes before collecting an arterial blood sample.
• Be sure to indicate on the laboratory request the amount and type of oxygen therapy the patient is receiving. Also note the patient's current temperature, most recent haemoglobin level, current respiratory rate and, if he's on a ventilator, fraction of inspired oxygen and tidal volume.
• If the patient isn't receiving oxygen, indicate that he's breathing room air (21%).
• If the patient has just received nebulizer treatment, wait about 20 minutes before collecting the sample.

Numbing effect

• Consider such use of local anaesthetic carefully as it must be applied 30 minutes pre-procedure to be effective. In an emergency situation this would be contraindicated as a delay in treatment would occur and the resulting vasoconstriction may prevent successful puncture.

Peripheral I.V. catheter insertion

A peripheral line is inserted to allow administration of fluids, medication, blood and blood components.

Peripheral I.V. line insertion involves selection of an appropriate device and an insertion site, application of a tourniquet, preparation of the site, and venepuncture. Selection of a cannulation device and site depends on the type of solution to be used; frequency and duration of infusion; patency and location of accessible veins; the patient's age, size, past medical history and current condition; and, when possible, the patient's preference.

What you need

Sterile field ✳ 70% alcohol pads or other approved antimicrobial solution as per local policy ✳ non-sterile gloves ✳ latex-free

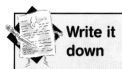

Write it down

Document-ing arterial puncture

In your notes, record:

• results of Allen's test
• time the sample was drawn
• patient's temperature
• arterial puncture site
• amount of time pressure was applied to the site to control bleeding
• type and amount of oxygen therapy the patient was receiving
• any resulting complications
• your name, signature and designation.

disposable tourniquet (or non-porous tourniquet which can be cleaned between uses) ✳ appropriate I.V. access cannula ✳ 10 ml syringe primed with 0.9% sodium chloride ✳ sharps container ✳ sterile 5 cm × 5 cm gauze pads ✳ polyurethane film I.V. dressing and date label ✳ appropriate needle-free extension port primed with 0.9% sodium chloride ✳ optional: pillow, protective pad for pillow/bed, warm packs, anaesthetic gel, scissors.

Commercial cannulation kits come with all of the above. In many clinical areas, cannulation equipment is kept on a tray or trolley, allowing a choice of correct access devices and easy replacement of contaminated items.

Getting ready

Prior to collecting equipment, assess the need for line insertion—is it required? What type and how much/many fluids are to be administered? This will allow you to assess which cannula (14 G to 27 G) and extension set (1 port to 3 port/anti-siphon) to select. Wash your hands, prepare a sterile field, select equipment, check use-by dates and sterility of the equipment and open on to the sterile field using a non-touch technique. Prime the 10 ml syringe and extension set with 0.9% sodium chloride. Take all equipment to the patient's bedside or room.

How you do it

• Check identification of the patient for 'right patient, right procedure', explain the procedure to the patient, allow the patient to ask questions, in order to gain consent and cooperation.
• Wash your hands thoroughly using soap, rinse and dry thoroughly (social hand wash), or using alcohol gel. Apply non-sterile gloves.

Selecting the site
• Place the patient in a comfortable, reclining position, leaving the arm in a dependent position to increase capillary fill of the lower arms and hands. If the patient's skin is cold, warm it by rubbing and stroking the arm, or cover the entire arm with warm packs for 5–10 minutes.
• Select the puncture site.
• If long-term therapy is anticipated, start with a vein at the most distal site so that you can move proximally as needed for subsequent I.V. insertion sites.

Applying the tourniquet

• Apply a tourniquet about 15 cm above the intended puncture site of the non-dominant arm, to dilate the vein. Check for a radial pulse. If it isn't present, release the tourniquet and reapply it with less tension to prevent arterial occlusion.

• Lightly palpate the vein with the index and middle fingers of your non-dominant hand. Stretch the skin to anchor the vein. If the vein feels hard or rope-like, select another.

Open sesame

• If the vein is easily palpable but not sufficiently dilated, one or more of the following techniques may help raise the vein. Place the extremity in a dependent position for several seconds, gently rub or stroke the skin upward toward the tourniquet to create friction and thus heat, or have the patient open and close his fist several times.

• Leave the tourniquet in place for no longer than 3 minutes. If you can't find a suitable vein and prepare the site in that time, release the tourniquet for a few minutes. Then reapply it and continue the procedure. Select a vein 2–3 cm in length.

Preparing the site

• Clip the hair around the insertion site if needed. Clean the site with 70% alcohol pads or another antimicrobial solution, (according to local policy) for 30 seconds and allow to dry. Work in a circular motion outward from the site to a diameter of 5–10 cm.

• If ordered, administer a local anaesthetic. Preferably 4% tetracaine gel as this has further benefits (antibacterial and vasodilation). Make sure the patient isn't sensitive to the gel used.

Round, firm and resilient

• Lightly press the vein with the thumb of your non-dominant hand about 4 cm from the intended insertion site. The vein should feel round, firm, fully engorged and resilient.

• Grasp the access cannula. If you're using a winged infusion set, hold the short edges of the wings (with the needle's bevel facing upward) between the thumb and forefinger of your dominant hand. Then squeeze the wings together. If you're using an over-the-needle cannula, grasp the plastic hub with your dominant hand, remove the cover, and examine the cannula tip. If the edge isn't smooth, discard and replace the device.

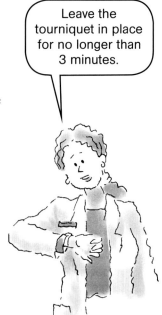

Leave the tourniquet in place for no longer than 3 minutes.

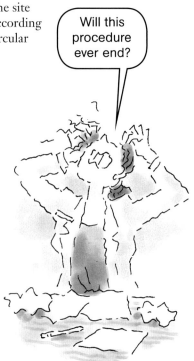

Will this procedure ever end?

Operation stabilization

- Using the thumb of your non-dominant hand, stretch the skin taut below the puncture site to stabilize the vein, and tell the patient that you're about to insert the device.
- Hold the needle bevel up and enter the skin parallel to the vein and push the needle directly through the skin and into the vein in one motion. Check the flashback chamber behind the hub for blood return, signifying that the vein has been properly accessed. (You may not see a blood return in a small vein.)
- If using a winged-tip device, advance the needle, hold it in place, and release the tourniquet.
- For an over-the needle catheter, advance approximately 2–3 mm of the device to ensure that the cannula itself—not just the introducer needle—has entered the vein.
- Grasp the cannula hub to hold it in the vein, advance the cannula down the introducer needle until you meet resistance, place gauze pad under the cannula, then withdraw the needle and dispose of immediately in the sharps container. The patient will bleed, this is normal—do not panic and do not press the artery above the insertion site as this may cause unnecessary trauma to the artery and failure of the cannulation attempt.
- Remove the hub from the end of the extension set using a non-touch technique and attach the extension set to the hub of the cannula to maintain a closed system and prevent infection. Do not use screw-on bungs or stopcocks.
- If the needle-free port on the extension set has become contaminated, clean using 70% alcohol.
- Inject the 0.9% sodium chloride solution to check patency of the cannula and observe for extravasation, pain and infiltration.

Dressing the site

- Use only an I.V.-appropriate dressing with a polyurethane window, to allow assessment of the site and to secure the device. (See *How to apply a transparent semi-permeable dressing.*) Put the date of insertion on the dressing, using the label provided.

Removing a peripheral I.V. line

- To remove the I.V. line, first clamp the I.V. tubing and gently remove the transparent dressing and all tape from the skin.
- Open a gauze pad and adhesive bandage and place them within reach. Put on gloves. Hold the sterile gauze pad over the puncture site with one hand, and use your other hand to withdraw the cannula slowly and smoothly, keeping it parallel to the skin. (Inspect the cannula tip; if it isn't smooth, assess the patient immediately, and notify the doctor.)

How to apply a transparent semi-permeable dressing

To secure the I.V. insertion site, you should apply a transparent semi-permeable dressing as follows:

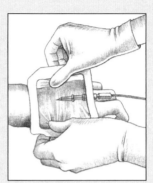

- Make sure the insertion site is clean and dry.
- Remove the dressing from the package. Using aseptic technique, remove the protective seal.
- Place the window of the dressing directly over the insertion site and the semi-permeable area of dressing down the sides of the hub, as shown. Don't cover the tubing or stretch the dressing.
- To remove the dressing, grasp one corner, and then lift and stretch it.
- If removal is difficult, try loosening the edges with alcohol or water.

• Using the gauze pad, apply firm pressure over the puncture site for 1–2 minutes after removal or until bleeding has stopped.
• Clean the site and apply an adhesive bandage or, if blood oozes, apply a pressure bandage and instruct the patient to restrict activity for about 10 minutes and to leave the dressing in place for at least 1 hour. If the patient experiences lingering tenderness at the site, apply warm packs and notify the doctor.
• Discard of cannula, fluid and administration set as per local policy. Do not reuse the administration set. If a new I.V. cannula is sited, obtain a new, sterile administration set.

Practice pointers

• Insertion is contraindicated in a sclerotic vein, an oedematous or impaired arm or hand, or a post-mastectomy arm, and in patients with a mastectomy, burns or an arteriovenous fistula. Subsequent insertions should be performed proximal to a previously used or injured vein.
• If you fail to see blood flashback after the needle enters the vein, remove the cannula and try again with a new device, or proceed according to your local policy.
• Be sure to rotate the I.V. site, usually every 72 hours.
• Change the dressing if it appears stained or unstuck.
• If the patient is to receive peripheral I.V. therapy at home, review teaching with him. (See *I.V. therapy in the home* and *Documenting peripheral I.V. catheter insertion*.)

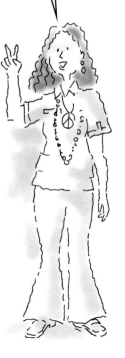

Flashback? I know just what you mean!

Home care connection

I.V. therapy in the home

If you're caring for a patient going home with a peripheral line, teach him how to care for the I.V. site and identify certain complications. If he must observe movement restrictions, make sure he understands them. Because the patient may have special drug delivery equipment that differs from the type used in hospital, be sure to demonstrate the equipment and have him give a return demonstration.

What's on the syllabus?

Teach the patient how to examine the site, and instruct him to notify the doctor or primary care nurse if redness, swelling or discomfort develop; if the dressing becomes moist; or if blood appears in the tubing. Also tell the patient to report any problems with the I.V. line; for instance, if the solution stops infusing or an alarm goes off on an infusion pump. Explain that the I.V. site will be changed at established intervals by the primary care nurse.

If the patient is using an intermittent infusion device, teach him how and when to flush it. Finally, teach the patient to document daily whether the I.V. site is free from pain, swelling and redness. Peripheral line complications can result from the needle or catheter (infection, phlebitis and embolism) or from the solution (circulatory overload, infiltration, sepsis and allergic reaction).

Write it down

Documenting peripheral I.V. catheter insertion

In the medical and nursing notes, record:

- date and time of the insertion
- needle type and gauge
- cannula length
- anatomical location of the insertion site
- reason the site was changed
- number of attempts (if you made more than one)
- type and amount of flush administered
- adverse reactions and nursing actions
- patient teaching and evidence of patient understanding
- your name, signature and designation.

Peripheral I.V. catheter maintenance

Routine maintenance of I.V. sites and systems includes regular assessment and rotation of the site. It also includes periodic changes of the dressing, tubing and solution. These measures help prevent complications, such as thrombophlebitis and infection. They should be performed according to locally used Phlebitis scale procedure/policy (*Phlebitis scale*, cited in the Royal College of Nursing (2005) *Standards for infusion therapy*).

What you need

For dressing changes

Non-sterile gloves and apron ✳ 70% alcohol pads ✳ sterile gauze pads ✳ transparent semi-permeable dressing.

For I.V. site change
Equipment as described above or commercial kits containing the equipment.

Getting ready

If you're changing the cannula and the administration set, prime the I.V. administration set and solution prior to insertion of cannula.

How you do it

- Explain the procedure to the patient and gain consent.
- Wash your hands.

Changing the dressing
- Loosen the old dressing, use hand gel, apply gloves and apron, open all packages.
- Hold the cannula in place with your non-dominant hand and assess the site for signs of infection (redness and pain at the puncture site), infiltration (coolness, blanching and oedema at the site), and thrombophlebitis (redness, firmness and pain along the path of the vein, and oedema). If any such signs are present, cover the area with a sterile 5 cm × 5 cm gauze pad and remove the catheter or needle. Apply pressure to the area until the bleeding stops, and apply an adhesive bandage or gauze. Then, using fresh equipment and solution start the I.V. in another appropriate site, preferably on the opposite extremity.
- If the site is intact, stabilize the cannula and carefully clean around the puncture site with an alcohol pad, working in a circular motion. Allow the area to dry completely.
- Cover the site with a transparent semi-permeable dressing as described above.

Changing the solution
- Wash your hands and, with a second appropriately qualified and registered colleague, inspect the new solution container for cracks, leaks and other damage. Check the solution for expiry date, discoloration and particulates.
- Clamp the tubing when inverting it to prevent air from entering the tubing, keeping the drip chamber half full.

Brand new bag

- If you're replacing a bag, remove the seal or tab from the new bag and remove the old bag from the pole. Remove the spike, insert it into the new bag, and adjust the flow rate.

- If you're replacing a bottle, remove the cap and seal from the new bottle and wipe the rubber port with an alcohol pad. Clamp the line, remove the spike from the old bottle, and insert the spike into the new bottle. Then hang the new bottle and adjust the flow rate.

Changing the tubing
- Stop the infusion. Using a non-touch technique, disconnect the infusion set from the cannula extension set.
- Using a non-touch technique, remove the old infusion set spike from the container and hang the container on the I.V. pole.
- Using a non-touch technique, unsheath the new spike and insert it into the I.V. container and prime the new infusion set.
- Clean the cannula extension port with 70% alcohol and allow it to dry.
- Uncap the infusion line and, using a non-touch technique, attach it to the extension port. Adjust the flow rate and observe the cannula site regularly.

Practice pointers

- Check the prescribed I.V. flow rate before each solution change to prevent errors. If you crack the adapter or hub (or if you accidentally dislodge the cannula from the vein), remove the cannula. Apply pressure and an adhesive bandage to stop any bleeding. Re-site the cannula and restart the I.V. (See *Documenting peripheral I.V. catheter maintenance*.)

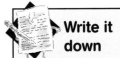

Write it down

Documenting peripheral I.V. catheter maintenance

Record the time, date, rate and type of solution (and any additives) on the patient's medicines administration record and fluid balance chart. Also record this information, dressing or tubing changes, and site appearance in the nursing care plan.

I.V. bolus injection

The I.V. bolus injection method allows rapid drug administration. It's used to administer drugs that can't be given intramuscularly, to achieve peak drug levels in the bloodstream, and to deliver drugs that can't be diluted.

The term 'bolus' usually refers to the concentration or amount of a drug. Bolus doses of medication are injected directly into the peripheral I.V. cannula.

What you need

The patient's medication administration record (MAR) ✳ gloves ✳ prescribed medication ✳ appropriate gauge needle and syringe ✳ diluent, if needed ✳ 70% alcohol swabs ✳ second 10 ml syringe filled with 0.9% sodium chloride solution, or heparin flush solution if used with a long-term device such as a peripherally inserted central catheter (PICC) or central venous catheter (CVC).

Getting ready

Check the prescription/direction in the MAR. Know the actions, adverse reactions and administration rate of the medication to be injected. Draw up the prescribed medication in the syringe and dilute with appropriate diluent as necessary. Remember that when drawing up from a glass, plastic or through a rubber bung, a 25 gauge or filter needle should be used to prevent administration of plastic polymers, glass shards or rubber polymers to the patient's venous system.

How you do it

• Confirm the patient's identity, wash your hands, put on gloves and explain the procedure.

If I.V. therapy is being administered
• Check the compatibility of the medication with any I.V. therapy solution being administered.
• Close the flow clamp of the I.V fluid therapy solution administration set and clamp the cannula extension line, to prevent reflux of the bolus injection into the I.V. therapy solution.
• Wipe the needle-free injection port on the extension set with 70% alcohol for 30 seconds and allow to dry.
• Connect the syringe containing the medication to the extension set and administer at the recommended rate (between 3 and 7 minutes) to prevent speed shock. Once the drug has been administered, disconnect the syringe and clean the port again with 70% alcohol.
• Unclamp the I.V. therapy solution extension port and recommence fluid at the prescribed rate.
• Observe the patient regularly for adverse reactions.

If no I.V. therapy is being administered
• Wipe the needle-free injection port on the extension set with 70% alcohol for 30 seconds and allow to dry.
• Using a non-touch technique, attach the 10 ml syringe containing 0.9% sodium chloride solution (flush solution) to the extension set and slowly administer 5 ml of the solution, while observing for signs of infiltration and blockage, and ensuring that the patient is not feeling any pain. Should any complications be noted, stop; remove the cannula and re-site.
• Disconnect the 'flush' solution, again using a non-touch technique, and maintain sterility of the syringe for future use, by either replacing the syringe into sterile packaging or using a sterile bung on the syringe tip.

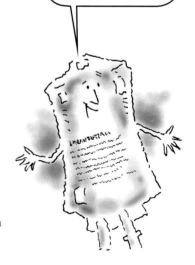

Remember to check my expiry date, lot number, colour and consistency before using me.

- Connect the syringe containing the medication to the extension set and administer at the recommended rate (between 3 and 7 minutes) to prevent speed shock. Once the drug has been administered, disconnect the syringe and maintain sterility of the extension set port.
- Reconnect the 'flush' solution and administer the last 5 ml of solution, slowly over 2–3 minutes, remove the syringe and clean the port with a 70% alcohol swab.
- Observe the patient regularly for adverse reactions.

Practice pointers

- Because drugs administered by I.V. bolus or push injections are delivered directly into the circulatory system and can produce an immediate effect, an acute allergic reaction, or anaphylaxis, can develop rapidly. If signs of anaphylaxis (dyspnoea, cyanosis, seizures and increasing respiratory distress) occur, notify the doctor immediately and begin emergency procedures, as necessary. Also watch for signs of extravasation (redness and swelling). If extravasation occurs, stop the injection, estimate the amount of infiltration, using an infiltration scale, and notify the doctor.
- Never leave an I.V. catheter or cannula *in situ* 'just in case you need it' (not being used) as this increases the risk of infection.

Sub for saline

- Flushing pre- and post-administration of the medication when no I.V. solution is being administered prevents overdose of the drug being administered.
- Excessively rapid administration may cause adverse reactions, depending on the medication administered. You need to know the drug you're administering and the rate at which to inject the drug. You also need to be aware of the intended effects, and monitor the patient as indicated by the medication given. If you are unsure, do not administer, check the BNF or with pharmacy. (See *Documenting I.V. bolus injections*.)

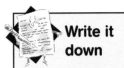

Write it down

Document-ing I.V. bolus injections

In the patient's MAR and the fluid balance chart, record:

- amount and type of drug administered
- time of injection
- appearance of the site
- duration of administration
- patient's tolerance of the procedure
- drug's effect and adverse reactions
- your signature.

I.V. infusion pump use

Various types of pumps regulate the flow of I.V. solutions or drugs electronically, with great accuracy.

Volumetric pumps, used for high-pressure infusion of drugs or for highly accurate delivery of fluids or drugs, have mechanisms to propel the solution at the desired rate under pressure. (Pressure is brought to bear only when gravity flow rates are insufficient to maintain preset infusion rates.) The peristaltic pump applies pressure to the I.V. tubing to force the solution through it. (Not all peristaltic pumps are volumetric; some count drops.) The piston-cylinder pump pushes the solution through special disposable cassettes. Most of these pumps operate at high pressures (up to 45 psi), delivering from 1 to 999 ml/hour with about 98% accuracy. (Some pumps operate at 10–25 psi.)

Specialty items

The portable syringe pump, another type of volumetric pump, delivers small amounts of fluid over a long period. It's used to administer fluids to infants and to deliver drugs such as opiates.

What you need

Pump ✳ I.V. pole ✳ I.V. solution ✳ sterile administration set ✳ alcohol pads ✳ adhesive tape.

Getting ready

To set up a volumetric pump

Ensure the pump is clean and has been maintained prior to use. Attach the pump to the I.V. pole. Then swab the port on the I.V. container with alcohol, insert the administration set spike, and fill the drip chamber completely to prevent air bubbles from entering the tubing. Next, prime the tubing and close the clamp. Follow the manufacturer's instructions for tubing placement.

How you do it

• Position the pump on the same side of the bed as the I.V. or anticipated cannula site. If necessary, perform the cannulation.
• Plug in the machine and attach its tubing to the catheter extension port.
• Turn it on and press the start button. Clear any previous patient data, including volume to be infused (VTBI) and volume infused data. Set the appropriate dials on the front panel to the desired infusion rate (ml/hour) and VTBI. Set the end of infusion alarm dial at 50 ml less than the prescribed volume, or 50 ml less than the volume in the container, so that you can hang a new container before the old one empties.
• Check the patency of the I.V. line and watch for infiltration.
• Turn on the alarm switches and explain the alarm system to the patient. If the patient is to go home using an I.V. pump, review teaching with him. (See *Using an I.V. pump in the home.*)

Home care connection

Using an I.V. pump in the home

Make sure the patient and his family understand the purpose of using the pump. Demonstrate how the device works and how to maintain the system (tubing, solution and site assessment and care) until you're confident they can proceed safely. Have the patient repeat the demonstration.

Discuss which complications to watch for, such as infiltration, and review measures to take if complications occur. Schedule a teaching session with the patient or family so you can answer questions they may have about the procedure before discharge. Refer patient to the primary care team and organize a meeting with them and the patient/family prior to discharge. Give the patient written instructions of his home care team's contact details prior to discharge.

Practice pointers

• Monitor the pump and the patient frequently to ensure the device's correct operation and flow rate and to detect infiltration and complications, such as infection and air embolism.
• Do not administer blood via a volumetric pump because it may cause haemolysis of the infused blood. (See *Documenting I.V. pump use*.)

Blood transfusion

Whole-blood transfusion replenishes both the volume and the oxygen-carrying capacity of the circulatory system. You may also transfuse packed red blood cells (RBCs), from which 80% of the plasma has been removed; this, however, restores only the oxygen-carrying capacity. Both types of transfusions treat decreased haemoglobin levels and haematocrit.

Two nurses must identify the patient and blood products before administering a transfusion, to prevent errors and a potentially fatal reaction. (See *Transfusion complications*.) If the patient is a Jehovah's Witness, a transfusion requires special written permission.

What you need

Blood administration set (tubing with drip chamber and filter) ✳ I.V. stand ✳ non-sterile gloves ✳ apron ✳ large-gauge cannula (20G or greater) ✳ whole blood or packed RBCs ✳ 250 ml of normal saline solution ✳ optional: face shield or goggles.

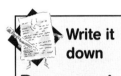

Write it down

Document-ing I.V. pump use

In addition to routine documentation of the I.V. infusion, record the use of a pump on the I.V. record and in your notes.

Warning!
Transfusion complications

Despite improvements in cross-matching precautions, transfusion reactions can still occur. Unlike a transfusion reaction, an infectious disease transmitted during a transfusion may go undetected until days, weeks or even months later, when it produces signs and symptoms. Hepatitis C accounts for most post-transfusion hepatitis cases. The tests that detect hepatitis B and C can produce false-negative results and may allow some hepatitis cases to go undetected.

When testing for antibodies to human immunodeficiency virus (HIV), keep in mind that antibodies don't appear until 6–12 weeks after exposure. The estimated risk of acquiring HIV from blood products varies from 1 in 40,000 to 1 in 153,000.

What else can go wrong?

Circulatory overload and haemolytic, allergic, pyrexial and pyrogenic reactions can result from any transfusion. Coagulation disturbances, citrate intoxication, hyperkalaemia, acid–base imbalance, loss of 2,3-diphosphoglycerate, ammonia intoxication and hypothermia can result from massive transfusion.

Getting ready

Avoid obtaining either whole blood or packed RBCs until you're ready to begin the transfusion. Prepare the equipment when you're ready to start the infusion.

How you do it

- Explain the procedure to the patient, and gain consent and cooperation. Record baseline vital signs.
- Obtain whole blood or packed RBCs from the blood bank and commence within 30 minutes. Observe the blood for abnormal colour, RBC clumping, gas bubbles and extraneous material. Return outdated or abnormal blood to the blood bank and document these findings.

ID issues

- Compare the name, hospital number and date of birth on the patient's wristband, medical notes and blood bank documentation with those on the blood bag label. Check the blood bag identification number, ABO blood group and Rh compatibility. Also, compare the patient's blood bank identification number, if present, with the number on the blood bag. Identification of blood and blood products is performed at the patient's bedside by two registered professionals, according to the local policy.

• Put on gloves, an apron and a face shield (if necessary). Using a blood administration set, close all the clamps on the set. Then insert the spike of the line into the blood bag. Hang the bag on the I.V. pole, open the clamp on the line, and squeeze the drip chamber until it's half full, then slowly adjust the line clamp until the line is primed with the blood.

• If the patient doesn't have an I.V. catheter/cannula in place, perform venepuncture, using a 20G or larger-diameter catheter. Avoid using an existing line if the needle or catheter lumen is smaller than 20G. Central venous access devices also may be used for transfusion therapy.

Shaken, not stirred

• If you're administering whole blood, gently invert the bag several times to mix the cells.

• Clean the cannula extension port with 70% alcohol and allow to dry, flush the cannula with 5 ml of 0.9% sodium chloride if the cannula has not been used for 4 hours or more, or has just been inserted, to check patency.

• Attach the prepared blood administration set to the cannula extension port using a non-touch technique. Then open the clamp between the blood bag and the patient. Adjust the flow clamp closest to the patient to deliver the blood at the calculated drip rate.

• Observe and record the patient's vital signs at 15-minute intervals for the first hour of transfusion and then half-hourly during the rest of the infusion, for signs of a transfusion reaction, such as pyrexia, chills, urticaria, increased respiratory rate or respiratory difficulty.

• If such signs develop, record vital signs and take action according to the 'track and trigger' system in place locally. Stop the transfusion. Infuse 0.9% sodium chloride solution at a moderately slow infusion rate, and notify the doctor at once.

• After completing the transfusion, you'll need to put on gloves, remove and discard the used infusion equipment as per local policy. Then remember to connect and commence any further I.V. therapy as per the direction in the patient's MAR, or discontinue the I.V. infusion and remove the peripheral cannula if not required for further use.

Write it down

Document-ing blood transfusions

In your notes, record:

• date and time of each transfusion
• type and amount of transfusion product
• patient's vital signs
• your check of all identification data
• patient's response
• transfusion reaction and nursing actions taken
• the names, signatures and designations of both nurses who have checked the product.

No PIN required

- Return the empty blood bag to the blood bank, and discard the tubing and filter as a single unit in a sharps container to prevent sharps injuries to colleagues.
- Record the patient's vital signs.

Practice pointers

- A unit of RBCs may be given over 1–4 hours as ordered.
- Although some microaggregate filters can be used for up to 10 units of blood, always replace the administration set if more than 1 hour elapses between transfusions.
- For rapid blood replacement, know that you may need to use a pressure infuser device.
- Never add any other products, such as antibiotics, to blood products (See *Documenting blood transfusions.*)

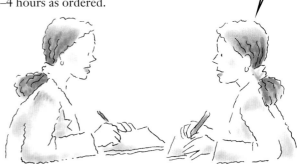

Two registered professionals must identify the patient and blood products before a transfusion.

Transfusion reaction management

A transfusion reaction typically stems from a major antigen–antibody reaction and can result from a single or massive transfusion of blood or blood products.

Although many reactions occur during the transfusion or within 96 hours afterward, infectious diseases transmitted during a transfusion may go undetected until days, weeks or months later, when signs and symptoms appear. A transfusion reaction requires immediate recognition and prompt nursing action to prevent further complications and, possibly, death.

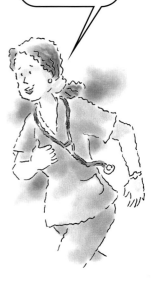

Every moment counts if your patient has a transfusion reaction.

What you need

0.9% sodium chloride solution ✻ I.V. administration set ✻ sterile urine specimen container ✻ evacuated blood sample tubes and needle device ✻ transfusion reaction report form ✻ oxygen ✻ non-rebreathe oxygen mask and tubing ✻ anaphylaxis treatment kit including adrenaline ✻ warming blanket or electronic air patient warming system.

Getting ready

As soon as you suspect an adverse reaction, stop the transfusion and start the saline infusion at a rate to-keep-vein-open (TKVO) and notify the doctor immediately. Monitor vital signs every 15 minutes, or as indicated by the 'track and trigger system' used locally, or by the severity and type of reaction.

How you do it

• Compare the labels on all blood containers with corresponding patient identification forms to verify that the transfusion was the correct blood or blood product.

• Notify the blood bank of a possible transfusion reaction and collect blood samples, as ordered. Immediately send the samples, all transfusion containers (even if empty) and the administration set to the blood bank. The blood bank will test these materials to further evaluate the reaction.

• Collect a urine specimen, mark the collection slip 'Possible transfusion reaction', and send it to the laboratory immediately. The laboratory tests this urine specimen for the presence of haemoglobin (Hb), which indicates a haemolytic reaction.

• Closely monitor intake and output. Note evidence of oliguria (less than 0.5 ml/kg/hour) or anuria (absence of urine) because Hb deposition in the renal tubules can cause renal damage.

• In an emergency situation always administer oxygen (without a prescription) using a non-rebreathe mask at a flow of 15 litres/minute when the signs and symptoms of hypoxia are present. Apply a hypothermia blanket to reduce fever, and administer adrenaline as required.

Practice pointers

• Treat all transfusion reactions as serious until proven otherwise. If the doctor anticipates a transfusion reaction, such as one that may occur in a leukaemia patient, he may order prophylactic treatment with antihistamines or antipyretics, such as paracetamol, to precede blood administration. (See *Documenting transfusion reaction management*.)

Chemotherapeutic medications

Specially trained nurses and doctors may administer chemotherapeutic drugs through a number of routes. Although the I.V. route (peripheral or central) is most common, these drugs may also be given orally, subcutaneously, intramuscularly, intra-arterially,

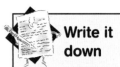

Write it down

Document-ing transfusion reaction management

In your notes, document:

• time and date of the transfusion reaction
• type and amount of infused blood or blood products
• clinical signs and symptoms of the transfusion reaction in order of occurrence
• patient's vital signs and actions taken
• specimens sent to the laboratory for analysis
• treatment given and patient's response
• complete the local transfusion reaction documentation
• patient's fluid intake, output and balance
• your name, designation and signature.

into a spinal or body cavity, or through an implanted device. They may also be administered into an artery, peritoneal cavity or pleural space. The administration route depends on the drug's pharmacodynamics and the tumour's characteristics.

What you need

The patient's MAR ✳ prescribed drug ✳ gloves ✳ apron and face mask ✳ 0.9% sodium chloride solution ✳ syringes and needle-less adapters ✳ infusion pump or controller ✳ impervious sharps and waste containers labelled 'Caution: Biohazard Cytotoxic Waste'.

Getting ready

Assess the patient's physical condition, and review his medical history and recent laboratory results. Make sure you understand what needs to be given and by what route, and provide the necessary teaching and support to the patient and his family.

Determine the best site to administer the drug. When selecting the site, consider drug compatibilities, frequency of administration, and vesicant potential of the drug. Check local policy before administering a vesicant as some policies request they be administered before or after other drugs.

History lesson

• Determine whether the patient has received chemotherapy before, and note the severity of any adverse effects. (See *Chemotherapy complications*.) Also, check his drug history for medications that might interact with chemotherapy. If you have questions or concerns, talk with the doctor or pharmacist before you give it.

• Next, double-check the patient's MAR for the complete chemotherapy protocol order, including the patient's name, the drug's name and dosage, route, rate and frequency of administration. See if the drug's dosage depends on certain laboratory results. Two registered professionals are required to check the drug and amount being administered.

• Check to see whether the doctor has requested any adjuvant therapies to be administered such as an anti-emetic, I.V. fluids, diuretics, or electrolyte supplements to be given before, during or after chemotherapy administration.

How you do it

• Evaluate the patient's and his family's understanding of chemotherapy, and provide information and teaching as required.

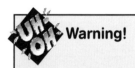 **Warning!**

Chemotherapy complications

Nausea and vomiting are the most common adverse reactions to chemotherapy. Another major complication is bone marrow suppression, leading to neutropenia and thrombocytopenia.

All the rest

Other adverse reactions include intestinal irritation, gastritis, pulmonary fibrosis, cardiotoxicity, nephrotoxicity, neurotoxicity, hearing loss, anaemia, alopecia, urticaria, radiation recall (if drugs are given with or soon after radiation therapy), anorexia, oesophagitis, diarrhoea and constipation.

I.V. issues

I.V. administration of chemotherapeutic drugs may lead to extravasation, causing inflammation, ulceration, necrosis and loss of vein patency.

- Next, put on gloves. Keep them on through all stages of handling the drug, including preparation, priming the I.V. tubing and administration.

Start fresh

- Gain I.V. access by cannulating the patient proximal to any previous site. Avoid giving chemotherapeutic drugs through an existing I.V. line.
- When an appropriate line is in place, infuse 5–10 ml of 0.9% sodium chloride solution to test vein patency, and then administer the drug as appropriate. Non-vesicants are given by I.V. bolus or as an additive to a bag of I.V. fluid; vesicants, by I.V. bolus through a Y-connection set connected to a rapidly infusing I.V. line.
- During I.V. administration, monitor the patient closely for signs of a hypersensitivity reaction or extravasation.

Saline smoothes the way

- After infusing the medication, infuse 5–10 ml of 0.9% sodium chloride solution and give the next agent, or discontinue the I.V. line.
- Dispose of used equipment—needles, syringes, infusion bags and infusion sets—as single units by placing them in an impervious container for incineration, labelled 'Cytotoxic Waste'. Dispose of personal protective equipment in a clinical waste bag, labelled 'Cytotoxic Waste'. Check local policy for colour and storage details.
- Wash your hands thoroughly with soap and water.

Practice pointers

- Observe the I.V. site frequently for signs of extravasation and an allergic reaction (swelling, redness and urticaria). If you suspect extravasation, stop the infusion, leave the I.V. catheter in place, and notify the doctor.
- When giving vesicants, avoid sites where damage to underlying tendons or nerves may occur (veins in the antecubital fossa, near the wrist or in the dorsal surface of the hand).

If nature calls

- If you're unable to stay with the patient during the entire infusion, use an infusion pump to ensure drug delivery within the prescribed time and rate.
- Observe the patient at regular intervals and after treatment for adverse reactions. Monitor his vital signs throughout the infusion to assess any changes during chemotherapy administration.

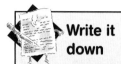

Write it down

Documenting chemotherapy

In your notes, document:

- location and description of the I.V. site before treatment
- drugs and dosages administered
- sequence of drug administration including time
- needle type and size used
- amount and type of flushing solution
- site's condition after treatment
- adverse reactions
- patient's tolerance of the treatment
- topics discussed with the patient and his family
- your name, designation and signature and the name of your colleague who performed safety checks.

- Maintain a list of the types and amounts of drugs the patient has received. This is especially important if he has received drugs that have a cumulative effect and that can be toxic to such organs as the heart and kidneys. (See *Documenting chemotherapy*.)

Epidural analgesics

Epidural analgesia helps manage acute and chronic pain, including moderate to severe post-operative pain. The epidural catheter, inserted near the spinal cord, eliminates the risks of multiple I.M. injections, minimizes adverse cerebral and systemic effects, and eliminates the analgesic peaks and valleys that usually occur with intermittent I.M. injections.

In this procedure, medication is injected or infused into the epidural space. The drug diffuses slowly into the subarachnoid space of the spinal canal and then into the cerebrospinal fluid (CSF), which carries it directly into the spinal area, bypassing the blood–brain barrier. In some cases, the doctor injects medication directly into the subarachnoid space. (See *Placement of a permanent epidural catheter*.)

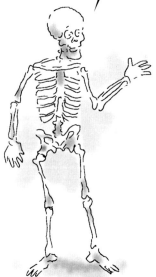

Delivering an analgesic near my spinal canal has impressive results.

What you need

Volumetric infusion device and epidural infusion tubing (appropriate to infusion device) ✳ patient's medication administration record and epidural care plan ✳ prescribed epidural solutions ✳ transparent dressing ✳ labels for epidural infusion line ✳ tape ✳ vital signs monitoring equipment.

Have on hand the following for emergency use: oxygen, including tubing and non-rebreathe mask ✳ resuscitation trolley and emergency drugs.

Getting ready

Prepare the infusion device according to the manufacturer's instructions and local policy. Check the medication concentration and infusion rate against the doctor's direction/prescription.

How you do it

- Explain the procedure and possible complications to the patient. Tell him that he'll feel some pain as the catheter is inserted. Make sure that a consent form has been properly signed and witnessed.

Placement of a permanent epidural catheter

An epidural catheter is implanted beneath the patient's skin and inserted near the spinal cord at the first lumbar (L1) interspace. For temporary analgesic therapy (less than 1 week), the catheter may exit directly over the spine and be taped up the patient's back to the shoulder. For prolonged therapy, it may be tunnelled subcutaneously to an exit site on the patient's side or abdomen or over his shoulder.

Dial down the dose

The most common complications of epidural infusions are numbness and leg weakness, which may occur after the first 24 hours, and are drug- and concentration-dependent. The doctor must titrate the dosage to identify the dose that provides adequate pain control without causing excessive numbness and weakness. Other possible complications include respiratory depression, pruritus, nausea and vomiting.

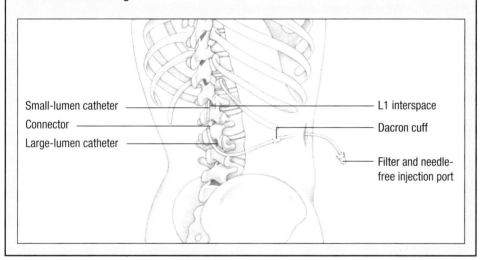

Small-lumen catheter
Connector
Large-lumen catheter

L1 interspace
Dacron cuff
Filter and needle-free injection port

- Position the patient on his side in the knee–chest position, or have him sit on the edge of the bed and lean over a bedside table.
- After the catheter is in place, prime the infusion device, confirm the appropriate medication and infusion rate, and then adjust the device for the correct rate.
- Help the anaesthetist or clinical nurse specialist to connect the infusion tubing to the epidural catheter. Then connect the tubing to the infusion pump.
- Secure all connection sites, and apply an epidural infusion label to the catheter, infusion tubing, and infusion pump to prevent accidental infusion of other drugs. Then start the infusion.

What's the score?

- Tell the patient to report any pain (according to a pain scale of 1–3). If the patient reports a high pain score, the infusion rate may need to be increased. Call the doctor/clinical nurse specialist/pain team or change the rate within the prescribed limits.
- Change the dressing over the catheter's exit site every 24–48 hours or as needed. The dressing is transparent to allow inspection of drainage and commonly appears moist or slightly blood-tinged.
- Change the infusion tubing every 48 hours or if disconnected from the epidural catheter, to prevent infection.

Removing an epidural catheter

- Typically, the anaesthetist inserts the catheter and prescribes analgesics; the anaesthetist or pain team nurse specialist will set up the initial infusion. However, local policy may allow a specially trained nurse to remove the catheter.
- If you feel resistance when removing the catheter, stop and call the doctor/pain team for further advice.

Practice pointers

- Epidural analgesia is contraindicated in patients who have local or systemic infection, known neurological disease, coagulation disorders, spinal arthritis or a spinal deformity, hypotension, marked hypertension, or an allergy to the prescribed medication, and in those who are undergoing anticoagulant therapy.
- Typically, the anaesthetist inserts the catheter and prescribes analgesics; the anaesthetist or pain team nurse specialist will set up the initial infusion.

Regular check-in

- Assess the patient's respiratory rate and blood pressure every hour for 8 hours and then every 4 hours for the rest of the infusion. Notify the doctor if the patient's vital signs are altered compared to the epidural care plan.
- Assess the patient's sedation level, mental status and pain-relief status every hour initially and then every 2–4 hours until adequate pain control is achieved. Notify the doctor if the patient appears drowsy, experiences nausea and vomiting, refractory itching or an inability to void, which are adverse reactions to certain opiate analgesics, or complains of unrelieved pain.

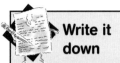

Write it down

Documenting epidural care

On the patient's MAR, record:

- administration of analgesics and adjuvant therapies, if any
- non-administration of medication prescribed, reason and actions taken
- the name, designation and signatures of registered professionals administering drugs.

On the epidural care plan, record:

- catheter patency
- condition of dressing and insertion site
- patient's vital signs and assessment results
- labelling of the epidural catheter
- changing of infusion bags
- patient's response and pain score.

Push and pull

- Assess the patient's lower-extremity motor strength every 2–4 hours. If sensory or motor loss occurs, large motor nerve fibres have been affected and the dose may need to be decreased.
- Keep in mind that drugs given via the epidural route diffuse slowly and may cause adverse reactions, including excessive sedation, up to 12 hours after the infusion has been discontinued.
- The patient should always have a peripheral I.V. line (with regular flushes being administered or continuous infusion) to allow immediate administration of emergency drugs. (See *Documenting epidural care*.)

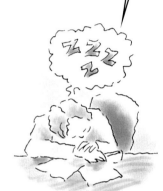

Epidurals can cause excessive sedation up to 12 hours after the infusion is discontinued.

Parenteral nutrition

When a patient can't meet his nutritional needs by oral or enteral feedings, he may require I.V. nutritional support, also known as parenteral nutrition.

Parenteral nutrition (PN) refers to any nutrient solution, including lipids, given through a central venous line. The most common delivery route for PN is through a central venous catheter (CVC) into the superior vena cava. Depending on the solution, it may be used to boost the patient's calorie intake, to supply full calorific needs or to surpass the patient's calorific requirements.

What you need

Bag of prescribed and prepared parenteral nutrition solution ✳ sterile I.V. tubing with integral micron filter ✳ tape ✳ 70% alcohol pads ✳ volumetric infusion pump ✳ scale ✳ fluid intake and output record ✳ sterile gloves ✳ 5 ml syringe filled with 0.9% sodium chloride or heparanized saline as directed for flush.

Getting ready

Make sure the solution, the patient and the equipment are ready. Remove the solution from the refrigerator at least 1 hour before use. Check the solution against the doctor or nutrition nurse specialist's direction for correct patient name, expiration date and formula components. Observe the bag for tears and leaks and the solution for cloudiness, turbidity and particles. If any of these are present, return the solution to the pharmacy.

When you're ready to administer the solution, explain the procedure to the patient. Check the name, hospital number and

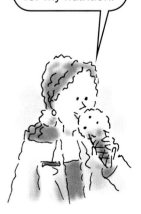

Personally, I prefer this delivery system for my nutrition.

date of birth on the solution label against the name on the patient's wristband and medicines administration record. Wash your hands thoroughly, put on apron and gloves.

There's an order to it

In sequence:
• Insert the spike of the administration set into the bag of solution using a non-touch technique.
• Squeeze then release the drip chamber to allow filling.
• Next, prime the tubing; open the roller clamp and let the solution fill the tubing. Continue to run the fluid through the line until there are no air bubbles trapped.
• Insert the administration set into the infusion pump, and prepare it according to the manufacturer's instructions. Remove and discard your gloves, wash your hands thoroughly.
• With the patient in the supine position, flush the catheter with appropriate solution and put on gloves. Clean the catheter Luer Lok extension port with a 70% alcohol swab (or as per local policy) and allow to dry.

How you do it

• If you'll be attaching the parenteral nutrition solution to a central venous (CV) line, clamp the CV line before disconnecting it, to prevent air from entering the catheter and associated air embolism.
• Using an aseptic technique, attach the tubing to the designated Luer-locking port and remove the clamp, if applicable.
• Set the infusion pump at the ordered flow rate, and start the infusion. Make sure the catheter junction is secure.
• Label the tubing with the date and time of change.

Starting the infusion

• Depending on the patient's tolerance, Parenteral nutrition can be initiated at a rate of 40–50 ml/hour and then advanced by 25 ml/hour every 6 hours (as tolerated) until the desired infusion rate is achieved. Alternatively, when the glucose concentration is low, you can initiate the rate necessary to infuse the complete 24-hour volume and discontinue the solution without tapering.

Changing solutions

• Prepare the new solution and I.V. tubing as described earlier and put on gloves.
• Turn off the infusion pump, close the flow clamps, remove the spike from the solution container that's hanging, and insert it into the new bag.

You don't need armour— just gloves and an apron.

Practice pointers

• Always infuse a parenteral nutrition solution at a constant rate without interruption, to avoid blood glucose fluctuations. If the infusion slows, consult the doctor or nurse specialist before changing the infusion rate.

Check points

• Monitor the patient's vital signs every 4 hours, or more often if necessary. Watch for an increased temperature, an early sign of catheter-related sepsis.
• Check the patient's blood glucose every 6 hours. Some patients may require supplementary insulin, which the pharmacist may add directly to the solution. The patient may also require additional subcutaneous doses.
• Change the dressing over the catheter according to local policy or whenever the dressing becomes wet, soiled or non-occlusive.
• Weigh the patient at the same time every morning. Maintain accurate intake and output records.
• Change the tubing every 24 hours (See *Documenting parenteral nutrition*.)

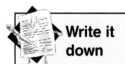

Write it down

Documenting parenteral nutrition

In your notes, document:

• times of the dressing, administration set, and solution changes
• condition of the catheter insertion site
• your observations of the patient's condition
• complications and interventions taken.

Papanicolaou test

Also known as the Pap test or Pap smear, the Papanicolaou test developed in the 1920s by George N. Papanicolaou allows early detection of cervical cancer. The test involves brushing secretions from the cervix, spreading them on a slide, and immediately coating the slide with fixative spray or solution to preserve specimen cells for nuclear staining. Cytology evaluation then outlines cell maturity, morphology and metabolic activity.

What you need

Bivalve vaginal speculum ✳ gloves ✳ Pap brush ✳ three glass microscope slides ✳ fixative (a commercial spray or 95% ethyl alcohol solution) ✳ adjustable lamp ✳ blanket ✳ laboratory request forms.

Getting ready

Select a speculum of the appropriate size, and gather the equipment in the examining room. Label each glass slide with the patient's name and an 'E', 'C' or 'V' to differentiate endocervical, cervical and vaginal specimens.

How you do it

- Introduce yourself to the patient, explain the procedure to gain cooperation and consent, and wash your hands (social hand wash).
- Instruct the patient to void to relax the perineal muscles.

Privacy, please!

- Provide privacy and maintain dignity, use of the examination room is best practice. Provide screens within the room and request that the patient undresses below the waist behind these screens. Then instruct her to sit on the examination couch and to cover herself with the blanket.
- Request the patient to lie in a semi-recumbent position with her knees drawn up, feet together and flat on the couch. Once this position has been achieved request that she allows her knees to flop out to the sides.
- Fold back the blanket to expose the genital area, adjust the lamp so that it illuminates the genital area.
- If you're performing the procedure, first put on gloves. Then take the speculum in your dominant hand and moisten it with warm water to ease insertion. Avoid using water-soluble lubricants, which can interfere with accurate laboratory testing.
- Warn the patient that you're about to commence the examination to avoid startling her. Then gently separate the labia with the thumb and forefinger of your non-dominant hand.

Promote relaxation

- Instruct the patient to take several deep breaths, and insert the speculum into the vagina. After it's in place, slowly open the blades to expose the cervix. Then lock the blades in place.

Fix immediately

- Insert a cotton-tipped applicator through the speculum 5 mm into the cervical os. Rotate the applicator 360 degrees to obtain an endocervical specimen. Then remove the applicator and gently roll it in a circle across the slide marked 'E'. Refrain from rubbing the applicator on the slide to prevent cell destruction. Immediately place the slide in a fixative solution or spray it with a fixative to prevent drying of the cells, which interferes with nuclear staining and cytology interpretation.
- Insert the brush end of the Pap brush through the speculum, and place it directly over the cervical os. Rotate the brush gently but firmly to pick up cells. Remove the brush, roll the brush and specimen across the slide marked 'C', and fix it immediately, as before.

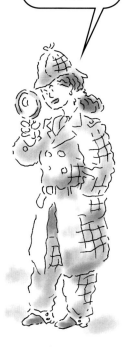

There's no speculation involved. You'll definitely need a speculum to perform a Pap test.

• Insert the cotton-tipped applicator through the speculum, and scrape the posterior fornix or vaginal pool, an area that collects cells from the endometrium, vagina and cervix. Remove the applicator, spread the specimen across the slide marked 'V', and fix it immediately.
• Unlock the speculum to ease removal and avoid accidentally pinching the vaginal wall. Then withdraw the speculum, inform the patient that the test is complete, dispose of the speculum in the clinical waste, remove your gloves and wash your hands.

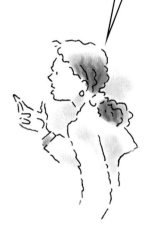

Rotate the Pap brush gently but firmly. That will collect cells.

Finish up

• If required assist the patient to a sitting position. Again provide privacy for her to dress.
• Fill out the appropriate laboratory request forms, including the date of last menstruation.

Practice pointers

• Many preventable factors can interfere with the Pap test's accuracy, so provide appropriate patient teaching beforehand. For example, use of a vaginal douche in the 48-hour period before specimen collection washes away cellular deposits and prevents adequate sampling. Sexual intercourse should be avoided for 24 hours prior to test and the instillation of vaginal medications in the same period makes cytology interpretation difficult. Collection of a specimen during menstruation prevents adequate sampling because menstrual flow washes away cells; ideally, such collection should take place 5–6 days before or 1 week after menstruation. Application of topical antibiotics promotes rapid, heavy shedding of cells and requires postponement of the Pap test for at least 1 month.
• If the patient has had a complete hysterectomy, collect test specimens from the vaginal pool and cuff. (See *Documenting a Pap test*.)

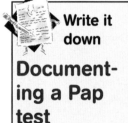

Write it down

Documenting a Pap test

In the patient's notes, record the date and time of specimen collection, complications and the nursing action taken.

Automated external defibrillation

Automated external defibrillators (AEDs) are commonly used today to meet the need for early defibrillation, which is currently considered the most effective treatment for ventricular fibrillation. Their use is also becoming common in such public places as shopping malls, sports stadiums, train and tube stations and airplanes. Instruction in using the AED is required for all registered nurses working in acute hospitals.

All in one package

The AED is equipped with a microcomputer that senses and analyses a patient's heart rhythm at the push of a button. Then it audibly or visually prompts you to deliver a shock. All devices record your interactions with the patient during defibrillation, in a solid-state memory module. Modern AEDs have an integral printer for immediate event documentation.

What you need

AED ✳ two pre-packaged electrodes. Training in either 'in-hospital basic life support' (BLS) or 'advanced life support'(ALS).

How you do it

• After discovering that your patient is unresponsive to voice and pain stimuli, pulseless, and apnoeic, follow either in-hospital BLS or ALS algorithms according to your level of training.
• Firmly press the device's ON button, and wait while the machine performs a brief self-test.
• Expose the patient's chest.

The machine talks

• The electronic voice recording will instruct you to 'connect electrodes'. Open the two foil packages, remove the backing film from the electrodes and, using the diagram on the packaging to assist you, place the electrodes on the patient's chest.
• The machine is ready to analyse the patient's heart rhythm once these are in place. Press the ANALYSE button when the machine prompts you to. Don't touch or move the patient while the AED is in analysis mode. (If the message 'Check electrodes' appears, verify correct electrode placement and a secure patient–cable attachment; then press the ANALYSE button again.)
• In 15–30 seconds, the AED will analyse the patient's rhythm. When the patient needs a shock, the AED displays a 'Stand clear' message and emits a beep that changes to a steady tone as it charges.

Just press the button

• When fully charged and ready to deliver a shock, the AED will prompt you to press the SHOCK button.
• Make sure that no one is touching the patient or his bed, oxygen is removed and call out 'Stand clear'. Then press the SHOCK

button on the AED. Most AEDs are ready to deliver a shock within 15 seconds.
• After the first shock, the AED will prompt you to continue cardio-pulmonary resuscitation (CPR). Replace oxygen therapy and commence CPR as instructed. The AED will continue to guide you through further analysis steps and shock delivery.

Continue until expert help takes over
• Continue following the instructions of the AED and the algorithm sequence until the resuscitation team leader arrives.
• After the arrest event, remove and transcribe the AED's computer memory module or tape, or prompt the AED to print a rhythm strip with code data. Follow your local policy for cardiac arrest auditing and storing data.

Practice pointers
• Defibrillators vary from one manufacturer to the next, so be sure to familiarize yourself with your equipment. Defibrillator operation should be checked and documented at least once per 8-hour shift (along with the rest of the cardiac arrest trolley and equipment) and after each use. (See *Documenting AED use*.)
• For further information on basic life support, advanced life support and AED use, visit the website of the United Kingdom Resuscitation Council (www.resus.org.uk).

Write it down

Documenting AED use

After using an automated external defibrillator (AED), give a verbal handover to the resuscitation team leader as soon as she arrives on scene. Remember to report:

- patient's name, age, medical history and reason for seeking care
- when you found the patient in cardiac arrest (be as time specific as possible)
- when you started cardiopulmonary resuscitation
- when you applied the AED
- how many shocks the patient received
- when the patient regained a pulse at any point
- what post-arrest care was given, if any
- physical assessment findings.

As soon after the vent as possible, be sure to document all of this information on both the cardiac arrest audit documentation and in the patient's medical and nursing notes.

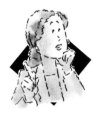

Quick quiz

1. What size needle should you use to draw up fluid from a glass vial?

    A. 25G (orange) or filter

    B. 20G (white)

    C. Insulin needle.

Answer: A. 25G or filter, to prevent administration of glass particles to the patient's vascular system.

2. When preparing I.V. fluids, how many registered professionals are required to perform safety checks?

    A. One.

    B. Two.

    C. Three.

Answer: B. Intravenous medications should be checked by two registered professionals, check local policy to ascertain which professionals are permitted.

3. When collecting a venous blood sample you should:

    A. Use a needle and syringe.

    B. Use an evacuated tube system.

    C. Use a central catheter.

Answer: B. Use an evacuated tube system, preventing associated complications of venepuncture, i.e. venous collapse.

4. When administered blood products you should record the patient's vital signs:

    A. Every 4 hours throughout transfusion.

    B. Every 15 minutes for the first hour of transfusion.

    C. Every hour during the transfusion.

Answer: B. To maintain patient safety and identify transfusion reactions quickly, vital signs should be recorded and acted upon every 15 minutes for the first hour and then half-hourly during transfusion.

Scoring

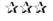 If you answered all four items correctly, splendid! You have certainly enhanced your ability to ace a quick quiz.

    If you answered three items correctly, fabulous! You're making solid progress on enhancing your knowledge and practice.

    If you answered fewer than three items correctly, don't miss a beat. Just review the chapter and try again.

9 Advanced clinical procedures: the nurse's role

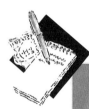

Just the facts

In this chapter, you'll learn:

♦ about common procedures performed in the clinical area by doctors and specialists

♦ what equipment preparation, care, complications and patient teaching are associated with each procedure

♦ about essential documentation for each procedure.

There are many more clinical procedures that can be undertaken either in the patient's own home, the primary care setting or within a hospital that have not been discussed in this book. These are procedures that are not undertaken specifically by a nurse, but where the nurse will be present in order to support the patient and assist with the procedure. Therefore this short chapter details how some of these procedures are undertaken in order that you, the nurse, can assist with both the pre-procedure and post-procedure care, and also the procedure itself.

Lumbar puncture

Lumbar puncture involves the insertion of a sterile needle into the subarachnoid space of the spinal canal, usually between the third and fourth lumbar vertebrae. This procedure is used to detect increased intracranial pressure (ICP) or the presence of blood in cerebrospinal fluid (CSF), to obtain CSF specimens for laboratory analysis, and to inject dyes or gases for contrast in radiological studies. It's also used to administer drugs or anaesthetics and to relieve ICP by removing CSF.

Proceed with caution

Performed by a doctor with a nurse present as the patient's advocate, lumbar puncture requires a sterile technique and careful patient positioning. This procedure is contraindicated in patients with lumbar deformity or infection at the puncture site. It should be performed cautiously in patients with increased ICP because the rapid reduction in pressure that follows withdrawal of CSF can cause tonsillar herniation and medullary compression.

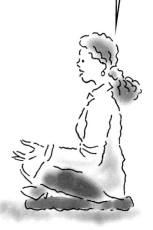

The nurse's role during lumbar puncture is to reassure the patient and act as his advocate.

What you need

Equipment trolley ✳ two pairs of sterile gloves of appropriate size for the doctor ✳ non-sterile gloves of appropriate size for you ✳ sterile gown for the doctor ✳ apron for the nurse ✳ iodine solution ✳ sterile gauze pads ✳ alcohol pads ✳ sterile drape ✳ 3 ml syringe for local anaesthetic ✳ 25G sterile needle for injecting anaesthetic ✳ local anaesthetic (usually 1% lidocaine (lignocaine))✳ 18G or 20G spinal needle with stylet (22G needle for children and adults below a weight of 60 kg) ✳ three-way tap ✳ manometer ✳ small adhesive bandage ✳ three sterile collection tubes with stoppers ✳ laboratory request forms ✳ labels ✳ light source.

Disposable lumbar puncture trays contain most of the sterile equipment needed.

Getting ready

Gather the equipment and take it to the patient's bedside.

How you do it

• Be with the patient while the doctor explains the procedure and assist in answering any questions the patient may have, this will ease the patient's anxiety and ensure his cooperation. Witness the giving of consent.
• Encourage the patient to cooperate during the procedure by providing verbal reassurance and agreeing a no-verbal 'stop' or 'rest' signal in order to minimize complications and side-effects such as a headache. (See *Perils of lumbar puncture*.)

Warning!

Perils of lumbar puncture

Headache is the most common adverse effect of lumbar puncture. Other adverse reactions may include:

- a reaction to the anaesthetic
- meningitis
- epidural or subdural abscess
- bleeding into the spinal canal
- cerebrospinal fluid leakage through the dural defect remaining after needle withdrawal
- local pain caused by nerve root irritation
- oedema or haematoma at the puncture site
- transient difficulty voiding, and fever.

The most serious complications of lumbar puncture, although rare, are tonsillar herniation and medullary compression.

- Check and confirm the patient's allergy status verbally, correlate with the medical notes, ID band and medicine administration record.
- Immediately before the procedure, provide privacy and ask the patient to void his bladder.
- Wash your hands thoroughly and put on an apron.
- Open the equipment tray on a dressing trolley, being careful not to contaminate the sterile field when you open the wrapper; open the iodine solution and pour into the galley pot.

Model behaviour

- Provide adequate lighting at the puncture site, and adjust the height of the patient's bed to allow the both the doctor and yourself to perform the procedure comfortably, without causing you back injury.
- Position the patient, and re-emphasize the importance of remaining as still as possible to minimize discomfort and trauma. (See *Positioning for lumbar puncture*.)
- Put on non-sterile gloves.

Careful preparation

- The doctor cleans the puncture site with sterile gauze pads soaked in iodine solution, wiping in a circular motion away from the puncture site; she uses three different pads to avoid contaminating spinal tissues with the body's normal skin flora. Next, she drapes the area with the fenestrated drape (drape with a hole) to provide a sterile field. (If the

Positioning for lumbar puncture

Have the patient lie on his side at the edge of the bed, with his chin tucked to his chest and his knees drawn up to his abdomen. Make sure the patient's spine is curved and his back is at the edge of the bed (as shown below). This position widens the spaces between the vertebrae, easing insertion of the needle.

To help the patient maintain this position, place one of your hands behind his neck and the other hand behind his knees, and pull gently. Hold the patient firmly in this position throughout the procedure to prevent accidental needle displacement.

Needle insertion site

Typically, the doctor inserts the needle between the third and fourth lumbar vertebrae (as shown below).

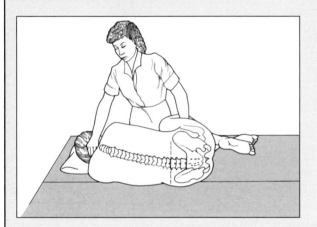

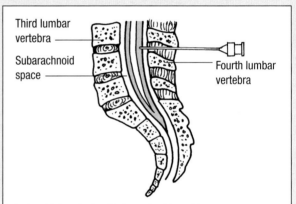

doctor uses iodine pads instead of sterile gauze pads, she may remove her sterile gloves and put on another pair to avoid introducing iodine into the subarachnoid space with the lumbar puncture needle.)
• Invert the vial of lidocaine to 45 degrees so that the doctor can insert a 25G needle and syringe and withdraw the anaesthetic for injection.
• Before the doctor injects the anaesthetic, tell the patient he'll experience a transient burning sensation and local pain. Ask him to report other persistent pain or sensations because they may indicate irritation or puncture of a nerve root, requiring repositioning of the needle.

Still and steady

• When the doctor inserts the sterile spinal needle into the subarachnoid space between the third and fourth lumbar vertebrae, instruct the patient to remain still and breathe normally. If necessary, hold the patient firmly in position to prevent sudden movement that may displace the needle.

• If the lumbar puncture is being performed to administer contrast media for radiological studies or spinal anaesthetic, the doctor injects the dye or anaesthetic at this time.

Meter reader

• When the needle is in place, the doctor attaches a manometer with a three-way stopcock to the needle hub to read CSF pressure. If ordered, help the patient extend his legs to provide a more accurate pressure reading.
• The doctor then detaches the manometer and allows CSF to drain from the needle hub into the collection tubes. When he has collected 2–3 ml in each tube, mark the tubes in sequence, insert a stopper to secure them, and label them.

Stop sign

• If the doctor suspects an obstruction in the spinal subarachnoid space, he may check for Queckenstedt's sign. After he takes an initial CSF pressure reading, compress the patient's jugular vein for 10 seconds as ordered. This increases ICP and—if no subarachnoid block exists—causes CSF pressure to rise as well. The doctor then takes pressure readings every 10 seconds until the pressure stabilizes.

Finishing touches

• After the doctor collects the specimens and removes the spinal needle, put on sterile gloves, clean the puncture site with iodine, and apply a small adhesive bandage. Remove gloves and wash your hands.
• Send the CSF specimens to the laboratory immediately, with completed laboratory request forms.

Practice pointers

• During lumbar puncture, watch closely for signs of adverse reaction: elevated pulse rate, pallor and clammy skin. Alert the doctor immediately to significant changes.
• The patient may be ordered to lie flat for 8–12 hours after the procedure. If necessary, place a patient-care reminder on his bed to this effect. (See *Documenting lumbar puncture*.)

Write it down

Documenting lumbar puncture

In your notes, record:

• how the consent was obtained
• initiation and completion times of the procedure
• patient's response to the procedure
• administration of drugs
• number of specimen tubes collected
• time of transport to the laboratory
• colour, consistency and other characteristics of the collected specimens
• any actions to be taken, i.e. lie flat for 12 hours, monitor vital signs 1 hourly, etc.
• your name, designation and signature.

Bone marrow aspiration and biopsy

A specimen of bone marrow—the major site of blood cell formation—can be obtained by aspiration or needle biopsy. The procedure allows evaluation of overall blood composition, including blood elements, precursor cells and abnormal or malignant cells.

Aspiration removes cells through a needle inserted into the marrow cavity of the bone; a biopsy removes a small, solid core of marrow tissue through the needle. Both procedures are usually performed by a doctor, but some specially trained chemotherapy nurses or nurse clinicians (who have achieved competency and confidence in the skill) can carry out the procedure with an assistant.

What you need

For aspiration
Pre-packaged bone marrow set, which includes: iodine pads ✳ two sterile drapes (one fenestrated, one plain) ✳ 10 cm × 10 cm gauze pads ✳ 5 cm × 5 cm gauze pads ✳ 10 ml syringe ✳ 22G or 19G needle ✳ scalpel ✳ sedative ✳ specimen containers ✳ bone marrow needle ✳ 70% alcohol ✳ 1% lidocaine ✳ 26G or 27G needle ✳ adhesive tape ✳ sterile gloves ✳ apron ✳ glass slides ✳ labels ✳ equipment trolley.

For biopsy
All equipment listed above ✳ Vim–Silverman, Jamshidi, Illinois sternal or Westerman–Jensen needle ✳ Zenker's fixative.

How you do it

• Inform the patient that the doctor would like to collect a bone marrow specimen, let the patient know the approximate time that this will be performed and explain the procedure in appropriate terms to him (use drawings if necessary) to ease his anxiety and ensure cooperation.
• Inform the patient that the procedure normally takes 5–10 minutes, that test results are usually available in 1 day, and that more than one marrow specimen may be required.
• Make sure the patient or a responsible family member understands the procedure, when the doctor has explained it again, and that written consent is gained.
• Alert the patient and his family that bleeding and infection are potentially life-threatening complications of aspiration or biopsy at any site and instruct them to alert a medical professional if this occurs (check local policy for outpatients regarding NHS Direct/GP or A&E).

Historically sensitive?

• Check the patient's medical history for hypersensitivity to the local anaesthetic. Inform him that he'll receive a local anaesthetic and feel heavy pressure from insertion of the biopsy or aspiration

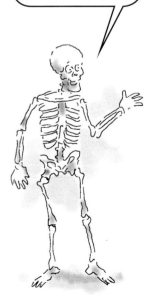

Only if you're specially trained, assessed to be competent and confident, and have permission from your employer can you perform bone marrow aspiration and biopsy.

needle as well as a brief, pulling sensation. Tell him that the doctor may make a small incision to avoid tearing the skin.

• Tell him which bone—sternum or posterior superior or anterior iliac crest—will be sampled.

• If the patient has osteoporosis, tell him that the needle pressure may be minimal.

• Administer any directed medication (see Chapter 5 for how to administer medication) before the test, e.g. sedation, analgesia.

• Assemble and prepare the equipment in the clinical treatment room (or prepare in a clinical room and take to patient's bedside if no treatment area is available); wash your hands, put on the apron, open the sterile pack, using only the outer corners, on to a clean surface; pour iodine solution into the galley pot.

• Position the patient according to the selected puncture site. (See *Common sites for bone marrow aspiration and biopsy*.)

Common sites for bone marrow aspiration and biopsy

The posterior superior iliac crest is the preferred site for bone marrow aspiration because no vital organs or vessels are nearby. The patient is placed either in the lateral position with one leg flexed or in the prone position.

For aspiration or biopsy from the anterior iliac crest, the patient is placed in the supine or side-lying position. This site is used with patients who can't lie in the prone position because of severe abdominal distension.

Aspiration from the sternum involves the greatest risk. However, it may be used because this site is near the surface, the cortical bone is thin, and the marrow cavity contains numerous cells and relatively little fat or supporting bone. This site is seldom used for biopsy.

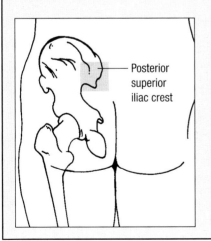

Posterior superior iliac crest

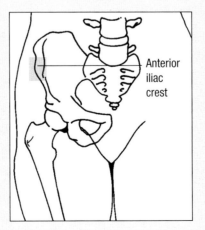

Anterior iliac crest

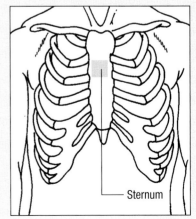

Sternum

Numbing needed

- Using sterile technique, the doctor will clean the puncture site with iodine pads and allow it to dry; then drape the area.
- To anaesthetize the site, the doctor infiltrates it with 1% lidocaine, using a 25G or 27G needle to inject a small amount intradermally and then a larger 22G needle to anaesthetize the tissue down to the bone.
- When the needle tip reaches the bone, the doctor anaesthetizes the periosteum by injecting a small amount of lidocaine in a circular area about 2 cm in diameter. The needle should be withdrawn from the periosteum after each injection.
- After allowing about 1 minute for the anaesthetic to take effect, a scalpel may be used to make a small stab incision in the patient's skin to accommodate the bone marrow needle. This technique avoids pushing skin into the bone marrow and also helps avoid unnecessary skin tearing, to help reduce the risk of infection.

Bone marrow aspiration

- The doctor inserts the bone marrow needle and lodges it firmly in the bone cortex. If the patient feels sharp pain instead of pressure when the needle first touches bone, the needle was probably inserted outside the anaesthetized area. If this happens, the needle should be withdrawn slightly and moved to the anaesthetized area.
- The needle is advanced by applying an even, downward force with the heel of the hand or the palm, while twisting it back and forth slightly. A crackling sensation means that the needle has entered the marrow cavity.
- Next, the doctor removes the inner cannula, attaches the syringe to the needle, aspirates the required specimen, and withdraws the needle.
- The nurse puts on gloves and applies pressure to the aspiration site with a gauze pad for 5 minutes to control bleeding, while an assistant prepares the marrow slides. The area is then cleaned with alcohol to remove the iodine, the skin is dried thoroughly with a gauze pad, and a sterile pressure dressing is applied.

Bone marrow biopsy

- The doctor inserts the biopsy needle into the periosteum and advances it steadily until the outer needle passes into the marrow cavity.
- The biopsy needle is directed into the marrow cavity by alternately rotating the inner needle clockwise and counter clockwise. Then a plug of tissue is removed, the needle assembly is withdrawn, and the marrow specimen is expelled into a properly labelled specimen bottle containing fixative or formaldehyde.
- The nurse puts on gloves, cleans the area around the biopsy site with alcohol to remove the iodine solution, firmly presses a sterile gauze pad against the incision to control bleeding, and then applies a sterile pressure dressing.

Practice pointers

- Faulty needle placement may yield too little aspirate. If no specimen is produced, the needle must be withdrawn from the bone (but not from the overlying soft tissue), the stylet replaced, and the needle inserted into a second site within the anaesthetized field.
- Bone marrow specimens shouldn't be collected from irradiated areas because radiation may have altered or destroyed the marrow.
- If a haematoma occurs around the puncture site, apply warm soaks. Give analgesics for site pain or tenderness. (See *Documenting bone marrow aspiration and biopsy.*)

Skin biopsy

Skin biopsy is a diagnostic test in which a small piece of tissue is removed from a lesion that's suspected of being malignant or from another dermatosis, while the patient is under local anaesthesia.

Pick one, any one . . .

One of three techniques may be used: shave biopsy, punch biopsy or excisional biopsy. Shave biopsy cuts the lesion above the skin line, which allows further biopsy of the site. Punch biopsy removes an oval core from the centre of the lesion. Excisional biopsy removes the entire lesion and is indicated for rapidly expanding lesions; for sclerotic, bullous or atrophic lesions; and for examination of the border of a lesion surrounding normal skin.

What you need

Gloves and apron ✳ scalpel for shave or excisional biopsy ✳ local anaesthetic ✳ specimen bottle containing 10% formaldehyde solution ✳ 4-0 sutures for punch or excisional biopsy ✳ adhesive dressing ✳ forceps.

Manufactured sterile packs containing all of the above may be used.

How you do it

- Explain to the patient that the biopsy provides a skin specimen for microscopic study. Describe the procedure and tell him who will perform it. Typically a doctor or an advanced practice nurse performs the biopsy and gains written consent for this invasive procedure. Answer questions he may have to ease anxiety, ensure cooperation and establish informed consent.

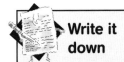

Write it down

Documenting bone marrow aspiration and biopsy

- Document the time, date, location, consent, patient response and the specimen obtained
- Record your name, designation and signature.

- Inform the patient that he need not restrict food or fluids.
- Tell him that he'll receive a local anaesthetic for pain and check the patient's history for hypersensitivity to the local anaesthetic.
- Inform him that the biopsy will take about 15 minutes and that the test results are usually available in 3 days (check local policy for receiving of results).
- Have the patient or an appropriate family member sign a consent form.
- Position the patient comfortably. Wash your hands, put on gloves and an apron. The doctor cleans the biopsy site before the local anaesthetic is administered.

Bleeding is a possible complication associated with any biopsy.

Shave . . .

- For a shave biopsy, the protruding growth is cut off at the skin line with a 15 scalpel.
- The tissue is placed immediately in a properly labelled specimen bottle containing 10% formaldehyde solution.
- Apply pressure to the area to stop the bleeding, assess the wound and apply an adhesive dressing.
- Remove and discard gloves and apron; wash your hands.
- Give the patient written and verbal information on how to care for the wound and advise on when further advice should be sought and from whom (check local policy).

. . . punch . . .

- For a punch biopsy, the skin surrounding the lesion is pulled taut, and the punch is firmly introduced into the lesion and rotated to obtain a tissue specimen. The plug is lifted with forceps or a needle and is severed as deeply into the fat layer as possible.
- The specimen is placed in a properly labelled specimen bottle containing 10% formaldehyde solution or in a sterile container if indicated.
- Closing the wound depends on the size of the punch. A 3 mm punch requires only an adhesive dressing, a 4 mm punch requires one suture, and a 6 mm punch requires two sutures.
- Apply pressure to the area to stop the bleeding, assess the wound and apply an adhesive dressing.
- Remove and discard gloves and apron; wash your hands.
- Give the patient written and verbal information on how to care for the wound and advise on when further advice should be sought and from whom (check local policy).

. . . or excisional . . .

- For an excisional biopsy, a 15 scalpel is used to excise the lesion; the incision is made as wide and as deep as necessary.

Write it down

Documenting skin biopsy

In the patient's notes, document:

- time and location where the specimen was obtained
- the name of the person who undertook the procedure
- the anatomical site of the biopsy
- use of local anaesthetic and skin preparation
- type and number of sutures, if applicable
- any complications that occurred and actions taken
- appearance of the site and specimen
- the type of dressing applied
- whether bleeding occurred at the biopsy site
- referral to community nurses/GP for aftercare, i.e. suture removal
- any medication given to take away
- time and date of specimen transfer to laboratory
- your name, designation and signature.

- The tissue specimen is removed and placed immediately in a properly labelled specimen bottle containing 10% formaldehyde solution.
- Apply pressure to the site to stop the bleeding.
- The wound is closed using a 4-0 suture.
- Check the biopsy site/wound for bleeding.
- Remove and discard gloves and apron; wash your hands.
- Send the specimen to the laboratory immediately.
- If the patient experiences pain, administer an analgesic.
- Apply an adhesive dressing.
- Give the patient written and verbal information on how to care for the wound and advise on when further advice should be sought and from whom (check local policy).

Practice pointers

- Support the patient pre-, during and post-procedure, ensure that reassurance and information are given to the patient, check his understanding of the explanation by asking questions regarding: what is to happen, when it will happen, who will be present, the side effects and complications, and the after care. (See *Documenting skin biopsy.*)

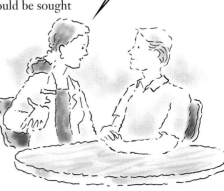

CVC insertion and removal

A central venous catheter (CVC) is a sterile catheter made of polyurethane, polyvinyl chloride or silicone rubber (Silastic). It's inserted through a large vein such as the subclavian vein or, less commonly, the jugular vein. A CVC line allows monitoring of central venous pressure, aspiration of blood samples and administration of I.V. fluids and parenteral nutrition solutions. It also preserves peripheral veins when a patient requires long-term venous access.

What you need

For insertion of a CVC
Sterile gloves and gowns * blanket * sterile towel and protective pad * sterile drape * masks * alcohol pads * iodine pads or other approved antimicrobial solution, such as 70% alcohol or 2% iodine * normal saline solution * 3 ml syringe with 25G needle * 1% or 2% injectable lidocaine * 5% dextrose * suture material * two 14G or 16G CVCs * I.V. solution with administration set prepared for use * infusion pump or controller, as needed * sterile gauze pads * sterile scissors * heparanized flushes as needed * portable X-ray machine * transparent semi-permeable dressing.

Special accessories

For flushing a catheter
0.9% sodium chloride solution or heparanized saline flush solution * 70% alcohol pad or other cleaning solution (check local policy).

For changing an injection cap
Alcohol pad or sterile gauze * injection cap.

For removal of a CVC
Clean gloves and sterile gloves * apron * mask * sterile drape * sterile suture removal set * alcohol pads * sterile gauze pads * forceps * tape * sterile, plastic adhesive-backed dressing or transparent semi-permeable dressing * sterile specimen bottle, if necessary for culture.

The type of catheter selected depends on the type of therapy to be used. Most clinical areas have prepared trays containing most of the equipment for catheter insertion.

Getting ready

Before insertion of a CVC, confirm catheter type and size with the doctor; usually, a 14G or 16G catheter is selected. Set up the I.V. solution and prime the administration set using a strict aseptic technique. Attach the line to the infusion pump or controller if ordered. Recheck all connections to make sure they're tight. As ordered, notify the radiology department that a portable X-ray machine may be needed if the patient is too acutely unwell to go to the radiology department.

How you do it

- Wash your hands thoroughly to prevent the spread of microorganisms. Put on the apron.

Inserting a CVC

- Reinforce the doctor's explanation of the procedure, and answer the patient's questions. Ensure that the patient has signed a consent form, if necessary, and check his history for allergies; offer reassurance.

Patient prep

- Position the patient with his head down (15–30 degrees), to dilate the veins and reduce the risk of air embolism.
- For subclavian insertion, place a rolled blanket lengthwise between the shoulders to increase venous distention. For jugular insertion, place a rolled blanket under the opposite shoulder to extend the neck, making anatomical landmarks more visible. Place a protective pad under the patient to prevent soiling the bed and causing him distress.
- Turn the patient's head away from the site.
- Prepare the insertion site by clipping hair or washing the skin as necessary, then establish a sterile field on a trolley, using a sterile towel or the wrapping from the instrument tray. Open all sterile equipment and place on the sterile field.

Bigger and bigger circles

- Wash your hands, put on a mask, non-sterile gloves and gown, and clean the area around the insertion site with pads soaked in 70% alcohol, followed by iodine solution or other approved antimicrobial solution, working in a circular motion outward from the site and maintaining non-touch technique. If the patient is sensitive to iodine, you may use a solution of 70% alcohol.

- Wash your hands and apply clean gloves.
- After the doctor puts on a sterile mask, gown and gloves, and drapes the area to create a sterile field, she will take the open 3 ml syringe and 25G needle and request the local anaesthetic.
- Wipe the top of a multi-dose lidocaine vial with an alcohol pad, allow it to dry, or open a new vial and invert it. The doctor then fills the 3 ml syringe and injects the anaesthetic into the site.
- The doctor will insert the catheter using aseptic technique.
- During this time, prepare the I.V. administration set for immediate attachment to the catheter hub.
- Attach the I.V. line to the catheter hub, set the flow rate at a keep-vein-open rate to maintain venous access. (Alternatively, the catheter may be capped and flushed with heparin or saline solution.) The doctor then sutures the catheter in place.

X marks the spot

- After an X-ray confirms correct catheter placement in the mid superior vena cava, set the flow rate as ordered.
- Use normal saline solution to remove dried blood that could harbour microorganisms. Secure the catheter with dressing, and apply a sterile CVC-appropriate dressing (sterile, plastic adhesive-backed dressing or transparent semi-permeable dressing). Expect some serosanguineous (serous) drainage during the first 24 hours. Label the dressing with the time and date of catheter insertion and catheter length, if not imprinted on the catheter.
- Place the patient in a comfortable position and reassess his status.

Flushing the catheter

- To maintain patency, flush the catheter routinely according to local policy.
- All lumens of a multi-lumen catheter must be flushed regularly. Some facilities use a heparin flush solution, available in premixed 10 ml multi-dose vials. Recommended concentrations vary from 10 to 100 units of heparin/ml. Use normal saline solution instead of heparin to maintain patency in two-way valved devices, such as the Groshong type, because research suggests that heparin isn't always needed to keep the line open.

How often?

- The recommended frequency for flushing CVCs varies from once every 12 hours to once weekly.

How much?

- The recommended amount of flushing solution also varies. Most policies recommend using 3–5 ml of solution to flush the catheter, although some policies call for as much as 10 ml of solution. Different catheters require different amounts of solution. Check policy first and ensure you are competent and confident to perform the procedure.
- To perform the flushing procedure, start by cleaning the needle-less port with an alcohol pad (using 70% alcohol solution). Allow the cap to dry.
- Access the port and aspirate to confirm the patency of the CVC, discard the aspirate then inject the recommended type and amount of flush solution.
- After flushing the catheter, maintain positive pressure by keeping your thumb on the plunger of the syringe while withdrawing the syringe for the port. This prevents blood backflow and clotting in the line.

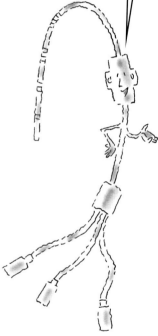

Changing the injection cap

- CVCs used for intermittent infusions have needle-free injection ports (similar to those used for peripheral catheters). These caps must be Luer Lok types to prevent inadvertent disconnection and an air embolism.
- The frequency of cap changes varies according to your local policy, the manufacturer's guidelines and how often the cap is used. Use a strict non-touch aseptic technique when changing the cap.
- Clean the connection site with an alcohol pad or an iodine pad.
- Close the catheter clamp, to prevent air from entering the catheter.

Removing a CVC

- If you'll be removing the CVC, first check the patient's record for the most recent placement (confirmed by an X-ray) to trace the catheter's path as it exits the body. Make sure that assistance is available if a complication (such as uncontrolled bleeding) occurs during catheter removal. Before you remove the catheter, explain the procedure to the patient.
- Place the patient in a supine position, wash your hands, and put on clean gloves and a mask.
- Turn off all infusions and prepare a sterile field, using a sterile drape.

- Remove and discard the old dressing, wash your hands and change to sterile gloves.
- Clean the site with an alcohol pad or a gauze pad soaked in iodine solution. Inspect the site for signs of infection.
- Clip the sutures and, using forceps, clamp the catheter ports and remove the catheter in a slow, even motion.

Make your mark

- Cover with a sterile gauze pad, and tape a transparent semi-permeable dressing over the gauze. Label the dressing with the date and time of the removal and your initials. Keep the site covered for 48 hours.
- Inspect the catheter tip and measure the length of the catheter to ensure that the catheter has been completely removed. If you suspect that the catheter hasn't been completely removed, notify the doctor immediately and monitor the patient closely for signs of distress. If you suspect an infection, send the tip of the catheter, in a sterile pot, to the laboratory for culture and sensitivity tests.
- Dispose of the I.V. tubing and equipment as per local policy.

Practice pointers

- While you're awaiting chest X-ray confirmation of proper catheter placement, infuse an I.V. solution such as 5% dextrose or 0.9% sodium chloride solution until correct placement is assured. Or cap the port and flush the line. Infusing an isotonic solution avoids the risk of vessel wall thrombosis.
- Change the dressing at least three times a week, according to your local policy, or whenever it becomes moist or soiled. Change the tubing and solution every 24–48 hours, or according to your local policy, while the CVC is in place. Dressing, tubing and solution changes for a CVC should be performed using an aseptic technique. Assess the site for signs of infection, such as discharge, inflammation and tenderness.
- To prevent an air embolism, close the catheter clamp each time the catheter hub is open to air. (A Groshong catheter doesn't require clamping because it has an internal valve.)
- If the patient is to go home with the CVC, provide education and make arrangements accordingly. (See *CVC therapy in the home* and *Documenting CVC insertion and removal*.)

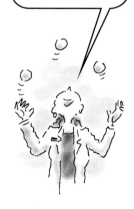

While you're waiting for X-ray confirmation of catheter placement, infuse with normal saline or another isotonic solution.

Home care connection

CVC therapy in the home

Long-term use of a central venous catheter (CVC) allows patients to receive potent fluids (i.e. chemotherapy agents, steroids and antibiotics such as vancomycin) and blood infusions at home. These catheters have a much longer life because they are less thrombogenic and less prone to infection than short-term devices.

Buddy system

A candidate for home therapy must have a family member, friend or care service provider who can safely and competently administer the I.V. fluids; a suitable home environment with access to a telephone and transportation; understanding of the risks and when to seek professional help; and the ability to prepare, handle, store and dispose of the equipment. The care procedures used in the home are the same as those used in the hospital environment.

Learning curve

The overall goal of home therapy is patient safety, so your patient teaching, as well as referral and set-up of home care provision, must begin well before discharge. After discharge, a primary care nurse will provide follow-up care until the patient or someone close to him can provide catheter care and infusion therapy independently. Many home therapy patients learn to care for the catheter themselves and infuse their own medications and solution.

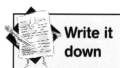

Write it down

Document-ing CVC insertion and removal

In your notes, record:

- and date of insertion
- length and location of the catheter
- solution infused
- doctor's name
- patient's response to the procedure
- time of the X-ray
- X-ray results and your notification of the doctor
- date of catheter removal
- type of antimicrobial ointment and dressing applied
- condition of the catheter insertion site
- collection of a culture specimen
- your name, designation and signature.

PICC insertion and removal

For a patient who needs central venous (CV) therapy for 1–6 months or who requires repeated venous access, a peripherally inserted central catheter (PICC) may be the best option. They're available in single- and double-lumen versions, with or without guide wires, and of varying diameters and lengths.

PICCs are being used increasingly for patients receiving home care. The device is easier to insert than other CV devices and provides safe, reliable access for drug administration and blood sampling. A single catheter may be used for the entire course of therapy with greater convenience and at reduced cost. If you have received theoretical and practical training, and have been assessed as competent and confident in the skill, and show sufficient knowledge of vascular access devices, you may insert a PICC.

What you need

Catheter insertion kit containing: three alcohol swabs or other approved antimicrobial solution ✳ iodine ointment ✳ 5 ml vial of heparin (100 U/ml) ✳ injection port with short extension tubing ✳ vial of 0.9% sodium chloride solution ✳ sterile gauze pads ✳ tape ✳ protective pad ✳ sterile drapes ✳ tourniquet ✳ sterile transparent semi-permeable dressing ✳ two pairs of sterile gloves ✳ sterile gown ✳ mask ✳ goggles ✳ clean gloves.

Getting ready

Gather the necessary supplies. If you're administering PICC therapy in the patient's home, bring everything with you.

How you do it

- Describe the procedure to the patient and wash your hands.

Inserting a PICC
- Select the insertion site, place the tourniquet on the patient's arm, and assess the antecubital fossa.
- Remove the tourniquet and determine the spot at which the catheter tip will rest after insertion. For placement in the superior vena cava, measure the distance from the insertion site to the shoulder and from the shoulder to the sternal notch, then add 7.6 cm to the measurement.
- Have the patient lie in a supine position with his arm at a 90-degree angle to his body and place a pad under his arm.
- Open the PICC tray and drop the rest of the sterile items on to the sterile field. Put on the sterile gown, mask, goggles and gloves.

- Using the sterile measuring tape, cut the distal end of the catheter according to specific manufacturer's recommendations and guidelines, using the equipment provided.
- Using a sterile technique, withdraw 5 ml of the sodium chloride solution and flush the extension tubing and the port. Attach the syringe to the hub of the catheter and flush.

Rub down

- Prepare the insertion site by rubbing it with alcohol or other approved antimicrobial solution, using a circular motion and working outward by about 15 cm. Allow the area to dry but be sure not to touch the intended insertion site.
- Take your gloves off and apply the tourniquet about 10 cm above the antecubital fossa.
- Put on a new pair of sterile gloves and place a sterile drape under the patient's arm and another on top of the arm. Drop a sterile gauze pad over the tourniquet.
- Stabilize the patient's vein and insert the catheter introducer at a 10-degree angle, directly into the vein.
- After successful vein entry, you should see a blood return in the flashback chamber. Without changing the needle's position, gently advance the plastic introducer sheath until you're sure the tip is well within the vein. Remove the tourniquet, using a sterile gauze pad to maintain a sterile technique.

Because you only need one catheter for the entire therapy, a PICC increases convenience and reduces costs.

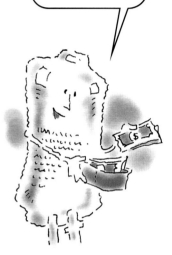

Pressure point

- Carefully withdraw the needle while holding the introducer still. To minimize blood loss, try applying finger pressure on the vein just beyond the distal end of the introducer sheath.
- Using sterile forceps, insert the catheter into the introducer sheath, and advance it into the vein 5–10 cm.
- Remove the tourniquet, using the gauze pad.
- When you have advanced the catheter to the shoulder, ask the patient to turn his head toward the affected arm and place his chin on his chest. This will occlude the jugular vein and ease the catheter's advancement into the subclavian vein.
- Advance the catheter until about 10 cm remain. Then pull the introducer sheath out of the vein and away from the venepuncture site.
- Grasp the tabs of the introducer sheath, and flex them toward its distal end to split the sheath, then pull the tabs apart and away from the catheter until the sheath is completely split. Discard the sheath.

- Continue to advance the catheter until it's completely inserted. Flush with sodium chloride solution followed by heparin, according to local policy.

Simon says: Hands down

- With the patient's arm below heart level, remove the syringe and connect the capped extension set to the hub of the catheter.
- Apply a sterile gauze pad directly over the site and a sterile, transparent semi-permeable dressing over that. Leave this dressing in place for 24 hours.
- After the initial 24 hours, apply a new sterile, transparent semi-permeable dressing. The gauze pad is no longer necessary. You can place Steri-Strips over the catheter wings. Flush with heparin, according to local policy.

Administering drugs

- As with any CVC line, be sure to check for blood return, and flush with sodium chloride solution before administering a drug through a PICC line.
- Clamp the extension tubing, and connect the empty syringe to the tubing. Release the clamp and aspirate slowly to verify blood return. Flush with 5 ml of sodium chloride solution, and then administer the drug.
- After giving the drug, flush again with 5 ml of normal saline solution in a 10 ml syringe. You should also flush the line between infusions of incompatible drugs or fluids.

Changing the dressing

- Change the dressing every 3–7 days, and more frequently if the integrity of the dressing becomes compromised. If possible, choose a transparent semi-permeable dressing, which has a high moisture-vapour transmission rate.
- Wash your hands and assemble the necessary supplies. Position the patient with his arm extended away from his body at a 45- to 90-degree angle so that the insertion site is below heart level, to reduce the risk of air embolism. Put on a sterile mask.

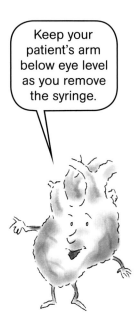

Keep your patient's arm below eye level as you remove the syringe.

Today's star: the thumb

- Open a package of sterile gloves, and use the inside of the package as a sterile field. Then open the transparent semi-permeable dressing and drop it on to the field. Put on clean gloves, and remove the old dressing by holding your left thumb on the catheter and stretching the dressing parallel to the skin. Repeat the last step with your right thumb holding the catheter. Free the remaining section of the dressing from the catheter by peeling toward the insertion site from the distal end to the proximal end, to prevent catheter dislodgment. Remove the clean gloves.
- Put on sterile gloves. Clean the area with alcohol, starting at the insertion site and working outward.
- Apply the dressing carefully. Secure the tubing to the edge of the dressing over the tape with 1 cm adhesive tape.

Removing a PICC

- Assemble the necessary equipment at the patient's bedside, explain the procedure to the patient, wash your hands, and place a pad under the patient's arm.
- Remove the tape holding the extension tubing and open two sterile gauze pads on a clean, flat surface. After putting on gloves, stabilize the catheter at the hub and remove the dressing by pulling it toward the insertion site.

Smooth move

- Next, withdraw the catheter with smooth, gentle pressure in small increments. If you feel resistance, stop and apply slight tension to the line by taping it down. Try to remove it again in a few minutes. If you still feel resistance, notify the doctor for further instructions. (See *PICC removal complications*.)
- After removing the catheter, apply pressure to the site with a sterile gauze pad for 1 minute.
- Measure and inspect the catheter. If any part has broken off during removal, notify the doctor immediately and monitor the patient for signs of distress.
- Cover the site with a gauze pad. Dispose of used items as per local policy, and wash your hands.

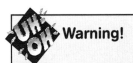 **Warning!**

PICC removal complications

If a portion of the peripherally inserted central catheter (PICC) breaks during removal, immediately apply a tourniquet to the upper arm, close to the axilla, to prevent advancement of the catheter piece into the right atrium. Then check the patient's radial pulse. If you don't detect the radial pulse, the tourniquet is too tight. Keep the tourniquet in place until an X-ray can be obtained, the doctor is notified and surgical retrieval is attempted.

What else can happen?

Catheter occlusion is also relatively common. Air embolism, always a potential risk of venepuncture, poses less danger in PICC therapy. Catheter tip migration may occur with vigorous flushing.

Practice pointers

• For a patient receiving intermittent PICC therapy, the catheter will need to be flushed with 5 ml of normal saline solution and 3 ml of heparin (100 U/ml) after each use, or according to local policy. For catheters that aren't being used routinely, flushing every 12 hours with 3 ml of heparin (100 U/ml) will maintain patency.

• If a patient will be receiving blood or blood products through the PICC, use at least an 18G cannula.

• Assess the catheter insertion site through the transparent semi-permeable dressing every 24 hours. Although oozing is common for the first 24 hours after insertion, excessive bleeding after that should be evaluated. (See *Documenting PICC insertion and removal*.)

Write it down

Documenting PICC insertion and removal

In your notes, document:

• the date and time of catheter placement
• the indication for placement
• the entire procedure, including problems with catheter placement
• size, length and type of catheter
• any medications administered, including flushes
• catheter insertion location
• your name, designation and signature.

10 Self-assessment guidelines

Introduction

A selection of self-audit/assessor checklists adapted from the intellectual property originals written by Jocelyn Hewitt, Clinical Skills Lead of the Clinical Skills Service, Whipps Cross University Hospital Trust, London is supplied in this chapter. These are for a variety (but not all) of the skills included in this text; some are for core skills and some are for enhanced skills. The purpose of these checklists is threefold:

- They standardize procedures for medical, nursing and allied health staff, in order that every healthcare professional follows the same principles and guidelines for care.
- They serve as an *aide memoir* for practitioners pre- and post-procedure.
- Finally, they standardize assessments by mentors.

Local policies and procedures specific to your host trust or employer must be followed; these assessments are included within this text for guidance and as examples only. Check whether your trust, university or employer has devised their own checklists/competency documents for you to use.

Whipps Cross University Hospital

NHS Trust

CLINICAL SKILLS SERVICE

Self-Audit Form/Assessor's Checklist: Social Handwash and Applying Sterile Gloves

Name…………………………….

Name & designation of assessor…………………………….…**Date**………..…………….

• All appropriate equipment was selected.	Yes ☐ No ☐
• He/she rolls up sleeves exposing forearm.	Yes ☐ No ☐
• Watches, rings or bracelets removed as appropriate.	Yes ☐ No ☐
• Gloves selected and laid out for use.	Yes ☐ No ☐
• Water set running and hands made wet.	Yes ☐ No ☐
• Adequate soap applied and worked into all aspects of hands.	Yes ☐ No ☐

- He/she demonstrates the 5 steps of hand washing, in any order:

> Backs of hands fingers interlaced,   Yes ☐ No ☐
> Fronts of hands fingers interlaced,
> Thumb wash,
> Backs of fingers interlocked,
> Fingertips to palms.

- Hands rinsed thoroughly with running water and taps turned off without re-contamination.   Yes ☐ No ☐

- Full hand wash performed for between 10 and 30 seconds.   Yes ☐ No ☐

- Hands dried with paper towels.   Yes ☐ No ☐

- Paper towel disposed of without re-contamination, by using foot pedal to lift the lid.   Yes ☐ No ☐

- Glove packet opened with out contaminating sterile gloves inside.   Yes ☐ No ☐

- First glove picked up by folded cuff, and applied correctly with out touching the sterile fingers.   Yes ☐ No ☐

- Second glove picked up with sterile gloved hand and preferably fingers inserted into cuff   Yes ☐ No ☐
fold to protect sterility of first gloves fingers while applying to ungloved hand.

- Second glove applied without sterile outer aspects of the glove becoming contaminated.   Yes ☐ No ☐

- If necessary, cuff folded back on to wrist by sliding sterile fingers between palm and cuff   Yes ☐ No ☐
and flicking back.

- Fingers adjusted in gloves with sterile gloved hand to assist in comfort and sensitivity for   Yes ☐ No ☐
procedure.

Whipps Cross University Hospital

NHS Trust

CLINICAL SKILLS SERVICE

<u>Self-Assessment Guideline: Recording a Blood Pressure</u>

Name......................................

Name & designation of assessor..**Date**...........................

• Wash hands with soap from a dispenser or use alcohol hand rub.	Yes ☐ No ☐
• Discuss and explain the procedure to the patient/assess for contraindications.	Yes ☐ No ☐
• Ensure the patient has time to relax.	Yes ☐ No ☐
• For non-routine monitoring, blood pressure in both arms should be measured. Be aware that 20 mmHg difference in systole or 10 mmHg in diastole requires that the greater blood pressure is used.	Yes ☐ No ☐
• Use the correct size cuff—if this is not possible, use a larger size. The bladder length should be at least 80% of the arm circumference.	Yes ☐ No ☐
• Apply the cuff around the arm—2.5 cm above the antecubital fossa.	Yes ☐ No ☐
• The 'artery' arrow on the cuff should be aligned to ensure that the centre of the bladder covers the brachial artery.	Yes ☐ No ☐
• If the patient is sitting or standing, the cuff should be placed at the heart level. If the patient is lying, the arm should rest next to the patient on a flat surface with the cuff in line with the mid axilla.	Yes ☐ No ☐
• Ensure that the sphygmomanometer is placed on a flat surface at eye level.	Yes ☐ No ☐
• The arm should be supported positioned at heart level with the palm of the hand uppermost.	Yes ☐ No ☐
• Palpate the brachial pulse and inflate the cuff to provide an estimate of the systolic pressure.	Yes ☐ No ☐
• Deflate cuff and wait for 15 seconds.	Yes ☐ No ☐
• Inflate cuff to approximately 30 mmHg higher than the estimated systolic.	Yes ☐ No ☐
• Place diaphragm of stethoscope over the brachial artery.	Yes ☐ No ☐
• Slowly deflate the cuff at 2–3 mmHg per second.	Yes ☐ No ☐
• Record the systolic when a <u>**minimum of two clear repetitive sounds is heard**</u> (Korotkoff's sound 1) and diastolic at the end of muffling just as the <u>**sound disappears**</u> (Korotkoff's sound 5).	Yes ☐ No ☐
• Record phases 4 and 5 of Korotkoff's sounds, if they are indistinct.	Yes ☐ No ☐
• Discuss the episode of care with the patient.	Yes ☐ No ☐
• Remove the equipment and cleanse stethoscope.	Yes ☐ No ☐
• Wash hands and dry thoroughly, or use alcohol hand rub.	Yes ☐ No ☐
• Complete appropriate documentation.	Yes ☐ No ☐

Whipps Cross University Hospital

NHS Trust

NHS

Self-Audit Form/Assessor's Checklist: Pulse Oximetry

Name.....................................

Name & designation of assessor...Date...............................

1. Describes indications for using pulse oximetry — Yes ☐ No ☐
   - Turns machine on and waits for calibration to end — Yes ☐ No ☐
   - Applies probe correctly, waiting for display/waveform — Yes ☐ No ☐
   - Reads oxygen saturation and heart rate — Yes ☐ No ☐
   - Checks alarms. — Yes ☐ No ☐
2. Discusses situations that might reduce waveform signal, such as: — Yes ☐ No ☐
   - Shaking/shivering — Yes ☐ No ☐
   - Cold peripheries — Yes ☐ No ☐
   - Nail varnish/extensions. — Yes ☐ No ☐
3. Aware of medical conditions that might affect the saturation reading, such as: — Yes ☐ No ☐
   - carboxyhaemaglobinaemia
   - methaemaglobinaemia.
4. Discusses at what percentage the low saturation alarm should be set. — Yes ☐ No ☐
5. Discusses what he/she would do if the saturation reading changed instantaneously from 99% to 80%, such as: — Yes ☐ No ☐
   - assess patient
   - check probe position.
6. He/she is aware that the pulse oximeter is not reliable for saturations below 70%. — Yes ☐ No ☐
7. He/she is aware that the pulse oximeter is not reliable in detecting type 2 respiratory failure. — Yes ☐ No ☐
8. He/she is aware that an arterial blood gas sample should be obtained to identify the presence of type 2 respiratory failure. — Yes ☐ No ☐

Whipps Cross University Hospital

NHS Trust

CLINICAL SKILLS SERVICE

Self-Audit Form/Assessor's Checklist: CVP Measurement

Name, designation..**Date**................................

Name & designation of assessor..

1. The procedure was explained to the patient, consent was established. **Yes** ☐ **No** ☐

2. The HP washed his/her hands or used alcohol hand rub. **Yes** ☐ **No** ☐

3. The equipment is checked to identify:

    a. 0.9% NaCl infusion fluid

    b. Administration set attached to distal lumen

    c. Lumen clamp opened

    d. 3-way taps turned off to other infusions if safe to do so. **Yes** ☐ **No** ☐

4. The patient is positioned with head elevated at a maximum 45%. **Yes** ☐ **No** ☐

5. The CVP manometer is zeroed and aligned with phlebostatic axis. **Yes** ☐ **No** ☐

6. Patency of the lumen is confirmed using saline infusion. **Yes** ☐ **No** ☐

7. Manometer is primed to a level 10 cmH$_2$O above previous reading. **Yes** ☐ **No** ☐

8. CVP recorded at end expiration and documented accurately on chart. **Yes** ☐ **No** ☐

9. Lumen is clamped/3-way tap turned off to patient at end of procedure and any infusion re-started if necessary. **Yes** ☐ **No** ☐

10. Washes hands or uses alcohol hand rub. **Yes** ☐ **No** ☐

11. Standard infection control procedures were achieved throughout the procedure. **Yes** ☐ **No** ☐

12. Discusses normal values and recognizes importance of actioning abnormal readings accompanied by other vital signs changes. **Yes** ☐ **No** ☐

Comments:

Whipps Cross University Hospital

NHS

NHS Trust

CLINICAL SKILLS SERVICE

<u>**Self-Audit Form/Assessor's Checklist: Recording an ECG**</u>

Name & designation of assessor...**Date**...........................

	Yes	No
• He/she is aware of current guidelines.	☐	☐
• He/she washed his/her hands.	☐	☐
• The patient's ID was confirmed, and the procedure explained, consent established and opportunity to ask questions provided.	☐	☐
• The patient's privacy and dignity were protected.	☐	☐
• He/she was correctly positioned and the patient's skin was prepared.	☐	☐
• He/she checked that the ECG machine was calibrated to 10 mm/millivolt and 25 mm/second.	☐	☐
• The electrodes were correctly applied.	☐	☐
• He/she attaches the 10 leads from the ECG machine to the electrodes.	☐	☐
• Ensures leads are not pulling or crossed over each other.	☐	☐
• Demonstrates a good standard of communication and professionalism with simulated patient and assessor.	☐	☐
• If the ECG is poorly recorded, he/she checks electrodes/connections, etc.	☐	☐
• Labels ECG with patient's name, hospital number, date and time.	☐	☐
• Informs patient when test is complete.	☐	☐
• Removes electrodes.	☐	☐
(a) Correctly interprets ECG and takes appropriate course of action, or	☐	☐
(b) on completion reports to a more senior colleague.	☐	☐
• He/she washed his/her hands or used alcohol hand rub.	☐	☐
• Episode documented.	☐	☐

Whipps Cross University Hospital

NHS Trust

NHS

CLINICAL SKILLS SERVICE

Self-Audit Form/Assessor's Checklist: ECG Interpretation

Name, designation...**Date**....................................

Name & designation of assessor...

- Mandatory safety checks were completed:

    Correct patient name   Yes ☐ No ☐

    Hospital number   Yes ☐ No ☐

    Date of birth.   Yes ☐ No ☐

- ECG defaults were checked:

    Chart speed 25 mm/sec   Yes ☐ No ☐

    ECG height 10 mm/1 cm   Yes ☐ No ☐

    Filter button off (first ECG).   Yes ☐ No ☐

- Rhythm strip:

    Correctly identifies the heart rate   Yes ☐ No ☐

    Correctly identifies the rhythm.   Yes ☐ No ☐

- Inferior leads (II, III and aVF):

    Assesses for evidence of ischaemia   Yes ☐ No ☐

    (ST segment/T wave changes and Q waves).   Yes ☐ No ☐

- Anterior leads (V_1–V_6 or C_1–C_6):

    Assesses for evidence of ischaemia   Yes ☐ No ☐

    (ST segment/T wave changes and Q waves)   Yes ☐ No ☐

    Comments on R-wave progression.   Yes ☐ No ☐

- The student correctly identified the abnormality.   Yes ☐ No ☐

- An appropriate and safe plan of care was discussed for the patient.   Yes ☐ No ☐

Whipps Cross University Hospital

NHS Trust

CLINICAL SKILLS SERVICE

Self-Audit form/Assessor's Checklist: Oxygen Therapy

Name..

Name & designation of assessor...................................**Date**..............................

• Correctly names each of the oxygen delivery devices shown.	Yes ☐ No ☐
• Correctly states oxygen concentration range delivered by each device.	Yes ☐ No ☐
• Selects appropriate device to give oxygen therapy to patient scenario 1.	Yes ☐ No ☐
• Checks valves intact on mask.	Yes ☐ No ☐
• Connects mask to oxygen cylinder and selects appropriate flow rate.	Yes ☐ No ☐
• Ensures non-rebreathe reservoir bag is fully inflated.	Yes ☐ No ☐
• Gives explanation, obtains consent and correctly places mask on patient.	Yes ☐ No ☐
• Prescribes oxygen on drug chart accurately with observation parameters.	Yes ☐ No ☐
• Requests nursing staff to carry out appropriate monitoring.	Yes ☐ No ☐
• States would obtain advice from relevant senior colleague.	Yes ☐ No ☐
• States would perform arterial blood gas.	Yes ☐ No ☐
• Demonstrates a good standard of communication and professionalism with assessor and 'simulated' patient.	Yes ☐ No ☐
• Documents episode in the patient's notes.	Yes ☐ No ☐
• Aware oxygen masks/tubing are single use only.	Yes ☐ No ☐

Whipps Cross University Hospital

NHS Trust

CLINICAL SKILLS SERVICE

Self-Audit Form/Assessor's Checklist: Venepuncture

Name/designation……………………………………..…….Date………..……………..….

Statements highlighted in **BOLD** are weighted. If they are not achieved, this will result in an unsatisfactory assessment (fail).

- He/she is aware of current guidelines for venepuncture. — Yes ☐ No ☐
- Has a clear understanding of indications/contraindications/risks of the procedure. — Yes ☐ No ☐
- **The patient's ID was confirmed and valid blood sample request form written/checked.** — Yes ☐ No ☐
- **Consent was obtained, explanation and opportunity to ask questions provided.** — Yes ☐ No ☐
- All appropriate equipment was selected (Vacutainer system). — Yes ☐ No ☐
- **He/she washed his/her hands prior to the procedure (social handwash) and applied gloves.** — Yes ☐ No ☐
- A tourniquet was applied and an appropriate vein was selected. — Yes ☐ No ☐
- The skin was cleansed with an 70% alcohol wipe and allowed to dry. — Yes ☐ No ☐
- **Insertion technique was satisfactory.** — Yes ☐ No ☐
- A blood sample was obtained. — Yes ☐ No ☐
- Asepsis was achieved throughout the procedure. — Yes ☐ No ☐
- **All equipment and sharps were disposed of correctly.** — Yes ☐ No ☐
- **Demonstrates a good standard of communication and professional values with patient/assessor.** — Yes ☐ No ☐
- He/she assessed the patient for complications. — Yes ☐ No ☐
- **Collection bottles were correctly labelled immediately at the bedside.** — Yes ☐ No ☐
- The procedure for specimen transfer to the laboratory was followed. — Yes ☐ No ☐
- He/she washed his/her hands (social handwash). — Yes ☐ No ☐
- Documentation completed. — Yes ☐ No ☐

Whipps Cross University Hospital

NHS

NHS Trust

CLINICAL SKILLS SERVICE

Self-Audit form/Assessor's Checklist: Blood Cultures

Name…………………………………..

Name & designation of assessor……………………………...………..**Date**………..……………..

- He/she is aware of current guidelines for blood cultures. **Yes** ☐ **No** ☐
- Has a clear understanding of indications/contraindications/risks of the procedure. **Yes** ☐ **No** ☐
- The patient's ID was confirmed and valid blood sample request form checked. **Yes** ☐ **No** ☐
- Consent was obtained, explanation and opportunity to ask questions provided. **Yes** ☐ **No** ☐
- All appropriate equipment was selected, including an aerobic and anaerobic culture bottle and their expiry dates checked. **Yes** ☐ **No** ☐
- He/she washed his/her hands prior to the procedure (social handwash) and applied non-sterile gloves. **Yes** ☐ **No** ☐
- An appropriate vein was selected. **Yes** ☐ **No** ☐
- The skin was cleansed with an 70% alcohol wipe, allowed to dry and the skin was not re-palpated. **Yes** ☐ **No** ☐
- He/she carried out the procedure correctly (blood was not injected). **Yes** ☐ **No** ☐
- Asepsis was achieved throughout the procedure. **Yes** ☐ **No** ☐
- The blood is mixed well with the culture media. **Yes** ☐ **No** ☐
- All equipment and sharps were disposed of correctly. **Yes** ☐ **No** ☐
- Demonstrates a good standard of communication and professionalism with assessor and 'simulated' patient. **Yes** ☐ **No** ☐
- He/she assessed the patient for complications. **Yes** ☐ **No** ☐
- Collection bottles were completed immediately (avoiding the bar code) at the bedside with ID, date, time and signed. **Yes** ☐ **No** ☐
- The procedure for specimen transfer to the laboratory was followed and relevant documentation completed in the patient's notes. **Yes** ☐ **No** ☐
- Clinical symptoms, such as pyrexia and current antibiotic therapy, were recorded on the request form. **Yes** ☐ **No** ☐
- He/she washed his/her hands (social handwash). **Yes** ☐ **No** ☐

Ref.:   Goodbourn, C. (2004) *Guidelines for blood cultures.* WXUH.

Whipps Cross University Hospital

NHS Trust

CLINICAL SKILLS SERVICE

Self-Audit Form/Assessor's Checklist: Blood Transfusion

Name......................................

Name & designation of assessor.................................**Date**..........................

1. Venepuncture for X match:
   - Discusses issues around consent and patient information   Yes ☐ No ☐
   - Checks patient identification from name bracelet   Yes ☐ No ☐
   - Labels specimen bottle at the bedside   Yes ☐ No ☐
   - Completes request form correctly   Yes ☐ No ☐
   - Cites correct process for transporting specimens.   Yes ☐ No ☐

2. On receiving the unit of blood:
   - Demonstrates an awareness of safe storage and care standards   Yes ☐ No ☐
   - Correctly prescribes transfusion   Yes ☐ No ☐
   - Discusses standard infection control and sharps management procedures   Yes ☐ No ☐
   - Performs ID checks prior to transfusing—laboratory documentation drug chart, transfusion report, and patient ID band)   Yes ☐ No ☐
   - Aware of written compliance for laboratory forms   Yes ☐ No ☐
   - Mentions two-person checking procedure   Yes ☐ No ☐
   - Selects correct infusion set   Yes ☐ No ☐
   - Discusses suitable cannula size   Yes ☐ No ☐
   - Discusses instruction/parameters for nursing staff   Yes ☐ No ☐
   - Confidently discusses signs and symptoms of Tx reaction   Yes ☐ No ☐
   - Describes appropriate action   Yes ☐ No ☐
   - Aware of safe disposal procedures (or who to ask)   Yes ☐ No ☐
   - Demonstrates a good standard of communication and professionalism with assessor and 'simulated' patient   Yes ☐ No ☐
   - Documents episode in the patient's notes.   Yes ☐ No ☐

Whipps Cross University Hospital

NHS Trust

CLINICAL SKILLS SERVICE

Self-Audit Form/Assessor's Checklist: Medicines management

Name…………………………………..

Name & designation of assessor………………………….………...Date………..……………...

No.	Standard	Yes/No	Comment
1.*	Ensures correct patient is identified.		
2.*	Aware of patient's diagnosis, past medical history and treatment regimes.		
3.*	Ensures the correct wristband is in place and is legible.		
4.*	Ensures the correct prescription chart is used if the patient has more than one.		
5.*	Ensures that the patient prescription is valid and legible.		
6.	Prepares appropriate equipment safely.		
7.	Demonstrates competent use of the BNF, special precautions and instructions noted.		
8.	Gives appropriate information to the patient prior to procedure.		
9.	Appropriately prepares the patient for administration of the medication.		
10.*	Selects appropriate route for the administration if prescription specifies a choice.		
11.	Follows Trust infection control practices as per policy.		
12.*	Allergy check made with patient, documentation and with prescription chart.		
13.*	Medication dose check, prescription within therapeutic range and appropriately timed.		
14.*	Demonstrates awareness of medication to be given, effects, side effect and incompatibilities.		
15.	Administers the medication correctly to the patient.		
16.*	Accurate and legible documentation of administration.		
17.	Correct management of drug refusal by patient.		
18.	Can identify and discuss common drug reactions and premonitory signs of anaphylaxis.		
19.*	Follows Trust drug administration policy throughout the procedure.		
20.*	Complete the medicines assessment in a reasonable and timely manner taking into consideration the medicines to be given and the patient's condition.		
21.*	Demonstrates the following practice values during the procedure: respect for the individual, consideration of differences of race, culture, religion, etc. Maintains privacy and dignity, maintains confidentiality and acts in a professional manner.		
Overall comment			

* These standards must be achieved in order to attain competency.

Whipps Cross University Hospital

NHS Trust

CLINICAL SKILLS SERVICE

Self-Audit Form/Assessor's Checklist: NG Tube Insertion

Name…………………………………..

Name & designation of assessor…………………..………….**Date**………..………………

- He/she is aware of the current guidelines for NG tube insertion and management.   **Yes** ☐ **No** ☐
- Has a clear understanding of indications/contraindications/risks of the procedure.   **Yes** ☐ **No** ☐
- The patient's ID was confirmed, consent obtained, explanation and opportunity to ask questions provided.   **Yes** ☐ **No** ☐
- All appropriate equipment was selected, including pH indicator strip **(litmus paper now withdrawn)**.   **Yes** ☐ **No** ☐
- He/she washed his/her hands prior to the procedure (social handwash) and applied gloves.   **Yes** ☐ **No** ☐
- Patient was assisted into the correct position, head supported.   **Yes** ☐ **No** ☐
- The distance that the tube is to be passed is correctly measured from the patient's ear lobe to the bridge of nose to the bottom of the xiphisternum.   **Yes** ☐ **No** ☐
- The nostrils were assessed and the tip of the tube lubricated.   **Yes** ☐ **No** ☐
- The 'patient' was communicated with again to promote trust and feeling of safety. A signal was arranged by which the patient could communicate if he/she wanted to stop.   **Yes** ☐ **No** ☐
- The tube was correctly inserted with the patient swallowing sips of water, if appropriate (not dysphagic).   **Yes** ☐ **No** ☐
- The patient was assessed for complications/distress which may indicate displacement.   **Yes** ☐ **No** ☐
- The position of the tube was checked **(no air/stethoscope check)** and correct placement assessed by establishing that gastric pH is between 0 and 5.   **Yes** ☐ **No** ☐
- If feeding tube was inserted, the guide wire was left in situ while the tube was aspirated and pH checked.   **Yes** ☐ **No** ☐
- The tube is secured appropriately, flushed with water and the guide wire removed (if feeding tube).   **Yes** ☐ **No** ☐
- He/she mentions that X-ray is necessary only in occasional circumstances, e.g. protein pump inhibitors/previous gastric surgery (leaves guide wire in).   **Yes** ☐ **No** ☐
- Drainage bag or spigot applied (if appropriate).   **Yes** ☐ **No** ☐
- Demonstrates a good standard of communication and professionalism with 'simulated' patient and assessor.   **Yes** ☐ **No** ☐
- Mentions documenting the procedure and fluid output.
- He/she washed his/her hands (social handwash).   **Yes** ☐ **No** ☐
- If indicated, the position of the tube was checked on X-ray and written instruction for nursing staff to commence feeding documented in the patient's notes.   **Yes** ☐ **No** ☐

Whipps Cross University Hospital

NHS Trust

CLINICAL SKILLS SERVICE

Self-Audit form/Assessor's Checklist: Female Catheterization

Name/designation……………………………………………Date…………..………………………………..

- The healthcare practitioner (HP) referred to the current guidelines. Yes ☐ No ☐
- The procedure was explained to the patient, consent was established. Yes ☐ No ☐
- The HP washed his/her hands (social handwash) and put on disposable apron. Yes ☐ No ☐
- The HP cleansed the trolley. Yes ☐ No ☐
- The HP selected appropriate equipment and materials and placed all on the bottom shelf of the trolley. Yes ☐ No ☐
- The HP took the trolley to the patient's bedside, disturbing the screens as little as possible. Yes ☐ No ☐
- He/she opened the pack and slid the pack out on to the trolley. Yes ☐ No ☐
- The HP used an aseptic technique, opening supplementary packs correctly. Yes ☐ No ☐
- Assists the patient to assume the correct position. Yes ☐ No ☐
- Cleans hands with alcohol hand rub. Yes ☐ No ☐
- Applies sterile gloves, placing sterile towel across the patient. Yes ☐ No ☐
- Effectively cleanses the area. Yes ☐ No ☐
- Inserts anaesthetic gel into the meatus—disposes of gloves. Yes ☐ No ☐
- Cleans hands and applies sterile gloves. Yes ☐ No ☐
- Introduces the catheter correctly, guarding against contamination. Yes ☐ No ☐
- Completes insertion, correctly inflates the balloon and connects to drainage bag. Yes ☐ No ☐
- Ensures patient comfort post procedure. Yes ☐ No ☐
- Disposes of equipment and washes his/her hands. Yes ☐ No ☐
- Demonstrates a good standard of communication and professionalism with patient and assessor. Yes ☐ No ☐
- Documents and fluid balance. Yes ☐ No ☐

Whipps Cross University Hospital

NHS Trust

CLINICAL SKILLS SERVICE

<u>**Self-Audit Form/Assessor's Checklist: Intravenous Drug Administration**</u>

Name/designation…………………………………………....Date………..………………………….

Statements highlighted in **BOLD** are weighted. If they are not achieved, this will result in an unsatisfactory assessment (fail).

1. General
   - The healthcare practitioner (HP) referred to the current guidelines/BNF. Yes ☐ No ☐
   - The procedure was explained to the patient, consent was established. Yes ☐ No ☐
   - The HP **washed his/her hands** (social hand wash). Yes ☐ No ☐
   - Cleanses port pre- and post-administration. Yes ☐ No ☐
   - Avoids inappropriate disconnection/opening of infusion system. Yes ☐ No ☐
   - Disposes of infusion set if it was disconnected from the cannula/port. Yes ☐ No ☐
   - Demonstrates awareness of standard infection control and sharps management procedures. Yes ☐ No ☐

2. Prescription
   - **Checks drug prescribed by generic name is legible, signed and dated.** Yes ☐ No ☐
   - **Checks correct strength, dose, route, frequency and time.** Yes ☐ No ☐
   - **Checks whether drug has already been administered.** Yes ☐ No ☐
   - **Checks for adverse medication reactions (box completed).** Yes ☐ No ☐

3. The drug
   - **The correct drug was selected.** Yes ☐ No ☐
   - Expiry date checked. Yes ☐ No ☐
   - **Checked that the drug is suitable for I.V. use.** Yes ☐ No ☐
   - If appropriate, checked whether a diluent was indicated. Yes ☐ No ☐
   - **Checked that the drug is compatible with other prescribed medication/infusions.** Yes ☐ No ☐
   - **Prepares 0.9% saline for I.V. flush.** Yes ☐ No ☐
   - **Correctly constitutes drug.** Yes ☐ No ☐
   - **Correctly calculates drug dosage (if appropriate).**
   - Aware of cautions/side effects. Yes ☐ No ☐

(Continued)

Whipps Cross University Hospital

NHS Trust

CLINICAL SKILLS SERVICE

__Self-Audit Form/Assessor's Checklist: I.V. Cannulation__

Name/designation……………………………………..Date………..……………………………….

Statements highlighted in **BOLD** are weighted. If they are not achieved, this will result in an unsatisfactory assessment (fail).

- Has a clear understanding of indications/contraindications/risks of the procedure.   Yes ☐ No ☐
- He/she is aware of current guidelines for intravenous cannulation.   Yes ☐ No ☐
- **The patient's ID was confirmed, the procedure was explained to the patient.**   Yes ☐ No ☐
- **Consent was obtained and opportunity to ask questions provided.**   Yes ☐ No ☐
- All appropriate equipment was selected.   Yes ☐ No ☐
- **He/she washed his/her hands prior to the procedure** (social handwash) and applied gloves.   Yes ☐ No ☐
- A tourniquet was applied and an appropriate vein was selected.   Yes ☐ No ☐
- The skin was cleansed with an 70% alcohol and allowed to dry.   Yes ☐ No ☐
- The appropriate cannula size was selected.   Yes ☐ No ☐
- **Insertion technique was satisfactory.**   Yes ☐ No ☐
- The vein was cannulated.   Yes ☐ No ☐
- The cannula was secured with a sterile transparent dressing and appropriate port selected and applied.   Yes ☐ No ☐
- **Asepsis was achieved throughout the procedure.**   Yes ☐ No ☐
- Vein patency was assessed (I.V. flush with N/saline).   Yes ☐ No ☐
- Cannula was secured.   Yes ☐ No ☐
- He/she assessed for complications.   Yes ☐ No ☐
- **All** equipment and **sharps** were **disposed of correctly.**   Yes ☐ No ☐
- He/she washed his/her hands (social handwash).   Yes ☐ No ☐
- **Demonstrates a good standard of communication and professionalism with patient and assessor.**   Yes ☐ No ☐
- Informs nursing staff of successful insertion (if appropriate).   Yes ☐ No ☐
- All relevant information was documented, dated, timed and signed.   Yes ☐ No ☐

Whipps Cross University Hospital

NHS Trust

CLINICAL SKILL SERVICE

<u>Self-Audit Form/Assessor's Checklist: Male Catheterization</u>

Name..**Date**..............................

Name & designation of assessor...

• Has a clear understanding of indications/contraindications/risks of the procedure.	**Yes** ☐	**No** ☐
• He/she is aware of current guidelines for catheterization.	**Yes** ☐	**No** ☐
• **The patient's ID was confirmed.**	**Yes** ☐	**No** ☐
• The procedure was explained, consent was established and opportunity to ask questions provided.	**Yes** ☐	**No** ☐
• **He/she washed his/her hands (social handwash) and put on a disposable apron.**	**Yes** ☐	**No** ☐
• He/she cleansed the trolley and selected all appropriate equipment and materials.	**Yes** ☐	**No** ☐
• **Mentions the importance of respecting the patient's privacy and dignity.**	**Yes** ☐	**No** ☐
• He/she used an aseptic technique, opening supplementary packs correctly.	**Yes** ☐	**No** ☐
• Ensures patient is assisted into a comfortable position and covered appropriately.	**Yes** ☐	**No** ☐
• Cleans hands with alcohol hand rub and applies sterile gloves, placing sterile towel across patient.	**Yes** ☐	**No** ☐
• Effectively cleanses the area.	**Yes** ☐	**No** ☐
• Inserts anaesthetic gel into the meatus.	**Yes** ☐	**No** ☐
• Cleans hands and changes sterile gloves.	**Yes** ☐	**No** ☐
• **Introduces the catheter correctly (satisfactory insertion technique), maintains asepsis.**	**Yes** ☐	**No** ☐
• Completes insertion, correctly inflates balloon and connects to drainage bag.	**Yes** ☐	**No** ☐
• Foreskin repositioned following procedure.	**Yes** ☐	**No** ☐
• Ensures patient comfort, post-procedure (foreskin), observes for complications.	**Yes** ☐	**No** ☐
• **Disposes of equipment, and washes hands.**	**Yes** ☐	**No** ☐
• Documents procedure (including device used, catheter size type) in the patient's notes.	**Yes** ☐	**No** ☐
• Ensures urinary output is recorded.	**Yes** ☐	**No** ☐
• **Demonstrates a good standard of communication and professionalism with 'simulated patient'/assessor.**	**Yes** ☐	**No** ☐

References and index

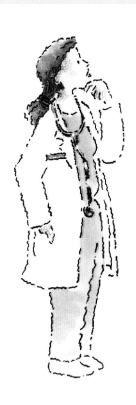

Selected references

Abrams, P., Cardozo, L., Fall, M., *et al.* (2002) Standardisation Sub-committee of the International Continence Society, The standardisation of terminology of lower urinary tract function; report from the Standardisation Sub-committee of the International Continence Society. *Neurourology and Urodynamics* 21: 167–168.

Bickley, L.S. and Hoekelman, R.A. (1999) *Bates' guide to physical examination and history taking*, 7th edn. Philadelphia: Lippincott Williams & Wilkins.

Chapple, A. and Rogers, A. (1999) '*Self-care*' *and its relevance to developing demand management strategies: a review of qualitative research. Health and Social Care in the Community* 17: 445–454.

Department of Health (1999) *Pressure ulcer treatment guildelines.*

Department of Health (2000) *The National Service framework for older people.*

Department of Health (2001) *Essence of Care: patient focused benchmarks for clinical governance.*

Diagnostics: An A-to-Z Guide to Laboratory Tests and Diagnostic Procedures. Springhouse, Pa.: Springhouse, 2001.

Elkin, M.K., *et al.* (2000) *Nursing interventions and clinical skills*, 2nd edn. St Louis: Mosby–Year Book.

Ellis, J.R. and Hartley, C.L. (2000) *Managing and coordinating nursing care*, 3rd edn. Philadelphia: Lippincott Williams & Wilkins.

Fortunato, N.H. (2000) *Berry & Kohn's operating room technique*, 9th edn. St Louis: Mosby–Year Book.

Goldman, L. and Bennett, J.C. (2000) *Cecil textbook of medicine*, 21st edn. Philadelphia: W.B. Saunders.

Hadaway, L.C. (1999) I.V. infiltration: not just a peripheral problem. *Nursing99* 29(9): 41–47.

Hess, C.T. (2002) *Clinical guide to wound care*, 4th edn. Springhouse, Pa.: Springhouse.

Horne, C. and Derrico, D. (1999) Mastering ABGs. The art of arterial blood gas measurement. *American Journal of Nursing* 99(8): 26–32.

Ignatavicius, D.D., *et al.* (2001) *Medical–surgical nursing: Critical thinking for collaborative care*, 4th edn. Philadelphia: W.B. Saunders.

Jagger, J. and Perry, J. (1999) Power in numbers: reducing your risk of bloodborne exposures. *Nursing99* 29(1): 51–52.

Joint Commission on Accreditation of Healthcare Organizations (2001) *Comprehensive accreditation manual for hospitals.* Oakbrook Terrace, Ill.

Lanken, P.N., *et al.* (2001) *The intensive care unit manual.* Philadelphia: W.B. Saunders.

Lynn-McHale, D.J. and Carlson, K.K. (eds) (2001) *AACN procedure manual for critical care*, 4th edn. Philadelphia: W.B. Saunders.

Maklebust, J. and Sieggreen, M. (2001) *Pressure ulcers: Guidelines for prevention and management*, 3rd edn. Springhouse, Pa.: Springhouse.

National Institute for Clinical Excellence (NICE) (2001) *Guidelines on pressure ulcer risk assessment and prevention.*

Nicol, M., *et al.* (2000) *Essential nursing skills.* St Louis: Mosby–Year Book.

Nursing Procedures, 3rd edn. Springhouse, Pa.: Springhouse, 2000.

Orem, D. (2001) *Nursing: concepts of practice*, 4th edn. St Louis: Mosby–Year Book.

Pancorbo-Hidalgo, P.L., *et al.* (2006) Risk assessment scales for pressure ulcer prevention: a systematic review. *Journal of Advanced Nursing* 54(1): 94–110.

Phillips, L.D. (2001) *Manual of I.V. therapeutics*, 3rd edn. Philadelphia: F.A. Davis.

Phippen, M.L. and Wells, M.P. (2000) *Patient care during operative and invasive procedures.* Philadelphia: W.B. Saunders.

Pierson, F.M. (1999) *Principles and techniques of patient care*, 2nd edn. Philadelphia: W.B. Saunders.

Shoemaker, W., Grenvik, A., *et al.* (2000) *Textbook of critical care*, 4th edn. Philadelphia: W.B. Saunders.

Smeltzer, S.C. and Bare, B.G. (2000) *Brunner and Suddarth's Textbook of Medical-Surgical Nursing*, 9th edn. Philadelphia: Lippincott Williams & Wilkins.

Stratton, R.J., Hackston, A., *et al.* (2004) Malnutrition in hospital outpatients and inpatients: prevalence, concurrent validity and ease of use of the 'malnutrition universal screening tool' (MUST) for adults. *British Journal of Nutrition* 92: 799–808.

Teasdale, G. and Jennett, B. (1974) Assessment of coma and impaired consciousness. *Lancet* ii: 81–84.

Young, L. (1991) The Clean Fight. *The Nursing Standard* 5(33): 54–55.

Useful websites and documents

British Dental Health Foundation: www.dentalhealth.org.uk

British Hypertension Society: www.bhsoc.org

British National Formulary: www.bnf.org

European Pressure Ulcer Advisory Panel: http://www.epuap.org

- Pressure ulcer treatment guidelines

National Institute for Clinical Excellence: www.nice.org.uk

- Recognition of and response to acute illness in adults in hospital (2007)

National Patient Safety Agency: www.npsa.nhs.uk

- Safer care for the acutely ill patient: learning from serious incidents
- Methods, evidence and guidance document
- Nutritional support for adults: oral nutrition support, enteral tube feeding and parenteral feeding

NHS Education for Scotland; http://www.nes.scot.nhs.uk/nursing

Nursing and Midwifery Council: nmc-uk.org

- Standards of proficiency for pre-registration nursing education (2004)
- Code of professional conduct (2004)
- Essential skills clusters (2007)
- Wipe it out campaign (2006)
- Standards for medicines management (2008)
- Review of fitness for practice at the point of registration (2006)

Royal College of Nursing: www.rcn.org.uk

- Standards for infusion therapy (2005)

The Scottish Government health Directorates Website, listing guidelines and consultation documents for NHS Scotland http://www.sehd.scot.nhs.uk

United Kingdom Resuscitation Council: www.resus.org.uk

Waterlow scoring: www.judy-waterlow.co.uk

Index

A

Abrasion, caring for, 129
Accountability and responsibility
    legislation, 160
    guidance and standards, 160–161
A-G of assessment, 37–39
Accuhaler, using, 186
AED. *See* Automated external defibrillators
Aerosol oxygen delivery systems, 193i
Aerosol sprays, 173, 175
Allen's test, 295i
Amputation, caring for, 129
Anaerobic specimen collector, 108i
Anaesthetized patients, latex reaction in, 10
Anti-embolism stockings
    applying, 147
    documenting application of, 148
    measuring for, 146i
    patient teaching for, 148
    special considerations for, 148–149
Apical pulse, how to take, 48–49
Apical-radial pulse, how to take, 49
Apnoea, 52t
Apnoeustic, 52t
Aprons, as PPE, 6
Arterial blood gas analysis, 294–298
Arterial puncture for ABG analysis
    Allen's test and, 295i
    documenting, 298
    performing, 295–298, 296i
    special considerations for, 298
    techniques for, 296i
Artificial fingernails, 3
Aseptic technique
    indications for use, 114
    non-touch technique, 116–117
    performing, 115–117
    special considerations for, 117
    sterile gloves, application, 116i
Automated external defibrillators, 323–325
    documenting use of, 325
    how to use, 324–325
Axillary temperature
    measuring, 45
    normal range for, 42

B

Bandaging techniques, 153i. *See also* Elastic
    bandage
Bed scale, how to use, 67

B (continued)

Behavioural responses, to pain, 79
Black wound, caring for, 119
Bladder irrigation, continuous,
    271–274
    documenting, 274
    performing, 273
    setup for, 271–272, 272i
    special considerations for, 273–274
Blood, in urine, 88
Blood culture, 291–293
    documenting, 293
    performing, 292–293
    special considerations, 293
Blood glucose tests
    documenting, 86
    ensuring accurate results of, 86
    performing, 84–86
    reading results of, 84
    reagent strips for, 84
    teaching patient to perform, 86
Blood pressure, 53–59
    choosing cuff for, 55
    diastolic, 53
    documenting, 59
    effects of age on, 53
    measuring, 54–55i, 55–57
        correcting problems of, 58
        special considerations for,
        57–58, 59
    positioning cuff for, 57
    pulse pressure on, 53
    systolic, 53
Blood transfusion, 309–312
    administering, 310–312
    complications, 310
    documenting, 311
    managing reactions to, 312–313
    special considerations for, 312
Bone marrow aspiration and biopsy
    assisting with, 332–334
    common sites for, 333i
    documenting, 335
    special considerations for, 335
Bradycardia, pulse pattern for, 48i
Bradypnoea, 52t
British National Formulary (BNF),
    The, 162–164
    guidelines to follow, 163–164
Buccal medications, 170–171
    administration, 172
    documenting administration of, 173
    problems with, 172

C

Capillary blood glucose (CBG). *See* Blood
    glucose tests
Cardiac monitoring, 74–78
    documenting, 78
    electrode placement for, 75, 76i
    hardwire, 75, 77
    special considerations for, 78
    telemetry, 77–78
    troubleshooting problems with, 77t
Catheter specimen of urine (CSU), 90–91
    documenting, 91
Central venous catheter
    changing injection cap for, 338, 341
    documenting insertion and removal, 343
    flushing, 338, 340–341
    home therapy with, 343
    inserting, 338–340
    removing, 338, 341–342
    special considerations for, 342
Central venous pressure (CVP), 67–70
    crystalloid fluids for, 68
    measuring, 68, 69–70i
Chair scale, how to use, 66–67
Chemical-dot thermometer, 43i, 44
Chemotherapeutic medications, 313–316
    complications of, 314
    documenting, 315
    performing, 314–315
    special considerations for, 315–316
Cheyne-Stokes respirations, 52t
Closed-wound drain
    complications of, 138
    documenting management of, 139
    managing, 137–139, 138i
    special considerations for, 139
Clostridium difficile, 5
Cognitive therapies, for pain, 80
Colour, of urine, 87
Colostomy
    applying pouch and skin barrier for,
        258–259
    caring for, 255–259
    documenting, 259
    emptying pouch for, 259
    fitting pouch and skin barrier for, 256
    ostomy pouching systems, 257i
    special considerations for, 259
Colour-top collection tubes, guide to, 286
Condom catheter, applying, 261i. *See also*
        Male urinary incontinence device

t refers to a table; i refers to an illustration